Lasers in Dentistry

Lasers in Dentistry

Edited by

Leo J. Miserendino, DDS, MS
Adjunct Assistant Professor
Department of Oral Biology
University of Illinois at Chicago
College of Dentistry
Chicago, Illinois

Senior Research Scientist
Wenske Laser Center
Chicago, Illinois

Robert M. Pick, DDS, MS, FACD, FICD
Clinical Associate Professor
Department of Periodontics
Northwestern University Dental School
Chicago, Illinois

Private Practice of Periodontics
Aurora, Illinois

quintessence books

Quintessence Publishing Co, Inc
Chicago, Berlin, London, Tokyo, São Paulo, Moscow, and Warsaw

Dedications

To my partner and wife, Cathy, whose patience, guidance, and support provided the inspiration necessary for the fulfillment of this project and who gives meaning to all my endeavors. —LJM

To my hero and grandfather, Archie Shore; my mother, Patricia; my father, Harold; and my partner, Ian. —RMP

Library of Congress Cataloging-In-Publication Data

Lasers in Dentistry / edited by Leo J. Miserendino, Robert M. Pick.
p. cm.
Includes bibliographical references and index.
ISBN 0–86715–282–6(hc)
1. Lasers in dentistry. I. Miserendino, Leo. II. Pick, Robert M.
[DNLM: 1. Mouth Diseases—therapy. 2. Lasers—therapeutic use.
3. Tooth diseases—therapy. WU 166 L343 1995]
RK685.L37L37 1995
617.6´05—dc20
DNLM/DLC
for Library of Congress 94-41152
CIP

Published by Quintessence Publishing Co, Inc
551 N. Kimberly Dr.
Carol Stream, IL 60188

Notice: The authors and the publisher of this work have made every effort to provide information that is reliable and complete. However, because of the possibilities of human error and developments in the field, neither the editors, contributors, nor the publisher of this work guarantees that the information contained herein is in every respect accurate or complete. Readers are encouraged to confirm the information contained herein with other sources, and they are advised to be aware of all pertinent governmental regulations and to review all manufacturer information.

Editor: Patricia Bereck Weikersheimer
Production Manager: Timothy M. Robbins
Production Assistant: Eric S. Przybylski
Printing and binding: Toppan Printing Co (S) Pte, Ltd, Singapore
Printed in Singapore.

Contents

Preface 11

Introduction 13

Part I The Scientific Basis of Laser Dentistry

Chapter 1 **The History and Development of Laser Dentistry** 17
Leo J. Miserendino

Chapter 2 **Laser Physics** 27
David M. Harris and Robert M. Pick

Chapter 3 **Laser Interaction with Biologic Tissues** 39
Leo J. Miserendino, Guy Levy, and Catherine A. Miserendino

Chapter 4 **Laser Effects on Dental Hard Tissues** 57
Hans J. Koort and Matthias Frentzen

Chapter 5 **Laser Effects on the Dental Pulp** 71
Charles Arcoria and Leo J. Miserendino

Part II Practical Considerations for Lasers in Dentistry

Chapter 6 **Laser Safety in Dental Practice** 85
Leo J. Miserendino, Robert M. Pick, and Richard J. Blankenau

Chapter 7 **Regulations, Standards, and Education for Lasers in Dentistry** 103
Harvey Wigdor and Leo J. Miserendino

Chapter 8 **Surgical Technique** 113
V. Kim Kutsch and Robert M. Pick

Part III Current Applications of Lasers in Dentistry

Chapter 9 **Surgical Applications of the Argon Laser** 129
V. Kim Kutsch and Richard J. Blankenau

Chapter 10 **Clinical Applications of the CO_2 Laser** 145
Robert M. Pick, M. Anthony Pogrel, and Hong Sai Loh

Chapter 11 **Er:YAG Effects Laser on Oral Hard and Soft Tissues** 161
Ulrich Keller and Raimund Hibst

Chapter 12 **Clinical and Investigative Research on the Excimer Laser** 173
Tim Liesenhoff

Chapter 13 **Clinical Applications of the Ho:YAG Laser** 187
Harvey Passes

Chapter 14 **Clinical Applications of the Nd:YAG Laser** 199
Alan Goldstein, Joel M. White, and Robert M. Pick

Chapter 15 **Clinical Applications of the Argon Laser in Restorative Dentistry** 217
Richard Blankenau, W. Patrick Kelsey, and V. Kim Kutsch

Chapter 16 **Laser Processing of Dental Materials** 231
Heidemarie Dobberstein, Herbert Dobberstein, Annegret Schwarz, Rainer Zuhrt, and Yoshiaki Tani

Chapter 17 **Biostimulation and Photodynamic Therapy** 247
Elliot Abt

Part IV Current Technology and Future Directions

Chapter 18 **Analysis of Excimer Laser Interactions with Hard Tissue** 261
Joseph Neev

Chapter 19 **Modern Optics and Dentistry** 283
Grigori B. Altshuler and Andrey V. Erofeev

Chapter 20 **New Concepts in Laser-Tissue Interaction** 299
Guy Levy and Ioana M. Rizoiu

Appendices

Appendix I **Glossary** 315

Appendix II **Units of Measurement, Equivalents, Formulas, and Constants** 320

Appendix III **Laser Precautions** 321

Appendix IV **Curriculum Guidelines and Standards for Dental Laser Education** 323

Index 333

Contributors

Elliot Abt, DDS, MS
Director, Dental Residency Program
Ravenswood Hospital Medical Center
Chicago, Illinois

Grigori B. Altshuler, PhD
Professor and Director, Laser Center
Chairman, Department of Quantum Electronics
Institute of Fine Mechanics and Optics
St. Petersburg, Russia

Charles Arcoria, DDS, MBA
Associate Professor
Department of Restorative Sciences
Baylor College of Dentistry
Dallas, Texas

Richard J. Blankenau, DDS
Professor
Department of Operative Dentistry
Creighton University School of Dentistry
Omaha, Nebraska

Heidemarie Dobberstein, Dr sci med
Private Practice
Berlin, Germany

Herbert Dobberstein, Dr sci med
Private Practice
Berlin, Germany

Andrey Erofeev, PhD
Institute of Fine Mechanics and Optics
St. Petersburg, Russia

Matthias Frentzen, DDS
Professor
University Dental Clinic, Bonn
Bonn, Germany

Alan Goldstein, DMD
Private Practice
New York, New York

David M. Harris, PhD
Assistant Professor
Department of Oral Biology
College of Dentistry
University of Illinois at Chicago
Chicago, Illinois

Raimund Hibst, PhD
Director
Department of Research
Institute for Laser Technology in Medicine
University of Ulm
Ulm, Germany

Ulrich Keller, DDS
Assistant Professor and Assistant Medical Director
Department of Dental Surgery and Radiology
University of Ulm Dental School
Ulm, Germany

W. Patrick Kelsey, DDS
Professor and Chairman
Department of Operative Dentistry
Creighton University School of Dentistry
Omaha, Nebraska

Hans J. Koort
Physicist
MedLas Medical Techniques
Bonn, Germany

V. Kim Kutsch, DMD
Private Practice
Albany, Oregon

Guy Levy, DMD, MS, PhD
Professor
Department of Endodontics
School of Dentistry
University of Marseille
Marseille, France

Tim Liesenhoff, Dr med
Clinic for Oral Surgery
Technical University of Munich
Munich, Germany

Loh Hong-Sai, DDS
Professor and Chairman
Department of Oral and Maxillofacial Surgery
Faculty of Dentistry
National University of Singapore
Singapore

Catherine A. Miserendino
Senior Research Scientist
Wenske Laser Center
Chicago, Illinois

Joseph Neev, PhD
Assistant Professor
Beckman Laser Institute and Medical Clinic
University of California, Irvine
Irvine, California

Harvey Passes, DDS
Director
Division of Laser Dentistry
Jamaica Hospital
Jamaica, New York

M. Anthony Pogrel, MB, ChB, BDS, FDS, RCS, FRCS
Associate Professor
Department of Oral and Maxillofacial Surgery
School of Dentistry
University of California, San Francisco
San Francisco, California

Ioana Rizoiu, MS
Senior Research Physicist
Biolase Technology, Inc
San Clemente, California

Annegret Schwarz, Dr med
Private Practice
Berlin, Germany

Yoshiaki Tani, DDS, D Med Sc, FADM
Professor and Director
Research Center for Biomedical Engineering
Kyoto University
Kyoto, Japan

Joel M. White, DDS, MS
Associate Professor
Division of Biomaterials and General Restorative Dentistry
School of Dentistry
University of California, San Francisco
San Francisco, California

Harvey Wigdor, DDS, MS
Chief of Dentistry
Ravenswood Hospital Medical Center
Chicago, Illinois

Rainer Zuhrt, Dr med dent
Professor
Department of Operative Dentistry
Center of Dentistry
Humboldt University
Berlin, Germany

Preface

Lasers in Dentistry is not just another dental textbook about a specialized aspect of dentistry. Because it is the first comprehensive publication about this new field, it is indeed unique, but to those who have been involved with lasers in dentistry over the past thirty years or more, it is much more. For those pioneering researchers and clinicians who have been involved with the development or evolution of laser use in dentistry, it represents a major step forward, or coming of age, for laser dentistry. The book documents the basic scientific and clinical applied research that substantiates the appropriate use of the laser as a dental instrument. *Lasers in Dentistry* marks a new stage of maturity for this growing technology.

For many, this book will serve as a reference on a subject that is new and unknown. To aid the reader in focusing on specific subjects of interest, the information in the book is organized into four sections. Part I addresses topics relevant to the scientific basis of lasers to familiarize those new to laser dentistry with principles of how lasers work and interact with oral structures. Part II identifies practical aspects of laser use in dentistry, such as regulation and safety concerns, which are essential for incorporating lasers in clinical practice. Part III is perhaps the core of the book. In this section, the technical aspects of practical applications and clinical procedures are described in detail for the various types of laser systems currently available for use in dentistry. Part IV examines advanced topics related to current research and future directions for lasers in dentistry. The appendices contain supplementary information, such as definitions of technical terms, standards of practice, and sample course outlines for educational purposes.

It is the goal of this text to help the clinician understand the important differences between lasers and their tissue interactions. In this way, those new to lasers can become laser-literate and begin using lasers where applicable. For those already familiar with lasers, this book will act as an all-encompassing guide to laser physics and tissue interaction, laser safety, and the current status of lasers in clinical practice.

It is important to recognize that since this book is intended for an international audience, some of the information and clinical applications contained herein may be considered experimental in certain jurisdictions. Acceptable treatment modalities and practice standards may vary based on regional norms and regulations. Therefore it remains the responsibility of the dental practitioner, in consultation with the patient, to select appropriate methods of treatment that apply within their specialty or area of practice. Dental practitioners should contact their local governing boards or authorities prior to any clinical use of lasers.

Although *Lasers in Dentistry* is the first book of its kind, it will not be the last. As technology advances and our understanding of laser light expands and its potential unfolds, it will be necessary to revise and update from time to time. Researchers and clinicians must continue to explore and search for more effective methods of treatment. We hope that this book will serve as a foundation upon which to build.

We wish to express our sincere gratitude to Peter M. Baker, Executive Director of the Laser Institute of America, and Robert Handren, President of the Laser Institute of America, for their assistance in the development of this book.

This book is not the product of any one individual's efforts, but rather the combined contributions of many individuals from around the world. One needs only to glance through the list of contributors to recognize the names of experts who have distinguished themselves in the field of laser dentistry. We wish to thank the contributors for their unending efforts.

Introduction

Lasers range from those activated by natural gases, elements, molecules, or manmade crystals to those that measure distances to the moon, create laser-guided warfare, and record the price of our groceries. Over the past several years, we have seen the strong emergence of lasers in the field of dentistry. Lasers are not, however, new to the field; some of the first reports, on in-vitro studies, date back to the late 1960s. It was not until the early 1980s, however, that lasers truly saw their first use in clinical practice.

Early pioneering teams such as Fisher and Frame in the United Kingdom, Pecaro and Pick in the United States, and Melcer in France began using CO_2 lasers for soft tissue surgery. Melcer also initiated hard tissue applications with the CO_2 laser. Shortly thereafter, pioneering teams began exploring Nd:YAG lasers for soft tissue procedures and hard tissue applications, including Myers and Myers in the United States, Midda in the United Kingdom, and Yamamoto in Japan. Other important early contributors were Powell and Blankenau, Miserendino, White, Featherstone, Wigdor, Abt, Pogrel, Mungo, and Rempfer from the United States, Dederich and Zakariasen from Canada (and now the U.S.), Levy from France, and Hibst and Keller from Germany.

When used efficaciously and ethically, lasers are an exceptional modality of treatment for many clinical conditions that dentists or dental specialists treat on a daily basis. For some procedures in dentistry, such as the maxillary midline frenectomy, lasers are so clinically effective that they should become the standard of care, as they have in certain medical procedures.

Regardless of the wavelength used, lasers in dentistry offer a variety of advantages. Because lasers seal blood vessels, they offer a dry operating field and excellent visibility, reducing operative time. In addition, lasers seal lymphatic vessels, which yields minimal postoperative swelling. Lasers offer the ability to negotiate curves and folds in the oral cavity, and depending on power settings and mode of delivery, they can vaporize, coagulate, or cut tissue.

With the use of lasers, pain is reduced-to-absent 90% of the time, probably due to the sealing of nerve fibers. The other 10% of the time, patients will have pain of various intensities and durations. In some procedures, such as the maxillary midline frenectomy, it is almost certain that there will be no postoperative pain. Lasers offer little chance for mechanical trauma, they cause minimal scarring, and sutures are rarely needed. They cause reduction in bacterial counts, and in some areas they may sterilize the field as well. Therefore, for patients at risk for bacteremias, the use of lasers may be especially beneficial.

In daily clinical practice, how many times do we not perform or, worse yet, not recommend therapy that is efficacious and yields more esthetic results because we are afraid that the treatment modality and postoperative course are not acceptable to the patient? One of the greatest advantages of laser use in dentistry is a high rate of patient acceptance. Patients today are aware of lasers and their advantages. For example, a patient with an unesthetic smile line due to excess gingival soft tissue can be informed that the tissue can be removed without flap reflection, sutures, or dressings and assured that with a laser procedure the postoperative course will be relatively comfortable.

Most dental laser users report increased referrals and greater practice income. When used ethically and efficaciously, these increases come from greater patient acceptance of certain treatments. Furthermore, patients who experience minimal postoperative discomfort and appreciate state-of-the-art therapy will lead to referrals of new patients.

Some clinicians are wary of entering this exciting field because of the equipment's size and cost. The original lasers were not only large but had six-figure price tags. Lasers will, however, continue to get smaller and less expensive, as have computers and calculators. Dental lasers today are small, lightweight, highly portable, and increasingly affordable. One can wait for cheaper lasers and smaller lasers, but it is possible to invest so late that technology has passed one by.

The future of dental lasers is bright. Some of the newest ongoing research addresses the use of dental lasers for guided tissue regeneration, connective tissue attachment, and tissue welding. Dental lasers of the future may make incisions, reflect flaps, perform osseous surgery, and weld the flaps into position. Multiple wavelengths (some of them perhaps not yet known) may be incorporated into a single unit.

Dentistry has entered an exciting era of high technology. The dental laser offers the dentist not only a window, but a door into this high-tech, rewarding, and potentially profitable arena.

Part I

The Scientific Basis of Laser Dentistry

Chapter One

The History and Development of Laser Dentistry

Leo J. Miserendino

Light has been used as a therapeutic agent for many centuries. In ancient Greece, the sun was used in heliotherapy, or the exposure of the body to the sun for the restoration of health (Daniell and Hill, 1991). The Chinese used the sun to treat such conditions as rickets, skin cancer, and even psychosis. The beneficial effects of the sun in the treatment of rickets became apparent in the late 1700s. This use of light for treatment of various pathologies is referred to as *phototherapy*. In 1903, a Danish physician named Niels Finsen developed a technique known as carbon arc phototherapy for the treatment of lupus vulgaris that employed the use of ultraviolet rays.

The earliest use of photochemotherapy, or the use of an exogenous photosensitizer to absorb light and render a therapeutic effect, dates back to 1400 B.C. Indians used a drug called *psoralens*, obtained from plants, to treat vitiligo. A lotion was applied to the skin, which was then exposed to sunlight. The Egyptians also used psoralens to treat the skin disease leukoderma. In 1974, it was found that psoralens combined with exposure to ultraviolet A radiation (PUVA) was indeed effective in the treatment of psoriasis and vitiligo.

Discovery of the Maser

The first laser, or "maser" as it was initially called, was developed by Theodore H. Maiman of Hughes Aircraft Corporation in 1960 (Maiman, 1960). "Maser," like the more familiar term "laser," is an acronym for "Microwave Amplification by Stimulated Emission of Radiation," which describes the basic principle by which all lasers operate. According to Goldman (Goldman, 1991), these principles were first reported in 1958 by Schawlow and Townes of the Massachusetts Institute of Technology, but the Nobel Prize for the development of the laser was awarded to Townes, Basov, and Prokhorov in 1964. Credit for the development of the theory of spontaneous and stimulated emission of radiation, however, is generally given to Einstein for his treatise, "Zur Quantum Theorie Der Stralung," which was initially published in 1916 (Einstein, 1916).

Early Dental Laser Research

The first laser constructed by Maiman was a pulsed ruby laser, which emitted light of 0.694-μm wavelength (Maiman, 1960). Surprisingly, the second laser to be developed was the neodymium laser, which followed only one year later (Snitzer, 1961). Nearly all of the early dental laser research was performed with the ruby laser, which may have resulted in a delay in the development of laser dentistry (Table 1.1). Had dental researchers focused on the neodymium laser sooner, laser dentistry may have progressed to its present status some 10 years earlier. The following synopsis of the progression of basic and applied clinical laser research in the field of dentistry over the past 30 years may support this concept.

The Ruby Laser

Dental laser research began in 1963 at the University of California at Los Angeles School of Dentistry with the investigations of Ralph H. Stern and Reidar F. Sognnaes. Like most of the early dental laser researchers, interests centered around the thermal effects of the ruby laser on the dental hard tissues (enamel and dentin) and restorative materials. They reported the development of cratering and glasslike fusion of enamel, and the penetration and charring of dentin following a single millisecond pulse of the ruby laser at 500 to 2,000 J/cm^2 (Stern, 1964). In further experiments they observed that under specific parameters of exposure to the ruby laser there occurred an increased resistance to acid penetration into enamel, suggesting a possible role for the laser in caries prevention (Stern, 1974).

The first report of laser exposure to a vital human tooth appeared in 1965 when Leon Goldman, MD, applied two pulses of a ruby laser to the tooth of his brother, Bernard, who was a dentist. According to their report (Goldman et al, 1965), the first dental laser patient experienced no pain with only superficial damage to the crown. Ironically, the first laser dentist was a physician and the first dental laser patient was a dentist.

Unfortunately, the results of other early dental research with the ruby laser were not as promising. Most experiments involving the application of this laser to teeth

Table 1.1. Early Dental Laser Research

Date	Investigators	Laser	Subject	Results
1963	Stern & Sonnaes	Ruby	Enamel and dentin effects	Unfavorable
1965	Goldman et al	Ruby	Vital tooth (case report)	Promising
1965	Taylor et al	Ruby	Oral tissue effects (in vivo)	Unfavorable
1968	Lobene et al	CO_2	Enamel and dentin effects	Promising
1971	Adrian et al	Ruby	Pulp effects (in vivo)	Unfavorable
1972	Stern et al	CO_2	Enamel effects	Favorable
1972	Kantola	CO_2	Enamel and dentin effects	Favorable
1974	Yamamoto & Ooya	YAG	Caries prevention	Favorable
1977	Lenz et al	Argon	Surgical application (case report)	Promising
1977	Adrian	Nd:YAG	Pulp effects (in vivo)	Questionable
1977	Adrian & Huget	Nd:YAG	Welding	Favorable
1980	Yamamoto & Sato	Q-switched YAG	Caries prevention	Favorable

produced unfavorable results, which may be attributed to the destructive interaction of the 6.943-nm wavelength with dental hard tissue. The histologic effects of the ruby laser on the dental pulp were first reported by Taylor and associates (Taylor et al, 1965). In an early in vivo experiment, they observed extensive hemorrhagic necrosis and disruption of the odontoblastic layer in the incisors of laboratory animals, which had been exposed to a 3-millisecond pulse of the ruby laser ranging from 35 to 55 J. Damage to adjacent teeth and surrounding structures was also reported as a result of scattering of the laser beam. This first report of extensive pulpal injury and destruction with the ruby laser was later confirmed by Adrian and others (Adrian, 1971) even at greatly reduced power levels. These reports and others tended to contribute to the opinion that the ruby laser showed little promise as a dental tool. By the end of the 1960s most dental researchers agreed that excessively high energy levels were required for the removal of tooth structure by ruby laser, which would result in severe thermal damage to vital tissues in the oral cavity.

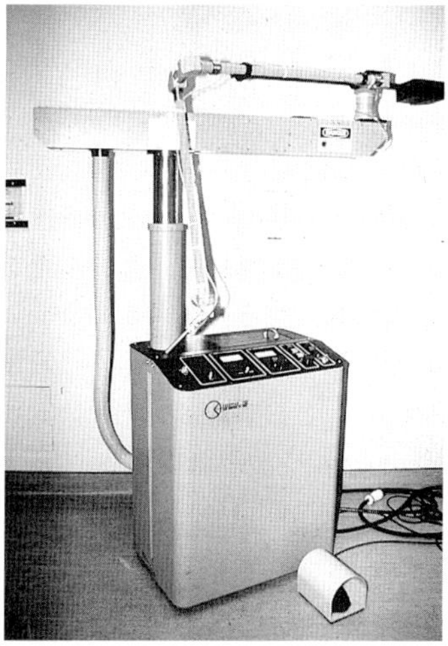

Fig 1.1 Early CO_2 surgical lasers: Sharplan surgical laser.

The Carbon Dioxide Laser

From the 1960s to the early 1980s, dental researchers continued to search for other types of lasers that might be more effective for application to hard tissue. In the United States, Stern at UCLA and Lobene at the Forsyth Dental Center in Boston shifted their attention to the carbon dioxide laser. Because its wavelength of 10.6 µm is well absorbed by enamel, it was thought that the carbon dioxide laser (Fig 1.1) might be suitable for selected surface applications to teeth, such as the sealing of pits and fissures; the welding of ceramic materials to enamel; or the prevention of dental caries (Lobene and Fine, 1966; Lobene et al, 1968; Stern et al, 1972).

During this time, a significant amount of work was also being performed with the carbon dioxide laser in Finland by Kantola and others. In a series of studies employing scanning electron microscopy, X-ray diffraction, and electron probe microanalysis techniques, they determined the chemical and physical transformations that resulted from exposure of enamel (Fig 1.2) and dentin by this wavelength (Kantola, 1972; Kantola et al, 1973). While these studies confirmed the ability of the carbon dioxide laser to induce resistance to acid penetration of enamel, attempts to use this laser for the sealing of pits and fissures and for the welding or fusion of materials such as hydroxyapatite to enamel (Fig 1.3) were unsuccessful due to the excessively high surface temperatures generated during the process (Stewart et al, 1985). During this same period, Melcer and others were actively involved in the clinical application of the carbon dioxide

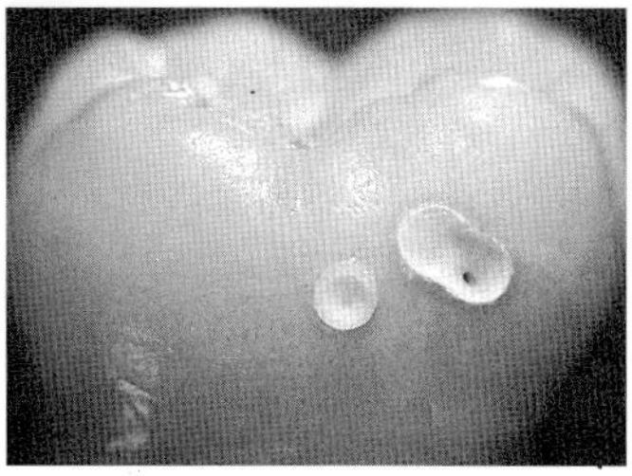

Fig 1.2 CO_2 laser effects on enamel. Recrystallized (white) area represents amorphous crystalline hydroxyapatite.

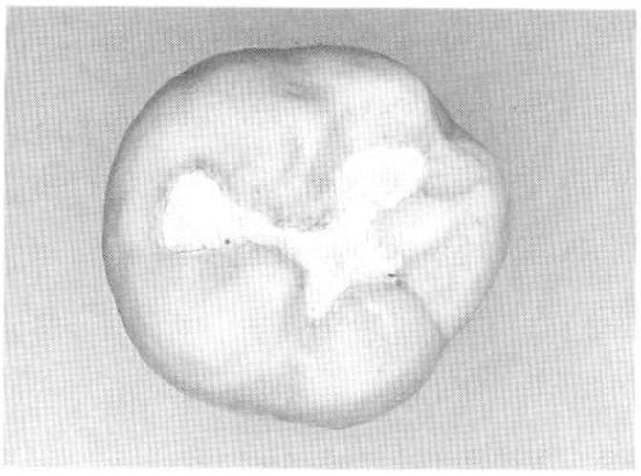

Fig 1.3 CO_2 laser-assisted fusion of hydroxyapatite to enamel.

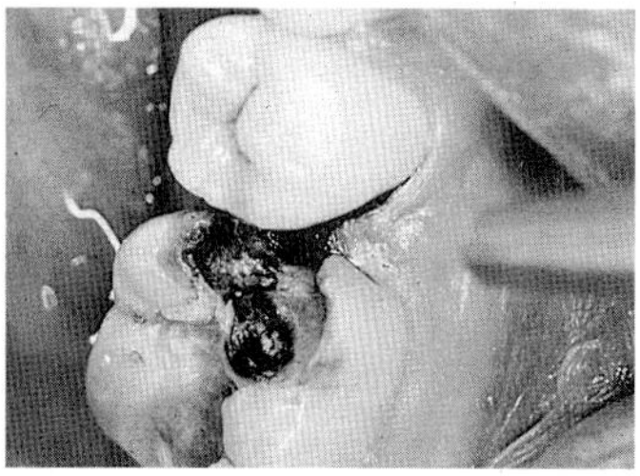

Fig 1.4 Caries removal by CO_2 laser. (Courtesy of Dr Harvey Wigdor.)

laser for the vaporization of caries. They reported the successful treatment of over 1,000 human patients in clinical trials of caries removal by the laser (Melcer et al, 1984). They further concluded by in-vivo animal studies (Melcer et al, 1987) that the laser could induce secondary dentin formation and sterilization of dentin and the exposed pulp (Fig 1.4).

The Neodymium Laser

The first report of dental application of the neodymium laser to vital oral tissue in experimental animals was that of Yamamoto and others from Tohoku University School of Dentistry in Japan (Yamamoto and Ooya, 1974). In a series of experiments, Yamamoto determined that the Nd:YAG laser was an effective tool for inhibiting the formation of incipient caries both in vitro and in vivo (Yamamoto et al, 1974; Yamamoto and Sato, 1980). During this same time, Adrian, who was working at the U.S. Army Institute of Dental Research at Walter Reed Medical Center, began to consider the neodymium laser for use on teeth and for laser welding of dental alloys (Adrian, 1977; Adrian and Huget, 1977). However, it would not be until much later that the first Nd:YAG laser would become available for use in dentistry, and remarkably the application of the laser to dental hard tissues has not been approved to date.

Clinical Application of Lasers in Dentistry

The Laser and Soft Tissue Surgery

While dental researchers continue their quest for the ideal wavelength or search for some unknown parameter that will open the door to hard tissue laser dentistry, enormous strides have been made in the field of dental laser surgery of oral soft tissue. Within the field of medicine, ophthalmology was the first specialty to apply the ruby laser successfully for surgical treatment of the retina in the early-to-mid 1960s (AMA Council on Scientific Affairs, 1986). Use of argon, carbon dioxide, and neodymium lasers by other medical surgical specialties did not occur until the 1970s (Polanyi, 1982). Extensive investigations involving the experimental use of the carbon dioxide laser for various surgical procedures were reported in the medical literature throughout the 1960s and early 1970s. By the mid 1970s, laser surgery in medicine, although not routine, became more commonplace.

Introduction of the laser for soft tissue oral surgery undoubtedly came through the interaction of oral and maxillofacial surgeons with otolaryngologists and other head and neck surgeons. According to Willenborg (Willenborg, 1991), the first reported application of a laser for maxillofacial surgery was by Lenz, who used an argon laser to create a nasoantral window (Lenz et al, 1977). An extensive account of the benefits of the carbon dioxide laser in oral and maxillofacial surgery was presented by Pecaro and Garehime of Northwestern University Dental School in Chicago (Pecaro and Garehime, 1983). In January 1987, the Food and Drug Administration gave the first marketing approval for laser use in oral surgery to the Pfizer Laser Company for a 10-W portable carbon dioxide laser unit (Fig 1.5). Shortly afterward, a number of important papers were presented by Fisher and Frame of England on the treatment of benign and premalignant oral lesions with the carbon dioxide laser during the 1980s (Fisher et al, 1983; Fisher and Frame, 1984; Frame et al, 1984; Frame, 1985).

According to most authorities, the list of advantages derived through application of the carbon dioxide laser in particular for surgical procedures in the mouth is quite extensive. It includes excellent hemostasis; improved visibility during the procedure; minimal damage to adjacent tissues; reduced swelling, pain, and infection postoperatively; and a relative absence of scarring and wound contracture (Hall, 1971; Fisher et al, 1983; Pecaro and Garehime, 1983; Frame et al, 1984; Frame, 1985) The cited benefits have been attributed to the ability of the carbon dioxide laser to seal small blood vessels and lymphatics and thereby circumvent some of the early manifestations of the inflammatory process as occurs in wound healing.

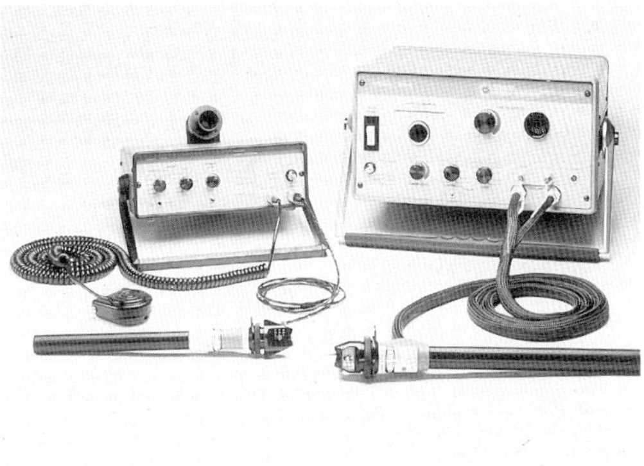

Fig 1.5 First FDA marketing clearance for dental use of lasers. Office tabletop lasers. Ten-watt (left) and 20-W (right) CO_2 laser units (Pfizer Laser Systems, Irvine, CA).

The properties of improved hemostasis afforded through tissue ablation with the carbon dioxide laser were first recognized and applied to periodontal surgery by Pick (Pick et al, 1985). The technique that he developed for a nearly bloodless gingivectomy in patients with bleeding disorders was perhaps the first step toward expansion of laser use into procedures that are more commonly encountered in general dental practice (Fig 1.6). Once lasers were in the hands of the periodontist, a multiplicity of surgical procedures evolved, which demonstrated to the profession the unquestionable superiority of the laser related to the previously mentioned advantages. Periodontal applications of the laser remained limited to those procedures that could be performed via optical lens delivery systems, that is, treatment of soft tissue surface lesions that could be easily accessed by direct vision in the mouth. Other limitations of early carbon dioxide laser systems can be attributed to its inability to be applied to vital hard tissue, namely bone, and for those procedures that require contact with dentin and cementum.

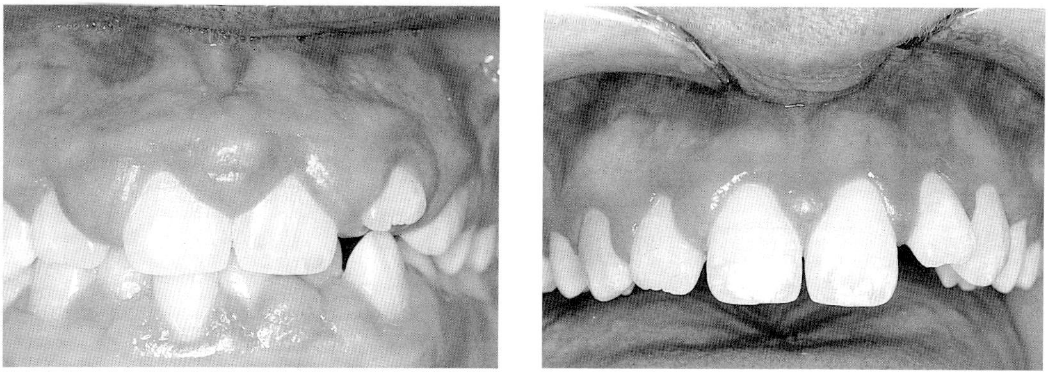

Fig 1.6 Laser gingivectomy: **(a)**, Dilantin hyperplasia pretreatment; **(b)**, 1 month postoperative appearance.

Early attempts to apply carbon dioxide laser light to enamel and dentin revealed that this laser was perhaps not destined to replace the drill for routine operative dental treatment. The thermal effects of radiant energy within the infrared range, such as ruby (0.693 μm) and CO_2 (10.6 μm) at energy levels sufficient to remove or ablate enamel or dentin, result in extensive damage to hard tissue and are equally injurious to the dental pulp (Taylor et al, 1965). Other attempts to use low-energy carbon dioxide laser exposure for surface treatments such as sealing of pits and fissures (Stewart et al, 1985), caries prevention (Nelson et al, 1986), enamel etching (Cooper et al, 1988; Leiberman et al, 1984), and dentin desensitization failed to stimulate widespread acceptance of this laser in general dental practice.

The Search for Better Wavelengths

The desire for laser systems that could offer broader application in routine dental practice perhaps was the stimulus for one general dentist from Michigan, to look at other wavelengths that might offer some advantages over CO_2. The fact that Dr Terry Myers and his brother, William, an ophthalmologist, selected the Nd:YAG laser for their experiments on removal of incipient caries should come as no surprise due to the widespread use of this type of laser in ophthalmology by the mid 1980s (Myers and Myers, 1985). Soon afterward, they began the development of the first true dental laser system, which undoubtedly could be considered the spark that ignited the laser revolution in dentistry. Not only did the introduction of the D-lase 300 (Fig 1.7) provide dentistry with its first dedicated dental laser system, designed specifically for dental application, but the resultant marketing effort that followed brought an awareness of lasers to dentistry and to the public, which was equally remarkable. Shortly after marketing clearances were approved by the Medical Device Division of the Food and Drug Administration in the United States, groups of laser dentists joined together to form local study clubs, societies, and diverse organizations for the purpose of gathering and sharing information related to their use (Goal, 1989).

Concurrent with the increasing acceptance of lasers by dentists for a growing number of laser dental procedures was an equal if not greater acceptance by patients for dental laser treatment. It is conceivable that patient demand for this new technol-

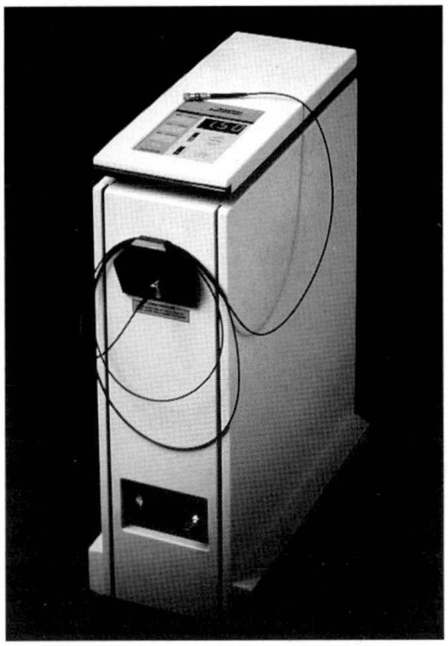

Fig 1.7 First dedicated dental laser unit, American Dental Laser DL-300 (Sunrise Technologies Inc, Sunnyvale, CA). Laser unit and fiber delivery system (oblique view).

ogy would alone be sufficient force to drive laser dentistry forward. The perception of the public, already cognizant of the advantages of laser surgery in medicine, particularly ophthalmology, was that this new high-tech modality was not only painless but superior to conventional methods. Whether fact or fiction, patient acceptance of laser dentistry would undoubtedly play a significant role in its development.

Facing decreasing demand for their services due to a decline in the incidence of dental caries and other economic pressures, many dentists recognized that the laser could be effective not only as a precision instrument, but also as a powerful marketing tool. Reports appeared in the dental literature (Shulkin, 1991) of increased practice productivity resulting from the addition of the laser. This increase was attributed to the addition of new patients desirous of laser treatment and to the addition of new laser procedures. The net result for many dentists was the successful incorporation of the laser into the general dental practice.

Lasers and Hard Tissue Applications

At this time, clinical applications of lasers in the United States have essentially been limited to soft tissue procedures. The Food and Drug Administration serves as the regulatory body by allowing marketing of devices such as lasers for specific purposes within the dental and medical professions. To date, only a limited number of investigational uses have been approved for the purpose of gathering the necessary information to ensure the safety and efficacy of laser application to hard tissues. These studies are closely monitored and structured to determine the appropriate use of lasers in the dental profession for specific procedures.

Regulation of the practice of dentistry within the United States is generally governed by state dental licensing boards or local government agencies. Outside the United States, clinical application of lasers to hard tissue is already taking place where permitted. The dentist is therefore obligated to recognize the restrictions that apply to his or her particular circumstance. Numerous clinical applications of lasers to dental hard tissues are either currently in practice or are being developed as newer wavelengths of lasers and methods of laser emission are being applied in the field of dentistry.

Sufficient research exists to predict that current laser systems such as erbium:YAG, holmium:YAG, Nd:YAG, and excimer have the potential to replace the dental drill for a number of uses (Fig 1.8).

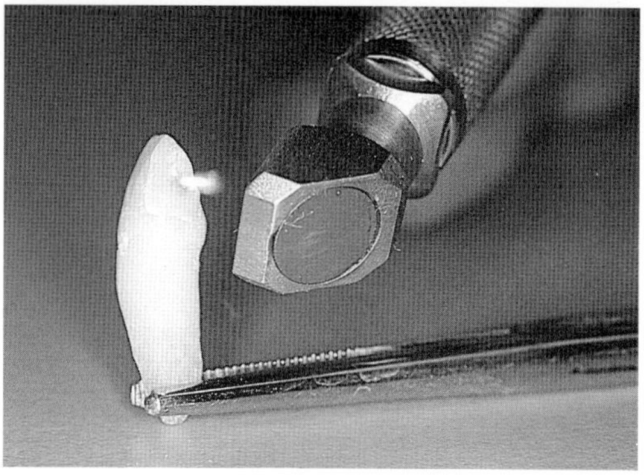

Fig 1.8 Nd:YAG laser impact on incipient caries.

The list of potential clinical applications of lasers to hard dental tissues includes but is not limited to the following: caries detection, prevention, and removal; cutting of enamel, dentin, and bone; desensitization of dentin; enamel etching; osteoplasty and ostectomy. Therapeutic uses of lasers may be beneficial for all aspects of dentistry, especially endodontics, oral surgery, periodontics, and restorative dentistry.

Future Directions

While great advances have already been made in the application of lasers to dental materials, there is even greater potential for further development in dental materials processing. Dental materials scientists and researchers will only need to look to industry to see the possibilities. Industrial use of lasers for cutting, welding, fusing, and handling of materials is just the beginning. Military and commercial applications of lasers for positioning, communications, measurement, and detection are only a few of the many possible uses that may be explored. Medical science is already taking advantage of lasers in diagnostics and therapeutics far beyond current clinical use in dentistry (Table 1.2). While some have stated that the laser is just another gadget in search of an application, others may counter that the limitations of the laser are only those imposed by the limited imaginations of its users.

Table 1.2. Medical and Industrial Applications of Lasers

Application	Industrial	Medical
Material processing	Cutting, drilling, etching, metal welding, fusion of ceramics, photopolymerization	Photopolymerization of composite resins (dental)
Imaging	Interferometry, stereolithography, holography, nondestructive testing	Holographic and video endoscopy, biomedical interferometry, pattern recognition
Detection and diagnostics	Laser-assisted sensing, positioning, surveying, spectroscopy, scanning	Laser doppler flowmetry, fiberoptic and fluorescent sensing, biomedical spectroscopy
Communication and information	Optical data storage (laser disk), fiberoptic telecommunication	Data storage on optical laser disks
Phototherapy		Photodynamic therapy, biostimulation, desensitization, wound healing, pain control, photosensitization

References

Adrian JC. Pulp effects of neodymium laser. A preliminary report. Oral Surg Oral Med Oral Pathol 1977;44:301–305.

Adrian JC, Bernier JL, Sprague WG. Laser and the dental pulp. J Am Dent Assoc 1971;83:113.

Adrian JC, Huget EF. Laser welding of nickel-chromium alloy. Milit Med 1977;141:299–301.

American Medical Association, Council on Scientific Affairs. Lasers in medicine and surgery. JAMA 1986;256:900–910.

Cooper LF, Myers ML, Nelson DG, Mowery AS. Shear strength of composite bonded to laser-pretreated dentin. J Prosthet Dent 1988;60:45–49.

Daniell MD, Hill JS. A history of photodynamic therapy. Aust NZ J Surg 1991;61:340–348.

Einstein A. Verk Deutsch Phys Ges 1916;18:318.

Fisher SE, Frame JW. The effect of the CO_2 laser surgical laser on oral tissues. Br J Oral Maxillofac Surg 1984;22:414–425.

Fisher SE, Frame JW, Browne RM, Tranter R. A comparative histological study of wound healing following CO_2 laser and conventional surgical excision of canine buccal mucosa. Arch Oral Biol 1983;28:287–291.

Frame JW. Carbon dioxide laser surgery for benign oral lesions. Br Dent J 1985;158:125–128.

Frame JW, Das Gupta A, Dalton G, Rhys Evans P. Use of the CO_2 laser in the management of premalignant lesions of the oral mucosa. J Laryngol Otol 1984;98:1251–1260.

Goal VP. A new drill: painless dentistry isn't here yet, but technology has brought it a lot closer. Wall Street J, November 13, 1989:11.

Goldman L. Background to laser medicine—history, principles, and safety. In Goldman (ed): Laser Non-surgical Medicine. Lancaster, PA: Technomic Publishing Co, Inc;1991.

Goldman L, Gray JA, Goldman J, Goldman B, Meyer R. Effects of laser impacts on teeth. J Am Dent Assoc 1965;70:601–606.

Hall RR. The healing of tissue by a carbon dioxide laser. Br J Surg 1971;58:222–225.

Kantola S. Laser induced effects on tooth structure 6 and 7. Acta Odontol Scand 1972;30:463–484.

Kantola S, Laine E, Tarna T. Laser induced effects on tooth structure 6 and 7. Acta Odontol Scand 1973;31:369–388.

Leiberman RR, Segal T, Nordenberg D, Serebro L. Adhesion of composite materials to enamel: comparison between use of acid and laser as pretreatment. Laser Surg Med 1984;4:323–327.

Lenz HJ, Eichler G, Schaffer J, Bettges G. Production of a nasoantral window with the argon laser. J Maxillofac Surg 1977;5:314–318.

Lobene RR, Bhussry R, Fine S. Interaction of CO_2 laser with enamel and dentin. J Dent Res 1968;47:311–317.

Lobene RR, Fine S. Interaction of CO_2 laser radiation with oral hard tissues. J Prosthet Dent 1966;16:589.

Maiman TH. Stimulated optical radiation in ruby. Nature 1960;187:493–494.

Melcer J, Chaumette F, Melcer F. Dental pulp exposed to the laser beam. Laser Surg Med 1987;7:347–352.

Melcer J, Chaumette F, Melcer F, Dejardin J. Treatment of dental decay by CO_2 laser beam: preliminary results. Laser Surg Med 1984;4:311–321.

Myers TD, Myers WD. The use of the laser for debridement of incipient caries. J Prosthet Dent 1985;53:776–779.

Nelson DGA, Shariati M, Glena R, Shields CP, Featherstone JDB. Effect of pulsed low energy infrared laser irradiation on artificial caries-like lesion formation. Caries Res 1986;20:289–299.

Pecaro BC, Garehime WJ. The CO_2 laser in oral and maxillofacial surgery. J Oral Maxillofac Surg 1983;41:725–728.

Pick RM, Pecaro BC, Silberman CJ. The laser gingivectomy. J Periodont 1985;56:492–494.

Polanyi TG. History of the CO_2 laser in surgery. In Andrews AH, Polanyi TG (eds): Microscopic and Endoscopic Surgery with the CO_2 Laser. Boston: J Wright Publishing Inc; 1982:1–25.

Shulkin NH. The American dental laser: initial patient response. Dent Today 1991;10:60–61.

Snitzer E. Optical maser action of Nd+3 in Ba crown glass. Phys Rev Letter 1961;7:444.

Stern RH. Dentistry and the laser. In Wolbarsht ML (ed): Laser Applications in Medicine and Biology, v 2. New York: Plenum Press; 1974:361–388.

Stern RH, Sognnaes RF. Laser beam on dental hard tissues. J Dent Res 1964;43:873.

Stern RH, Vahl J, Sognnaes RF. Laser enamel: ultrastructural observations of pulsed carbon dioxide laser laser effects. J Dent Res 1972;51:455–460.

Stewart L, Powell GL, Wright S. Hydroxyapatite attached by laser: a potential sealant for pits and fissures. Oper Dent 1985;10:2–5.

Taylor R, Shklar G, Roeber F. The effects of laser radiation on teeth, dental pulp, and oral mucosa of animals. Oral Surg Oral Med Oral Pathol 1965;19:786.

Willenborg GC. Lasers and electro-optics in dentistry. In Goldman L (ed): Laser Non-surgical Medicine. Lancaster, PA: Technomic Publishing Co Inc; 1991: 253–291.

Yamamoto H, Ooya K. Potential of yttrium aluminum garnet laser in caries prevention. J Oral Pathol 1974;3:7–15.

Yamamoto H, Ooya K, Matsuda K, Okabe H. YAG laser effects for acid resistance on tooth enamel (abstract 7). J Dent Res 1974;53:1093.

Yamamoto H, Sato K. Prevention of dental caries by acousto-optically Q-switched Nd:YAG laser irradiation. J Dent Res 1980;59:137.

Chapter Two

Laser Physics

David M. Harris and Robert M. Pick

When surgical lasers are used to incise soft tissues, little or no bleeding occurs and patients experience less postoperative discomfort than with traditional surgery. In addition, with proper parameters, a laser will produce less collateral thermal damage than will an electrocautery. Because of these and other advantages, many practitioners are replacing cold steel and electrosurgical devices with surgical lasers. But a laser is more than a fancy scalpel. Very precise control of laser output allows the tuning of the space, time, and wavelength to optimize the outcomes of specific clinical procedures. Some types of lasers are useful for processing dental materials, and some are useful for measuring blood flow (laser doppler). Research laser systems can discriminate normal from carious dentin spectrographically, and new and experimental systems hold the promise of a hard tissue "laser drill."

This chapter emphasizes those laser types currently in use and under investigation for dental applications. Dental lasers are simply surgical lasers (Fuller, 1987) used in dentistry. Surgical lasers are basically the same as scientific and industrial lasers (Hitz, 1991) with certain modifications to meet FDA standards and ergonomics of the clinical environment. Unique to most surgical systems are the specialized delivery devices that carry laser energy to living tissue (see Chapter 8).

Lasers are unique and versatile instruments by virtue of their physical characteristics. Properties such as collimation, coherence, and monochromaticity are generated in the high-energy processes occurring inside the optical cavity (Maiman, 1960). The laser beam that is projected from this cavity and onto the patient's tissues retains these characteristics. Therefore, if one is to learn how to apply laser energy to obtain a desired clinical effect, then one must understand laser fundamentals.

For most clinicians, laser fundamentals are not intuitively obvious. Because lasers did not exist in our childhood environment, we did not gain a feel for laser-tissue interactions the same way we understand knife-tissue effects. This chapter provides an overview of the basic concepts and characteristics of surgical lasers. It is suggested that the reader refer to a good text-

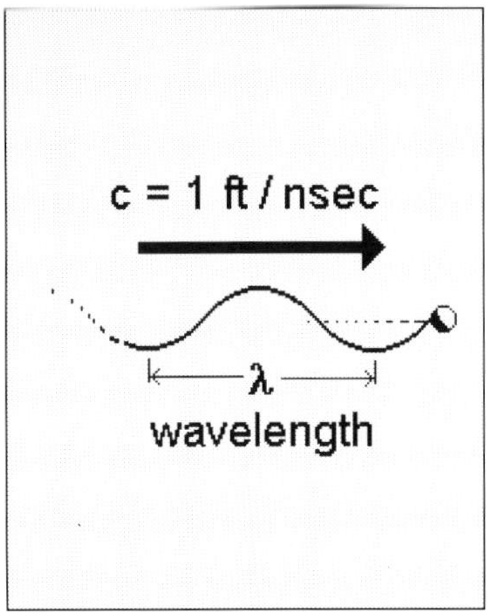

Fig 2.1a Schematic photon showing the approximate speed of light (1 ft/nsec) and the definition of wavelength. As a photon moves through space, the electric field oscillates in a plane. The distance a photon travels through one complete oscillation is its wavelength. A magnetic field, not shown, oscillates perpendicular to the electric field (in and out of the page). Thus, photons represent quanta of electromagnetic energy.

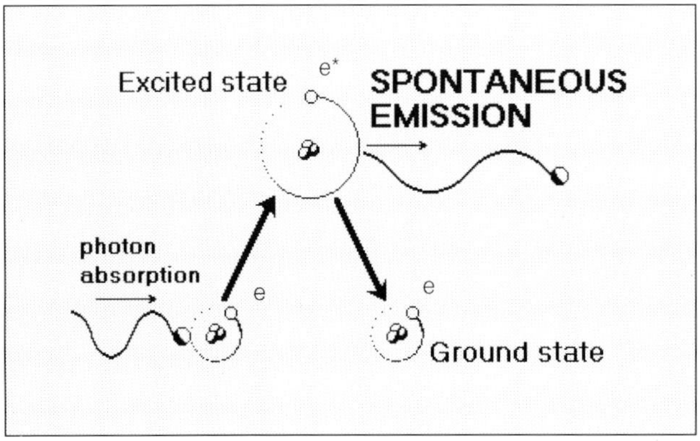

Fig 2.1b An atom absorbs a quantum of energy and is pumped up to an excited state. Spontaneous emission occurs when the atom decays from the excited state to a lower energy state. The excess energy is released as a photon.

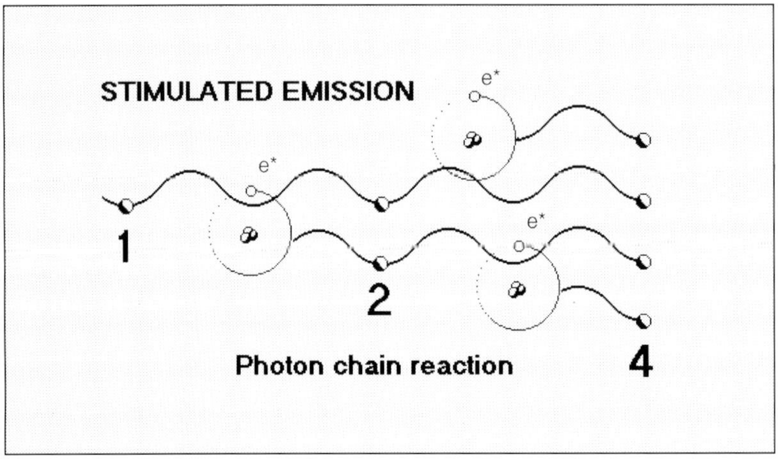

Fig 2.1c Stimulated emission occurs when an excited atom is stimulated to release stored energy. The exciting photon and the released photon stimulate two more excited atoms, and so on, producing a photon chain reaction.

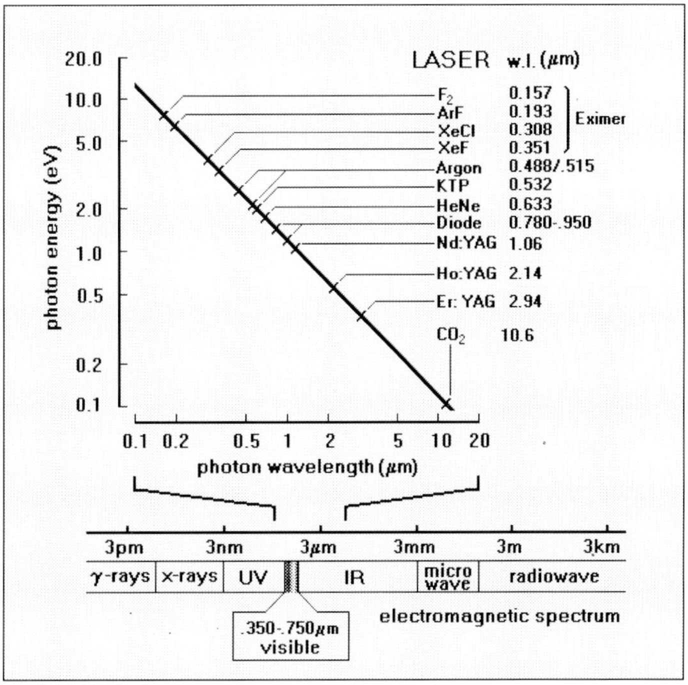

Fig 2.2 The electromagnetic spectrum extends from short wavelength, high-energy particles (γ-rays) to long-wavelength, low-energy particles (radiowaves). Common laser types are listed according to their wavelengths.

book on physical chemistry (eg, Atkins, 1986) for a more in-depth discussion of electromagnetic energy and atomic and molecular energy dynamics.

What Are Photons?

The basic units, or quanta, of light are called photons. Sometimes it is useful to think of them as particles, like little nano-BBs careening through space at 186,000 miles per second. From another perspective, photons behave like tiny wavelets similar to sound wave pulses (Fig 2.1a). A quantum of light can be depicted as an electromagnetic wave with an electric field oscillating up and down in the plane of the page. The photon moves across the page from left to right at 1 foot/nanosecond (1 ns = 1 billionth of a second). There is also a magnetic field associated with the photon that moves in and out of the page (not shown).

Quanta of electromagnetic energy are classified as cosmic rays, gamma rays, x-rays, light, microwaves, or radio waves (Fig 2.2). Light may be ultraviolet, visible (violet, blue, green, yellow, orange, red), or infrared. The physical property that determines this classification of electromagnetic energy is wavelength: the distance a photon travels while the electric field completes one complete oscillation (see Fig 2.1a). Cosmic rays have extremely short wavelengths (10^{-12} m), whereas radio waves have very long wavelengths (10^3 m). With current technology, laser light covers the range from about 0.1 to 10 μm. Most of the current types of clinical lasers plotted according to their wavelengths are shown (see Fig 2.2). Notice that short wavelength ultraviolet light is more energetic than long wavelength infrared.

Light Absorption and Emission

When light encounters matter, it can be deflected (reflected or scattered) or absorbed. If a photon is absorbed, its energy is not destroyed but rather used to increase the energy level of the absorbing atom or molecule. This idea is central to both laser physics and laser-tissue interactions.

An atom can absorb a photon (see Fig 2.1b). The photon then ceases to exist, and an electron (e) within the atom jumps to a higher energy level (e*). This atom is thus pumped up to an excited state from the resting ground state. In the excited state, the atom is unstable and will soon spontaneously decay back to the ground state, releasing the stored energy in the form of an emitted photon. This process is called *spontaneous emission*. The interval between absorption and re-emission is usually very short and defines the fluorescence lifetime of the atom. Notice in Fig 2.1b that the spontaneously emitted photon has less energy (a longer wavelength) than the absorbed photon. The difference in energy is usually turned into heat.

In any given atom, only certain orbits (energy levels) are allowed. When a photon is absorbed, the atom jumps to one of the allowable energy levels. This means that each type of atom or molecule can absorb only photons of exactly the right energy (or wavelength). The result is that each species of atom or molecule has a unique absorption spectrum.

Light Amplification by Stimulated Emission of Radiation

The process of lasing occurs when an excited atom can be stimulated to emit a photon before the process occurs spontaneously (see Fig 2.1c). When a photon of exactly the right energy (wavelength) enters the electromagnetic field of an excited atom, the incident photon triggers the decay of the excited electron to the lower energy state. This is accompanied by the release of the stored energy in the form of a second photon. The first photon is not absorbed but continues on to encounter another excited atom.

Stimulated emission can only occur when the incident photon has exactly the same energy as the released photon. Thus, the result of stimulated emission is two photons of identical wavelength traveling in the same direction. The release of the second photon is time-locked to the oscillations of the first photon, so that the two photons oscillate together in phase.

If a collection of atoms includes more that are pumped up into the excited state than remain in the resting state, a population inversion exists. This is a necessary condition for lasing. Now, the spontaneous emission of a photon by one atom will stimulate the release of a second photon in a second atom, and these two photons will trigger the release of two more photons; these four then yield eight, eight yield sixteen, and so on. In a small space at the speed of light, this photon chain reaction produces a brief, intense flash of monochromatic (same wavelength) and coherent (same phase) light.

Laser Components and Beam Generation

The basic components of a laser are actually quite simple. They include a lasing medium placed within an optical cavity, a pump energy source, and a cooling system (Fig 2.3). To contain and amplify the photon chain reaction that results from stimulated emission in a population of excited atoms, it is necessary to place this reaction within an optical cavity. An optical cavity consists of two parallel mirrors placed on either side of the laser medium. In this configuration, photons bounce off the mirrors and re-enter the medium to stimulate the release of more photons. If some form of energy is provided to continuously pump atoms up to the excited state, the population inversion can be maintained and high-intensity light circulating back and forth between the two mirrors can be generated. The mirrors collimate the light, that is, photons exactly perpendicular to the mirrors re-enter the active medium, while those off axis leave the lasing process. Because the process is not 100% efficient and some energy is converted into heat, it is necessary to provide some form of cooling.

If one mirror is totally reflective (see Fig 2.3, M2) and the other mirror partially transmissive (M1), the light that escapes through M1 becomes the laser beam. If our circulating power is 1,000 W and M1 is 10% transmissive, then the power returning from M1 is 900 W, and the exiting beam is 100 W. A round trip through the lasing medium brings the power back up to 1,000 W.

The active medium contains the homogeneous population of atoms or molecules that are pumped up to the excited state and are stimulated to lase. The exact species of atom or molecule determines the wavelength of the output beam. The active medium is suspended in the optical cavity as a gas, a liquid, or distributed in a solid state (eg, a crystal).

Thus, stimulated emission within an optical cavity generates a collimated, coherent, and monochromatic beam of light. The laser is named for the contents of the active medium and their state of suspension, eg, CO_2 gas laser or argon-ion gas laser.

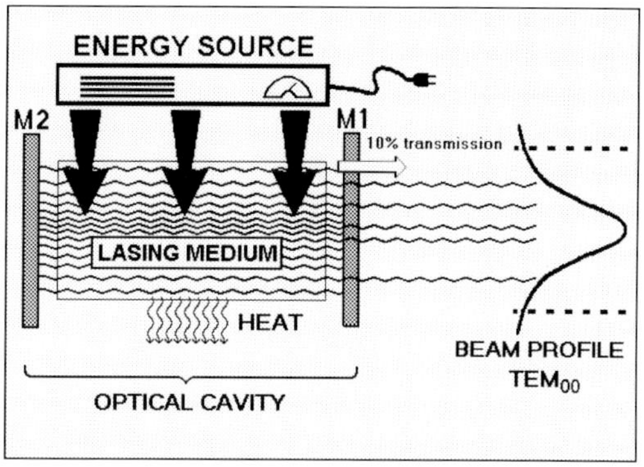

Fig 2.3 Schematic diagram of a laser. M1 and M2 are mirrors that define the optical cavity. Elements of the lasing medium (eg, CO_2, neodymium, or argon ions) are pumped up to an excited state by applying an external energy source. The laser beam exits the optical cavity via the partially transmissive mirror, M1.

The CO_2 Laser

The CO_2 laser works on a slightly different principle than outlined above. The CO_2 molecule stores energy in vibrational modes as well as electronic modes. That is, atoms have energy states based on the orbits that electrons occupy. Molecules have, in addition, discrete (and quantal) modes in which they vibrate, each mode having a different energy level. However, the basic concept as outlined above is the same. CO_2 molecules are pumped up to higher energy vibrational states and decay back to the ground state, releasing photons of specific wavelengths. The decay can be spontaneous or stimulated.

The lasing medium in a CO_2 laser actually contains a mixture of CO_2, nitrogen (N_2), and helium gases. In the CO_2 laser, the process becomes quite efficient if nitrogen molecules are pumped up with en-

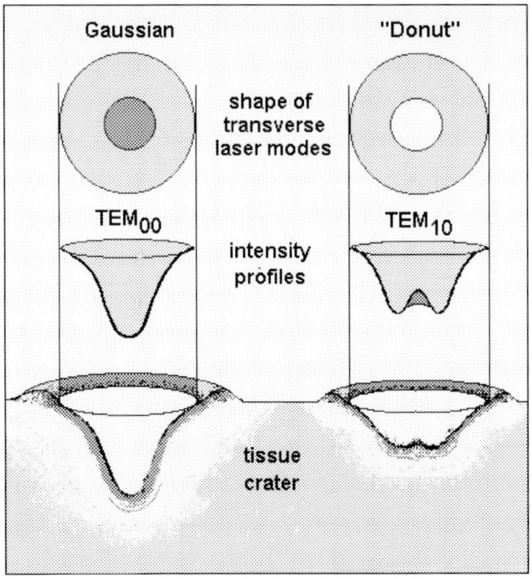

Fig 2.4 Two examples of beam geometry: (left) the TEM_{00}, Gaussian, or "fundamental" mode; (right) the TEM_{10}, or "Donut" mode. Schematized at the bottom are the crater geometries expected from each type of beam. This diagram illustrates that the physical processes occurring in the optical cavity influence the final tissue effects.

ergy from an electric discharge applied to the laser tube (pump source). Direct current (dc) can be passed through the lasing medium, or the medium can be pumped with an intense radiofrequency (rf) electric field. The electric current pumps N_2 up to the excited state. Nitrogen transfers this stored energy by colliding with ground-state CO_2. The pumped-up CO_2 then emits an infrared photon (10.6 μm) and returns to the ground state. Helium is also added to the gas mixture of N_2 and CO_2 to facilitate heat transfer from the lasing medium to the walls of the laser cavity. Some type of circulating coolant is used to remove the excess heat.

If the electric current is maintained through the lasing medium, the molecules are pumped up as soon as they decay. In this way, a population inversion and a continuous laser output are maintained. The energy that exits from the laser tube is an attenuated version of the energy circulating in the optical cavity, the attenuation being determined by the transmission of the output mirror. The width of the beam, determined by cavity cross section, is typically 0.5 to 2.0 cm for the CO_2, Nd:YAG, and argon lasers. This collimated beam will continue to propagate through space over extremely long distances with little dispersion.

Beam Profile and Spot Geometry

Notice in Fig 2.3 that there are more photons concentrated in the core of the beam and that the light intensity diminishes at the edges. Often in a well-tuned cavity the transverse cross section (profile) is the normal gaussian curve. This is referred to as the TEM_{00} (transverse electromagnetic mode: 00), also called the "fundamental mode." Other modes are possible such as the "Donut" mode (TEM_{10}), which has a cold spot in the center (Fig 2.4).

This beam profile can be seen in the effect it has on a target. As an experiment, lase a dry wooden tongue depressor at about 10 W for 0.1 sec. Look closely at the shape of the crater; the more concentrated the photons, the deeper the burn. The same experiment can be done on a pad of paper. In this case, photon concentration is proportional to the number of pages burned through. The projection of the beam on the target is called the spot. A cross section of the beam is called the beam profile, a common way of describing spot geometry. The diameter of the spot is called the spot size. As the pages of the pad are turned to examine the size of the burn hole below the surface layers, it is

Table. Power Densities (W/cm)

Power (W)	Spot Size Diameter (mm)		
	0.05	0.2	2.0
1.0	50,900	3,180	32
5.0	255,000	15,900	159
10.0	509,000	31,800	318
50.0	2,550,000	159,000	1,590

clear that the hole's diameter gets progressively smaller at greater depths. This simple experiment helps illustrate the shape of the laser beam.

Power Density

The previous experiment introduces the concept of power density (PD). Power density is simply the concentration of photons in a unit area. Photon concentration is measured in watts and area in square centimeters. Therefore,

$$PD = W/cm^2$$

To compute PD, the cross-sectional area of the beam is needed. This is obtained from the formula for the area of a circle (A) given the radius ($r = \frac{\text{diameter}}{2}$):

$$A = \pi r^2$$
$$\text{Where } \pi = 3.14$$

If 10 W in the beam exits the CO_2 laser, and the beam diameter is 1.0 cm:

$$\begin{aligned} PD &= 10 / 3.14\ [(0.5)\ 1]^2 \\ &= 10 / 0.79 \\ &= 12.7\ W/cm^2 \end{aligned}$$

This is the average PD. Notice from the beam profile that the PD in the center of the spot is higher and that at the edge of the spot it approaches 0.

Power density can be increased significantly by placing a lens in the beam path. Remember the experiment you did as a child on a sunny summer day, using a magnifying glass and an unsuspecting ant? By focusing the parallel beam of light from the sun, you increased the PD from warm to hot!

Because the light from the laser is collimated and monochromatic, it is possible to focus the power down to micrometer diameter spots. Lenses usually will not alter the beam profile, only change the power density. If 10 W is focused into a spot that is 0.05 mm (50 μm) in diameter, a PD of 509,000 W/cm^2 is created. Spot area is actually a better indicator of tissue effect than is spot diameter, but conventionally the spot size is described by the diameter.

Different power densities are achieved from different combinations of power and spot size (Table). Notice that 10 W in a 2.0-mm spot produces a power density of 318 W/cm^2. If the spot size is decreased by a factor of ten to 0.2 mm, power density increases by a factor of one hundred (10^2) to 31,800 W/cm^2. However, changing power by a factor of ten only changes power density by a factor of ten.

The size and shape of the lens determines the focal length and the spot size at the focal point. Beyond the focal point, the beam diverges and the power density or intensity decreases. The terms *focused* and *defocused* when working with lasers refers to the position of the focal point in relation to the tissue plane. When working on tissue, the laser should always be used either with the focal point positioned at the tissue surface (in focus) or positioned above the tissue surface (defocused or out of focus). The laser should never be positioned with the focal spot deep or within tissue (prefocused) as this can lead to deeper thermal damage and undesirable tissue effects (Fig 2.5).

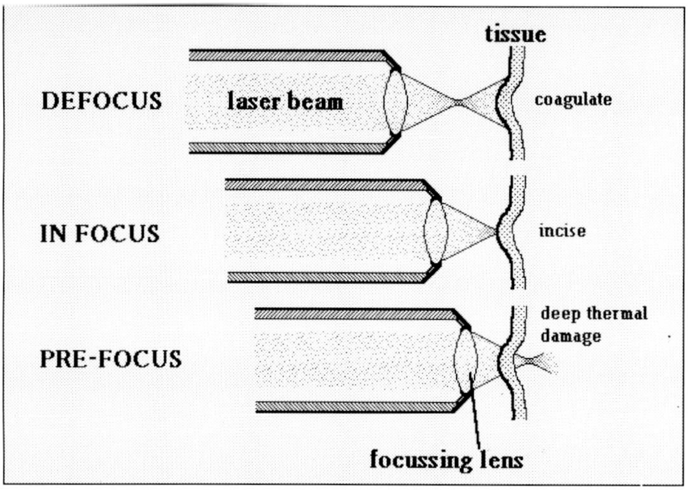

Fig 2.5 A lens placed in the beam path will focus the laser energy in a small spot at the focal point. Beyond the focal point, the beam diverges. Maximum power density is achieved when the beam is in focus at the target, producing rapid tissue vaporization. Pulling the laser handpiece back from the tissue defocuses the beam, and the lower power density achieves tissue coagulation. The prefocused mode is to be avoided clinically since it produces deep thermal damage.

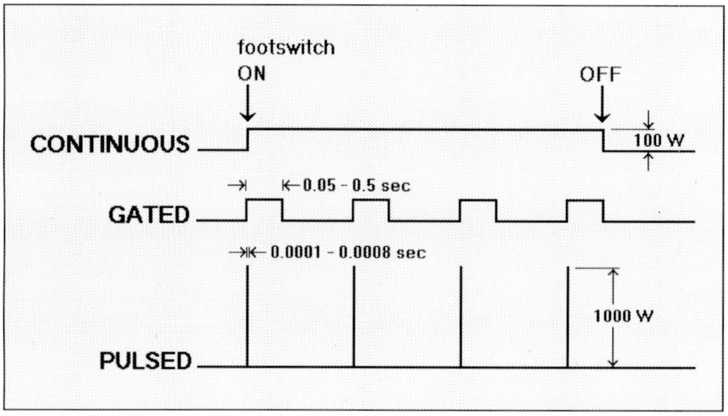

Fig 2.6 Timing schemes and relative peak powers for continuous, gated, and pulsed laser outputs.

Gating and Pulsing

Surgical lasers have a mechanical shutter positioned in the beam path (like a camera). The opening and closing of the shutter is controlled by a timing circuit. Timing values are set by controls on the front panel console. The time sequence is activated when the user steps on the foot pedal, or in some units, presses the button on the handpiece. Single pulses can have durations such as 0.05, 0.1, 0.2, 0.5, and 1.0 sec, or the shutter can remain open as long as the pedal is depressed (continuous). Timing circuits vary in sophistication. Usually pulse duration can be set and the time between pulses can be varied independently, changing the repetition rate. On some units, bursts of pulses can be delivered (Fig 2.6).

Even shorter duration pulses can be produced by pulsing the pump source. Recall that the pump source drives stimulated emission by pumping molecules up into the excited state. In a CO_2 laser, we can modulate the rf or dc pump energy and produce a train of pulses having durations of tens to hundreds of μsec (millionths of a second). The peak power of these superpulses may be over 1,000 W, although the average power delivered over 1 sec may only be 10 to 30 W. This train of superpulses may be gated with the mechanical shutter as described.

Energy and Energy Density

For very short duration pulses, it is often more practical to talk about the amount of *energy* per pulse in Joules (J), rather than the average output *power* in watts. Energy is actually the work that is done, or power applied for a period of time. A unit of energy, 1 J, is equal to one unit of power (1 W) times one unit of time (1 sec). Thus 100 J equals 100 W applied for 1 sec, or 10 W applied for 10 sec, etc:

$$1 \text{ J} = 1 \text{ W} \times 1 \text{ sec}$$

Most clinical pulsed lasers deliver less than 1 J per pulse. Here the unit millijoule is used:

$$1 \text{ J} = 1{,}000 \text{ mJ}$$

A similar concept to power density is energy density. This is simply the amount of energy per unit area. Or, stated another way, energy density is power density applied over time (Fig 2.7).

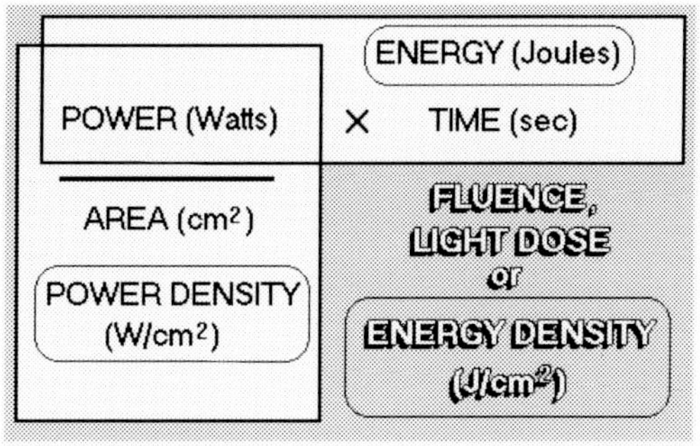

Fig 2.7 Diagram illustrating the relationships among power (W), area (cm^2), and time (sec). Power into area is power density. Power times time is energy. Energy into area is energy density.

Solid-State Lasers

In a CO_2 gas laser, the lasing medium (N_2 and CO_2) is dispersed in the optical cavity in the form of a gas. In solid-state lasers, the lasing medium is suspended in a transparent crystal. A garnet crystal made from yttrium and aluminum is commonly used in a variety of surgical lasers called YAG lasers.

In the past, YAG laser was used to refer to the neodymium:YAG (Nd:YAG). However, three types of YAG lasers are currently being used or are under investigation for their dental applications. Although each uses a YAG crystal to suspend the lasing medium, they differ in terms of the rare earth elements, neodymium, holmium, and erbium, that are doped into the crystal. Each element has a different arrangement of electron orbitals, so that lasing occurs at different wavelengths for each. The energy transitions in YAG lasers are more energetic than those in the CO_2 so that wavelengths are shorter in the near infrared (see Fig 2.2): Nd transition, 1.06 μm; Ho transition, 2.1 μm; Er transition, 2.9 μm.

The 10.6-μm wavelength of the CO_2 laser must be delivered to tissue through a system of mirrors and lenses (see Chapter 8). One advantage of visible light (eg, argon) and near infrared (Nd:YAG and Ho:YAG) lasers is that they can be delivered through an optical fiber, therefore access within the oral cavity is improved. The fiber can be used either in contact with the tissue or withdrawn (defocused) and used in the noncontact mode. The Er:YAG wavelength is beyond the transmission window of conventional optical fiber technology.

At this time, there are research systems that combine all three crystals in a single multiwavelength system. In addition, there are optical elements called nonlinear

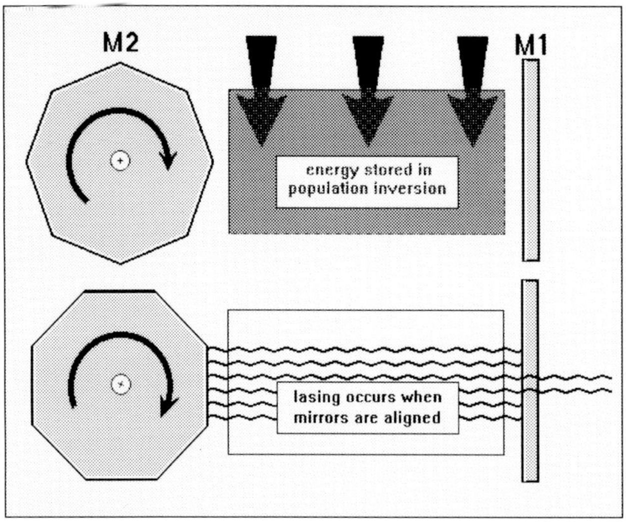

Fig 2.8 A Q-switch produces high-energy, short-duration pulses of laser energy. One type of Q-switch uses a rotating mirror to vary the quality of the optical cavity. During the very brief time when a facet of M2 is aligned with the surface of M1, the quality of the optical cavity is high, allowing lasing to occur. When the mirrors are not in alignment, energy is stored in the population inversion of the lasing medium.

crystals that can be placed in the optical cavity or in the beam path. The function of these crystals is to shift the wavelength of the light passing through them. The most common is the KTP (potassium titanium phosphate) crystal that shifts the 1.064-μm (near infrared) wavelength of the Nd:YAG to its first harmonic of 0.534 μm (green). One can imagine a multiwavelength system with multiple lasing crystals and a variety of nonlinear wavelength–shifting crystals. However, it will be several years before such versatile laser systems are practical for clinical use.

In the CO_2 laser, the pump source was described as an electric discharge from a dc or rf power supply. In YAG lasers, the lasing medium is pumped into higher energy states with light from an intense tungsten arc lamp, from a pulsed flash-lamp, or from another laser such as a diode laser. The optical cavity is surrounded with parabolic mirrors that focus the pump source into the YAG crystal.

A continuous output from a tungsten arc lamp can maintain a population inversion in a Nd:YAG crystal and maintain continuous power outputs of up to 100 W. This output beam can be shuttered as described for the CO_2 laser.

Flash-Lamp Pulsing

A popular system in dentistry is the pulsed YAG (neodymium, erbium, and holmium). In these systems, a flash-lamp is used to pump the lasing medium. As with the pulsed CO_2, peak powers are higher since the energy is confined to short duration pulses. The duration of the flash-lamp, typically 0.1 to 0.8 msec (100 to 800-μsec), determines the duration of the output pulse.

Q-Switching

Even shorter duration pulses are achieved with Q-switching. A simple Q-switch uses a rotating mirror as part of the optical cavity (Fig 2.8). Only when the rotating mirror is precisely aligned with the output mirror is lasing possible, so lasing is restricted to a very short time interval (1 to 10 nsec). Between alignments, energy is stored in the excited population. Thus, several hundred millijoules of energy can be squeezed into nanosecond pulses.

Diode Lasers

A much different type of solid-state laser is the diode laser. At this time, diodes are just finding application in surgery and are not yet used in dentistry. However, their small size and the promise of low cost suggest that they will soon find a place in the dental office.

The diode laser is a semiconductor chip that works like an electrical diode. The active region of the diode is a sandwich of different semiconductor materials consisting of a layer of p-type material (carrier of positive charge or electron holes), a nonconductive bandgap layer (junction), and a layer of n-type material (carrier of negative charge or free electrons). A negative voltage applied to the n-material and a positive voltage applied to the p-material makes charge carriers flow into the junction. At the junction, electrons fall into holes and energy is released. In most semiconductor materials, the energy is released as heat, but in materials such as gallium, aluminum, and arsenide, the energy is released as photons.

So far, we have described a light-emitting diode (LED). To make a diode laser, it is necessary to add a reflective surface at either end of the junction to establish an optical cavity. These optical cavities are very small—only a few millimeters long with a cross-sectional dimension of about 0.05 x 0.15 mm. Even on this scale some diode lasers can produce several watts of power.

Diodes have wavelengths in the red and infrared range (0.62 to 1.5 μm) that are determined by the semiconductor material and the operating temperature. Current clinical systems are in the range 0.8 to 0.9 μm. Intensive research is directed at producing 1 to 2 W at 0.63 μm for photodynamic therapy and biostimulation (see Chapter 17).

The geometry of the optical cavity results in a nonsymmetric beam. Special optics are necessary to recollimate the beam and focus it into fiberoptics. The output from several diodes in an array can be combined to boost output power up to 100 W.

Argon Laser

The argon laser is one of the rare-gas ion lasers capable of outputs of several watts continuous in the visible green and blue portion of the spectrum. These systems have found applications in the excitation of tissue fluorescence, in making diagnostic measurements, and in materials processing, such as polymerization and stereolithography. The surgical argon laser is most useful for the treatment of vascular disorders due to the selective absorption of hemoglobin in the green portion of the spectrum (see Chapter 9).

The active lasing medium is ionized argon gas. Molecular argon is inert, but ionized argon can undergo many energy conversions. In fact, 18 different wavelengths (or lines) are possible from argon ion transitions. Principal lines are at 0.514 μm (green) and 0.488 μm (blue).

Inside a vacuum tube, a high-current discharge is passed through a cloud of pure argon gas. An initial spike of several thousand volts ionizes the gas, then the voltage drops and current increases to sustain a population of excited argon ions. External magnets create a magnetic field that contains the lasing medium in a small diameter column in the center of the tube. Mirrors placed at each end of the tube provide an optical cavity.

A great deal of energy goes into ionizing the argon and, due to the low efficiency, a great deal of heat is produced and must be removed. High-power argon lasers (over 3 W) typically require water cooling and a 220 V power supply.

Because of the short wavelength of green and blue light (see Fig 2.2), it is possible to focus the argon beam into an extremely small spot. The laser microbeam is a device that focuses an argon beam through the optics of a microscope to perform surgery on single cells and even ablate single genes from chromosomes.

Conclusions

The process of lasing and the characteristics of most laser systems currently available to the dental practice have been examined. The physical processes occurring in the optical cavity determine the characteristics of the laser spot projected on the tissue. Therefore, an understanding of these processes improves the clinical judgment of a dentist performing a laser procedure.

There is another rationale for learning laser physics. New lasers are offered to the clinical community on a continuous basis. Laser dentistry is on the verge of expansion, with clinical trials in progress that are evaluating new laser procedures and devices for periodontics, endodontics, and hard tissue removal. An understanding of laser fundamentals gives the clinician a basis for making an informed judgment about whether or not a new system offers a real improvement over current technology.

References

Atkins PW. Physical Chemistry, ed 3. New York: WH Freeman, 1986.

Fuller TA (ed). Surgical Lasers: A Clinical Guide. New York: Macmillan, 1987.

Hitz CB. Understanding Laser Technology. Tulsa: Pennwell, 1991.

Maiman TH. Stimulated optical radiation in ruby. Nature 1960;187:493.

Chapter Three

Laser Interaction with Biologic Tissues

Leo J. Miserendino, Guy Levy, and Catherine A. Miserendino

Many of the basic principles governing laser-tissue interactions are relatively simple. The effects of laser emissions on biologic structures can, to some extent, be evaluated in terms of what occurs when radiant light energy reacts with matter. Other reactions of tissue to laser light involve biologic and physiologic processes of tissue, which are more complex in nature and reflect a more intricate interrelationship. Therefore, a practical knowledge of the biologic processes of tissue and the physical properties of laser light will provide the clinician with the ability to understand and control the outcome of laser treatment for a multitude of clinical applications.

In the previous chapter, the fundamental properties and parameters of laser light were identified. The essential elements of laser light that determine its interaction with matter are the *wavelength* of the radiant energy emitted by the laser; the *power density* of the beam; and the *temporal characteristics* of the beam energy, such as continuous vs pulsed delivery; pulse rate; and pulse duration. In addition to these factors, which are somewhat inherent to the particular type of laser, are other variables that relate to differences in the method of energy transfer attributable to instrumentation or delivery systems, such as contact vs noncontact optical fiber delivery, and focused vs unfocused beam.

The biologic factors that influence laser-tissue interactions are more extensive. Included among these are the optical properties of various tissue elements that govern how specific molecular and chemical components in tissue react with light energy. The optical properties of tissue elements determine the nature and extent of the tissue response through the processes of *absorption, transmission, reflection,* and *scattering* of the laser beam (Dederich, 1991). Other factors involve the various types of physiologic and mechanical processes that occur as a result of energy transformations within tissue. These include heat conduction and dissipation within the tissue mass, the inflammatory response of tissue to noxious stimuli, tissue vascularity, and repair mechanisms. The relationship between these biologic factors and processes, and the principles and properties of laser light energy will be described in greater detail in this chapter.

The extent of the interaction of laser light as a form of radiant energy with tissue will generally be determined by two dependent variables: the specific wavelength of the laser emission; and the optical characteristics of the particular target tissue (Dederich, 1991). Independent factors to be considered, which are under the control of the clinician, include the level of applied power (power density); the total energy delivered over a given surface area (energy density or fluence); the rate and duration of the exposure (pulse repetition rate and pulse duration); and the mode of delivery of the energy to the target tissue (ie, continuous vs pulsed; contact vs noncontact). Manipulation of these four variables (power output, spot size, fluence or total light dose, and mode of operation) will enable the operator to have precise control over the laser in the clinical setting to achieve the desired tissue effect when coupled with the ability to select the appropriate wavelength for the particular tissue target.

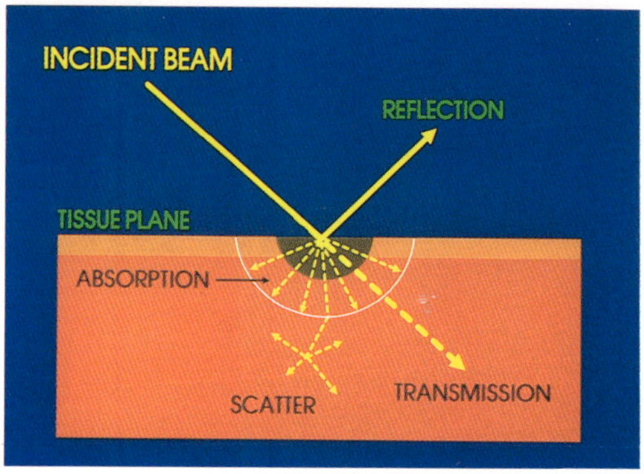

Fig 3.1 Four basic types of laser interaction with matter: reflection, absorption, transmission, scatter.

Optical Properties of Tissues and Wavelength Specificity

Radiant energy will interact with tissue in four ways (Fig 3.1). First, a portion of the incident beam may be reflected off the surface without penetration or interaction of the light energy with the tissue. Second, a portion of the light may be transmitted through the tissue unattenuated as if transparent to the laser beam. Third, some of the light may be absorbed into a component of the tissue, in which case there will be a transference of energy to the tissue. Fourth, the remaining light may penetrate the tissue and be scattered without producing a noticeable effect on the tissue. It is important to recognize that the previously mentioned laser-tissue interactions are not exclusive, but rather occur more commonly in varying proportions within tissue. This can be attributed to chemical and molecular variations found within composite biologic systems. In most cases the extent of the interaction will be proportional to the level of absorption of the particular wavelength by tissue.

In complex biologic systems composed of a great variety of cellular elements and tissue fluids, each with differing optical absorption characteristics, predicting the effect of specific laser emissions may at first appear to be problematic. Fortunately, oral soft tissue is largely composed of water, which predominantly controls the tissue effects of laser emissions within the infrared spectrum such as CO_2. This means that CO_2 laser energy at a wavelength of 10.6 μm is absorbed very efficiently by tissue fluids and has little penetration beyond the surface. On the other hand, water is comparatively transparent to the emission of the Nd:YAG laser, which accounts for its tendency to penetrate deeper into tissue. The transmission spectrum for water as it relates to specific wavelengths of radiant energy from 250 to 2,500 nm is illustrated in Fig 3.2.

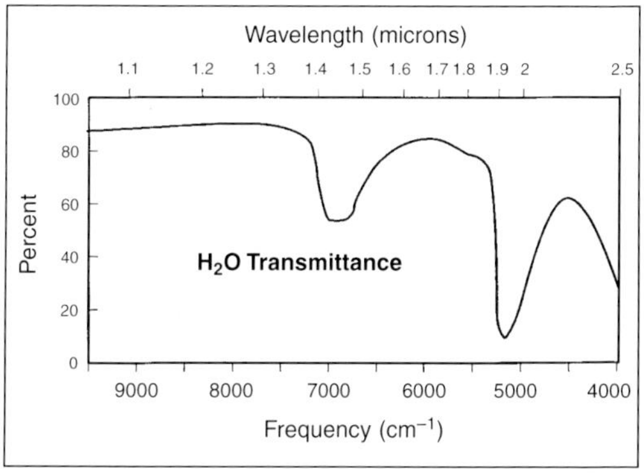

Fig 3.2 Transmission spectrum for water.

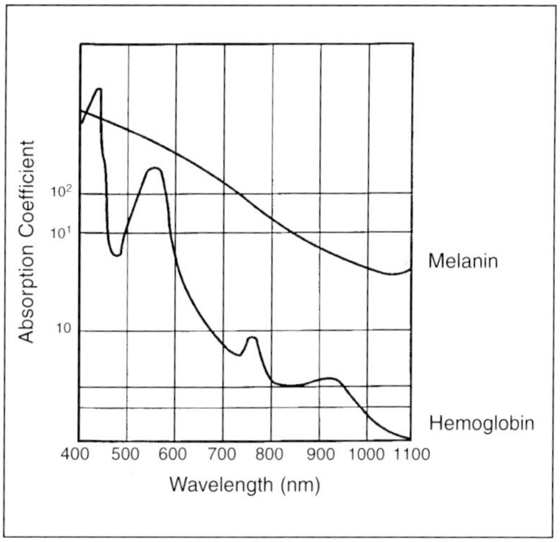

Fig 3.3 Absorption spectrum for hemoglobin and melanin pigment from 400 to 1,000 nm. (Adapted from Wright VC and Fisher JC. Laser Surgery in Gynecology. Philadelphia: WB Saunders, 1993;68.)

Tissue elements that exhibit a high coefficient of absorption for particular wavelengths or spectra of light energy are called chromophores. In fact, all matter has this property of absorption specificity, which controls how it will react to incident radiation. This characteristic of preferential absorption of specific wavelengths of radiant energy by chromophores within tissues allows for the unique interactions that occur between the monochromatic light energy of lasers and various tissue elements.

Other chromophores within tissues such as hemoglobin (Fig 3.3) and melanin pigments also exert a significant influence over the interaction of radiant energy and tissue. Hemoglobin readily interacts with 488- and 514-nm wavelengths, thus accounting for the greater ability of the argon laser for coagulation and hemostasis.

Spectrographic analysis of oral hard tissues such as enamel, dentin, bone (Figs 3.4 to 3.6), and synthetic hydroxyapatite (Fig 3.7) reveals some interesting findings. Although hydroxyapatite is a natural component of enamel, dentin, and bone, comparisons of the absorption, transmission, and scattering spectrographs of the four materials reveal marked dissimilarities between the pure synthetic and biologic materials. These differences may in part be attributed to variations in the percent composition of hydroxyapatite among the biologic materials or due to other more dominant soft tissue components affecting their optical behavior. Another theory, which is presented in more detail in Chapter 19, is that certain structural or morphologic interactions related to the direction of enamel rods and dentinal tubules are important.

A third very interesting observation that can be made by comparing the spectrographs for enamel, dentin, and bone is that all three biologic materials show favorable absorption, transmission, and scattering properties in the 2,000-nm region, which coincides with the emission wavelength for the thulium:YAG laser. This laser may prove to be the more ideal wavelength for dental hard tissue due to potentially more

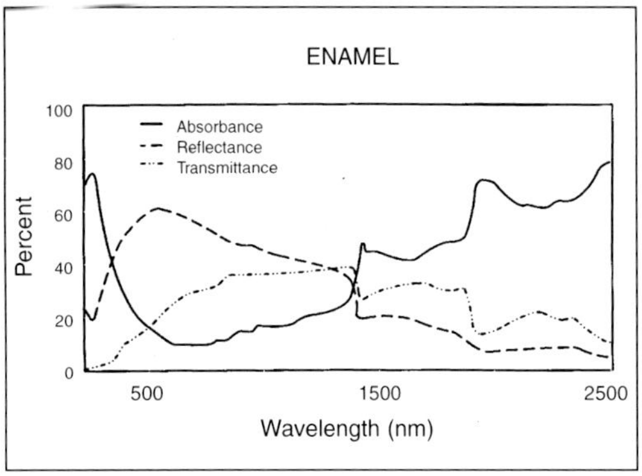

Fig 3.4 Spectrophotometric analysis of enamel (absorbance, reflectance, and transmittance) from 250 to 2,500 nm.

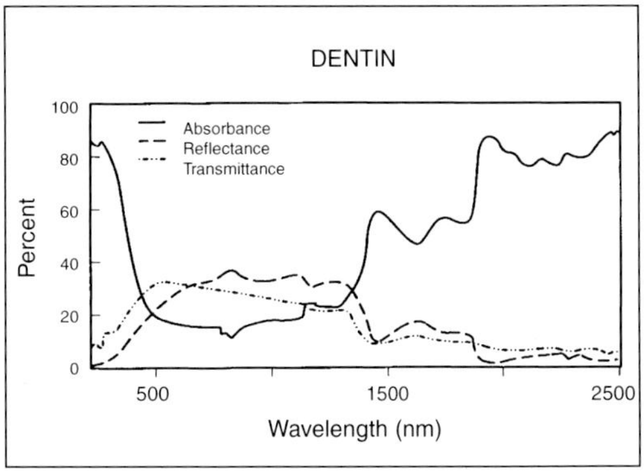

Fig 3.5 Spectrophotometric analysis of dentin (absorbance, reflectance, and transmittance) from 250 to 2,500 nm.

favorable hard tissue interaction and its ability to be transmitted (delivered) through optical fibers.

Therefore, in soft tissue, the effects of specific laser wavelengths are quite predictable due to the high absorption of energy of specific wavelengths by tissue elements or chromophores of differing optical properties. Preferential absorption by chromophores of particular laser wavelengths provides for a phenomenon of laser-tissue interaction known as wavelength or target specificity. Laser hard tissue interactions on the other hand are more unpredictable due to the limited amount of information presently available related to these types of interactions.

Tissue Effects of Laser Irradiation

When radiant energy is absorbed by tissue, four basic types of interactions or responses can occur: 1) photochemical interactions; 2) photothermal interactions; 3) photomechanical interactions; and 4) photoelectrical interactions. Because of the great number of clinical effects observed with these four types of interactions, they may be further subdivided according to how they manifest in clinical application as follows. Photochemical interactions include *biostimulation*, which describes the stimulatory effects of laser light on biochemical and molecular processes that normally occur in tissues such as healing and repair; *photodynamic therapy* (PDT), which is the therapeutic use of lasers to induce reactions in tissues for the treatment of pathologic conditions; and phosphorescent re-emission or tissue *fluorescence*, which may be used as a diagnostic method to detect light-reactive substances in tissue. Photothermal interactions manifest clinically as *photoablation*, or the removal of tissue by vaporization and superheating of tissue fluids; coagulation and hemostasis; and *photopyrolysis*, or the burning away of tissue. Photomechanical interactions include *photodisruption* or *photodisassociation*, which is the breaking apart of structures by laser light; and *photoacoustic* interactions, which involve the removal of tissue with shock-wave generation. Photoelectrical interactions include *photoplasmolysis*, which describes how tissue is removed through the formation of electrically

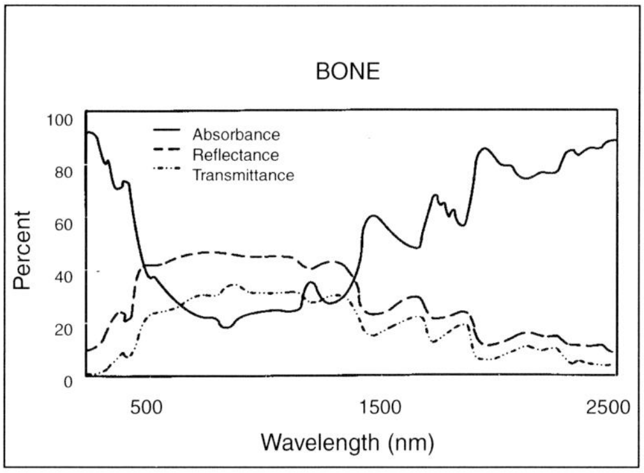

Fig 3.6 Spectrophotometric analysis of bone (absorbance, reflectance, and transmittance) from 250 to 2,500 nm.

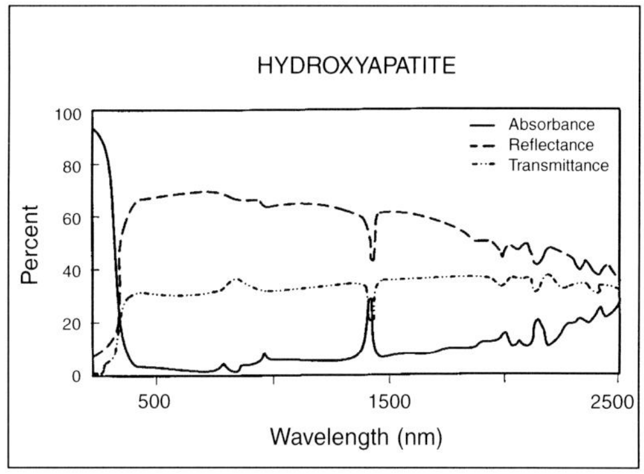

Fig 3.7 Spectrophotometric analysis of hydroxyapatite (absorbance, reflectance, and transmittance) from 250 to 2,500 nm.

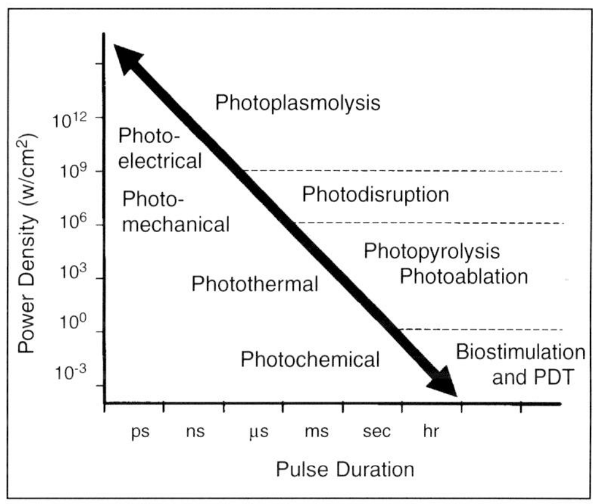

Fig 3.8 Relationship of power density and interaction time with the four mechanisms of light interaction: photoelectrical, photomechanical, photothermal, and photochemical, and their corresponding clinical manifestations in tissue. (Adapted from Harris and Werkhaven, 1989.)

charged ions and particles that exist in a semi-gaseous, high-energy state. Plasma is defined as the fourth state of matter, which is neither solid, liquid, or gas. The specific types of laser-tissue interactions previously mentioned above are explained later in this chapter.

The particular type of response that may occur when laser light interacts with tissue is not only wavelength-dependent, but is also strongly influenced by certain wavelength-independent variables or parameters, such as power density and exposure duration. Accordingly, tissue responses for a given light dose will vary based on whether the energy is delivered over a long duration or brief intervals. The nature of the tissue response to laser irradiation therefore is both wavelength- and time/rate-dependent.

Various types of tissue responses that result from exposure to laser energy, irrespective of wavelength, can be categorized over a theoretical range of exposure times and power densities (Fig 3.8). Generally, laser light emissions of relatively low intensity and long duration are less destructive and induce their effects at the cellular or molecular level, producing photochemical effects. One may surmise from this relationship between power density and exposure duration that potentially there could be a minimal level or threshold of energy required for specific types of interactions to occur.

Photochemical Interaction

The basic principle of the photochemical process is that specific wavelengths of laser light are absorbed by naturally occurring chromophores or wavelength-specific, light-absorbing substances that are able to induce certain biochemical reactions at the cellular level in both plants and animals. Investigative research has also shown that derivatives of naturally occurring chromophores or dyes can be used as photosensitizers to induce biologic reactions within tissue for both diagnostic and therapeutic applications.

A common example of a naturally occurring photochemical reaction is *photosynthesis*, where photons are absorbed by the chromophore, chlorophyll, to convert light energy into adenosine triphosphate (ATP). The process may be simplified by the chemical formula:

$$6\ CO_2 + 6\ H_2O \xrightarrow[\text{light energy}]{\text{chlorophyll}} C_6H_{12}O_6 + 6\ O_2$$

where carbon dioxide and water through a series of reactions are converted to glucose and oxygen. In the process, one electron of the chromophore, chlorophyll, absorbs light energy and becomes elevated to a higher energy level. The absorbed light energy becomes transformed into chemical energy by a process of photophorylation, which converts adenosine diphosphate (ADP) into ATP. The stored chemical energy is then used for the reduction of carbon dioxide and synthesis of glucose. This same principle is the basis for the type of photochemical reactions that occur in PDT and biostimulation (Harris, 1991). In PDT, the chromophore or photosensitizer is the drug, HpD, which is preferentially absorbed by malignant tumor cells. As the molecule of the photosensitizer, HpD, absorbs photons it becomes excited to a higher energy level. Once activated by laser light of specific wavelength, HpD promotes destruction of the tumor cells by release of singlet oxygen.

PDT has recently been applied for treatment of port wine stain. Here a photosensitizer and red laser light are used to induce photochemical destruction of subsurface blood vessels in the skin with a high degree of specificity. Another example of PDT is laser angioplasty for the treatment of atherosclerosis. In this application, the removal of arterial plaque is facilitated by laser irradiation delivered through an optical fiber. While still under development, the potential use of photosensitizers to induce selective absorption of the beam may reduce the risk of vessel perforation. The topics of photodynamic therapy and biostimulation are discussed in greater detail in Chapter 18.

Laser-induced photochemical reactions such as tissue fluorescence or phosphorescent re-emission may also be used for diagnostic purposes. Fluorescent tissue interaction or phosphorescent re-emission occurs when light energy is absorbed by specific molecules or tissue components that momentarily store and subsequently release the energy again as light. The absorbing tissue component acts as a biologic capacitor without undergoing any permanent transformation. The process of tissue fluorescence or phosphorescent re-emission is called photochemical decomposition. Certain oral tissues exhibit autofluorescence when stimulated by specific wavelengths. Generally, some energy is lost in the process during decomposition and therefore the re-emitted photon has a somewhat lower energy level than that of the incident radiation. This can be observed by the slightly longer wavelength of the fluorescent radiation. The entire process of phosphorescent re-emission occurs in less than 10^{-6} seconds. Recent research has demonstrated that laser-stimulated tissue fluorescence may be a viable method for the detection of caries. Other potential applications of tissue fluorescence include the use of photosensitizing dyes for the enhancement of absorption of particular wavelengths to induce destruction of microorganisms and for other tissue interactions.

Photothermal Interactions

At somewhat higher fluences (1 to 10,000 J/cm^2) and shorter exposure times (1 to 10^{-6} sec), photothermal interaction with tissue occurs. This class of interaction is the basis for most types of surgical laser applications. Because of its importance, extensive research has been performed to identify the biologic response of tissues attributed to the effects of heat generation from laser irradiation.

In photothermal interactions, radiant light energy absorbed by tissue substances and molecules becomes transformed into heat energy, which produces the tissue effect. The amount of laser light energy absorbed into tissue depends on a number of factors that include: the wavelength of the radiant energy from the laser; the laser parameters such as spot size, power density, pulse duration and frequency; and the optical properties and composition of the target tissue. It is important to recognize that each parameter of the laser beam significantly affects the nature and extent of the interaction with tissue. Thermal interactions are largely wavelength-dependent because the amount of heat generation in tissue is determined by the extent of preferential absorption of the beam attributable to wavelength and target specificity. Tissue pigments and other chromophores are selective absorbands for some specific wavelengths of laser emission, while other primary absorption regions for biologic molecules fall within the range of short wavelengths below 300 nm. Many biologic molecules have specific vibrational and rotational absorption bands for wavelengths within the infrared region (wavelengths > 1 μm), and in the visible spectrum. Additionally, the high water content of most oral soft tissues contributes to extensive absorption of radiant energy in the infrared region.

The CO_2 laser beam is highly attenuated by intracellular water within oral soft tissue. Because of this, 90% of the incident energy of the CO_2 laser is absorbed within the first 100 μm of penetration of the tissue surface (Carruth and McKenzie, 1986). The high absorption of the 10.6-μm wavelength by tissue fluids leads to rapid vaporization (boiling) of the water component and pyrolysis (charring and burning) of the organic matter within the target tissue. These types of thermal interactions are observed with the CO_2 laser even at moderately low power densities (>100 W/cm^2) when using a focused beam. The erbium laser has an even greater coefficient of absorption in water (8,000/cm) vs that of the CO_2 laser (770/cm) for comparison. Based on differences in water absorption alone, wavelengths such as Nd:YAG, with a coefficient of absorption in water of 0.18/cm, would have a calculated minimum boiling threshold of 42,800 W/cm^2 power density to achieve the equivalent clinical effect (Fisher, 1993). Other wavelengths such as Nd:YAG and argon however are more strongly absorbed by blood hemoglobin, melanin pigments, and other tissue components, which contribute to their thermal effects. With some wavelengths, exogenous dyes can be used to enhance absorption in tissue to induce interactions that otherwise might not occur. The mechanisms involved are not unlike those observed with endogenous pigments or other tissue chromophores.

Thermal interactions in tissue generally appear to take place almost instantaneously, however, a description of the temporal evolution of the thermodynamic processes occuring will provide additional insights into the mechanisms involved. Initially, absorbed laser light (photon energy) induces electronic or molecular excitation of structures in the tissue. An important condition for this to occur is that the absorbing molecules of the target tissue have an energy level structure similar to the wavelength of the incident laser beam. In later stages, heat energy within the tissue mass is dissipated to surrounding structures by processes of thermal diffusion and conduction. Heat dissipation or diffusion from the site is a function of the thermal conductivity of the tissue and will ultimately determine the extent of collateral damage observed adjacent to the wound. The time required for diffusion of heat or *thermal relaxation time* (TRT) for a given type of tissue is also related to its composition and vascularity and is another characteristic property of the type of tissue. Thermal relaxation time is defined as the time required for the accumulated heat energy within the tissue mass to cool to 37% of its original value (Harris and Werkhaven, 1989). The degree of heat conduction to adjacent tissue and rate of tissue cooling are two important factors in determining the extent of the thermally affected area and collateral tissue damage. This area is sometimes referred to as the *thermal damage envelope* for a given wavelength and tissue type.

The degree of collateral damage depends to a great extent on properties of the tissue that are related to its structure, composition, and water content. Other tissue factors that influence the extent of thermal damage are tissue vascularity, the volume of the irradiated tissue, and its surface area. These factors will have a direct influence on the rate at which heat is dissipated from the affected area by both passive and active mechanisms. For long laser exposures in particular, convection cooling by blood flow through regions adjacent to the target area plays an important role (Barnes, 1975). For shorter exposures on tissue surfaces, excess heat energy generated during the exposure is more easily released to the overlying air and surrounding tissue by passive conduction mechanisms.

Another important tissue factor influencing the extent of the thermal damage zone is the relative degree of absorption and scattering of the beam once it enters tissue. While much information has been gathered about the absorptive properties of the various types of tissue, little is known about scattering of the beam within tissue. Scattering can directly increase the extent of collateral tissue damage by spatial redistribution of the beam into a larger volume of surrounding tissue than would be affected by a more localized absorption. Much of the scattered energy from the beam is transformed into heat energy within the tissue since it has insufficient power density to induce vaporization. While the scattered component of the beam retains the same wavelength as the incident beam, the intensity or power density of the scattered radiation decreases with distance exponentially.

Tissue dehydration also plays a significant role in the thermal interaction of lasers with tissue. Laser-induced dehydration of tissue is a natural sequela of the heat generated within the thermally affected area. Laser-induced changes in the composition and other optical properties of tissue, such as charring, coagulation of blood elements, and protein denaturation, can thereby alter the nature of subsequent interactions that might occur. Carbon arcing is one example of a laser-induced modification of target tissue that interferes with further tissue ablation and contributes to excessive heat generation. Carbon arcing can occur as a result of photopyrolysis of organic matter. Carbon, which is the end product of the burning of tissue and a high absorber of all wavelengths, readily forms on the surface during the initial phase of laser tissue ablation. If lasing is continued, the carbonized layer that is formed will preferentially absorb the incident beam, preventing further tissue ablation. Instead the carbonized material, which burns at approximately 3,200°C, acts as a heat sink transferring thermal energy to surrounding tissue and thereby increasing the zone of collateral damage.

In most clinical situations it is desirable to minimize or control the extent of collateral damage to surrounding tissue. Extensive research has been performed to establish practical and effective methods to minimize and control the undesirable effects attributed to the thermal interactions of tissues. The size of the thermal damage envelope created by a laser in a particular tissue to some extent may be controlled by the laser operating parameters such as spot size, exposure duration, pulse repetition rate, and the duration of the pulse. If the thermal effects to tissue are controlled by spot size, then power density is the modified parameter. The focused laser beam in this case can be used to produce a well-localized hot spot, which may be essential for some applications such as incision and excision.

The temporal emission mode of lasers describes those parameters that control the time and rate of delivery of energy to the target such as exposure duration; pulse rate, pulse frequency, or pulse repetition rate; and pulse width or duration. For continuous wave laser emissions, the energy is deposited without any thermal relaxation time and therefore has a linear relationship directly proportional to the total time of the exposure (Miserendino et al, 1989). A pulsed beam is delivered in bursts or intervals, which provides brief moments for heat dissipation or cooling between pulses. Pulsing may be controlled over a wide variety of frequencies and durations to limit the extent of heat dispersion to surrounding tissues or to induce other types of tissue effects. Ultrashort pulses within the picosecond and nanosecond range compress the output of the laser beam to achieve very high peak powers that are capable of inducing other nonthermal types of interactions such as photoplasmolysis and photodisruption, which will be described later in this chapter. Superpulsing, Q-switching, and mode locking are some examples of the variety of lasers with the temporal emission modes necessary for inducing these types of nonthermal interactions.

The relationship between the various temporal emission modes (continuous, pulsed, superpulsed) and the level of heat dispersion to surrounding tissue can be illustrated by a theoretical graph of the expected temperature rise resulting from a 1-sec exposure for three modes of delivery of the same total energy. In general, it can be assumed that continuous wave exposures and longer pulse widths will result in a greater heat transfer to surrounding structures than that for shorter pulses. Conversely, longer intervals between pulses (lower pulse repetition rate) will produce less heat generation in adjacent tissue. While these generalities may hold true for laser interactions with oral soft tissue, the relationship with dental hard tissue such as enamel and dentin may differ substantially most likely due to the differing properties of heat conduction and diffusion between the two tissue types

(Miserendino et al, 1993). The effects of pulse width on heat transmission within soft tissue is described in an interesting study by Armon and Laufer (Armon and Laufer, 1985). They observed that longer pulse durations (> 1 sec) will produce a larger damage envelope adjacent to the crater than that produced by shorter pulses (1 millisecond) for the same energy of exposure (1 J).

Other methods used to limit or control the extent of collateral damage to hard tissue have been explored, such as cooling and precooling of the target area. According to theoretical models of thermal interactions with teeth (Boehm et al, 1977), once laser parameters have been fixed and the optical properties of the tissue are known, thermal distribution within tissue can be minimized by cooling or precooling of the irradiated area; but no clinical applications have been proposed. Wakaki studied the possibility of using nitrogen to cool and precool feline skin tissue that was irradiated with a CO_2 laser. When the thickness of the scars was measured, the results demonstrated an improvement in quality and period of healing for areas lased and cooled. However, this method has not been used.

In 1988, Levy (US patent no. 5,020,995) proposed another concept for hard and soft tissue applications by using an Nd:YAG (1,064 nm) pulsed laser beam in combination with an air-and-water spray as a transparent medium for the beam. This concept was applied in studies performed on soft and hard tissues (Levy, 1991). Rizoiu and Levy (1993) showed the benefits of using an air-and-water spray to cool the tooth structure during exposure with an Nd:YAG pulsed laser beam. They demonstrated that a spray of air and water as a coolant is more effective than only water or only air.

Thermal effects of laser irradiation range in intensity depending on the level of temperature rise within the target tissue (Table). Tissue changes may be either transient or more enduring. Temperatures below 60°C generally will manifest as tissue hyperthermia, which for short durations of exposure will not produce lasting or irreversible tissue effects. Between 45°C and 50°C, enzymatic changes occur and edema develops. Above 65°C, protein denaturation occurs accompanied by coagulation of blood elements with exposures of a few seconds duration or longer. Below 100°C, tissue dehydration or desiccation is observed, which clinically appears as a whitening or blanching of tissue. At temperatures above 100°C, superheating occurs producing rapid vaporization of tissue fluids resulting in tissue ablation and shrinkage or contracture of the adjacent area (Fig 3.9). Continued lasing of the area results in temperature elevation to several hundred degrees whereupon tissue vaporizes, carbonizes, and burns (Frank, 1989).

Table. Thermal Interactions of Tissue

Temperature (°C)	Tissue Effect
42–45	Hyperthermia (transient)
> 65	Desiccation, protein denaturation, and coagulation
70–90	Tissue welding
> 100	Vaporization
> 200	Carbonization and charring

The thermal response of tissue to a surgical laser exposure is best described with the CO_2 surgical laser wound as an example. When a single pulse of 15,000 W/cm^2 or greater is applied to oral mucosa, vaporization of water at the tissue surface occurs. Rapid expansion at the exposure site causes elevation of the superficial epithelium, which subsequently ruptures, releasing both vapor and tissue particles.

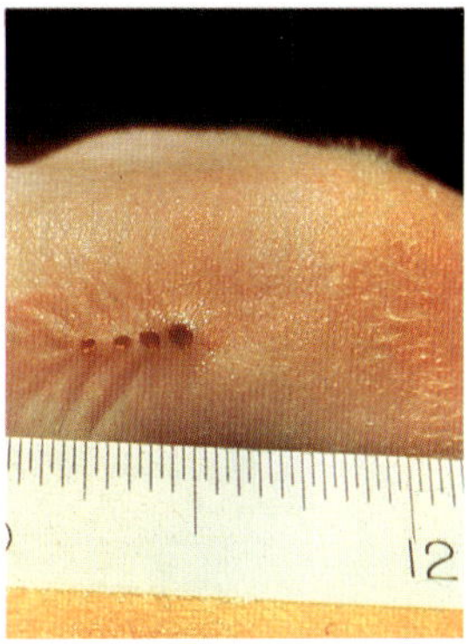

Fig 3.9 Example of relative wound contracture occurring from various CO_2 laser exposures in the skin of a nude mouse. (Courtesy of Dr David Harris.)

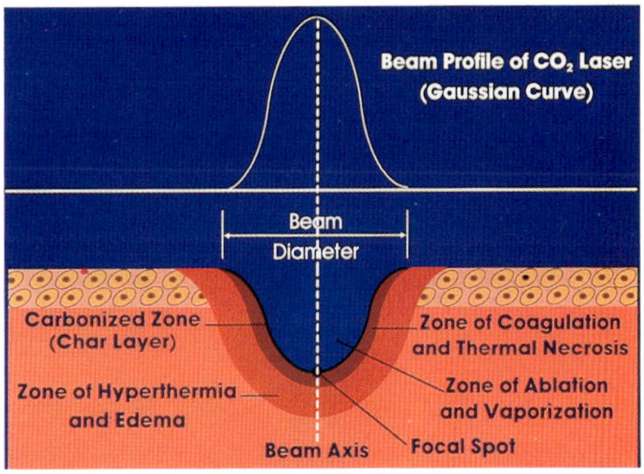

Fig 3.10 Laser crater. Shown is the relationship between beam profile and the crater produced in tissue by the CO_2 laser.

The net effect is ablation of tissue resulting in the formation of a craterlike defect on the tissue surface. Superficially, the laser crater appears as a circular hole. In cross section, the crater appears as an inversion of the gaussian beam profile (Fig 3.10). The greatest depth of penetration of the crater into tissue is represented by the center of the focal spot of the beam or point of greatest power density. Surrounding the defect are relative zones of tissue damage, which decrease in intensity toward the periphery. A diagrammatic section through the crater reveals the various zones of tissue interaction as they extend outward from the wall of the crater toward the unaffected tissues.

Lining the crater wall is a layer of carbonized tissue residue. Immediately adjacent to this carbonized zone is a layer of coagulation and thermal necrosis of approximately 0.5-mm thickness. Adjacent to this zone of thermal necrosis and extending outward is a zone of edema and hyperthermia, which will vary in thickness depending on the duration of the exposure or total light dose delivered to the tissue.

The depth of penetration of the beam will be a function of the physical properties of the particular target tissue, the wavelength, and the power density of the emitted beam. The degree or rate at which power density is diminished as the beam is projected deeper into tissue is determined by the *attenuation coefficient* (A) of the specific type of tissue. In most media, attenuation is an exponential function, that is the laser beam loses a constant fraction of its intensity as it travels through the medium. The attenuation coefficient for a particular medium can be derived from a mathematical formula known as Lambert's or Beer's Law, which states that the absorption of a medium is directly proportional to the concentration of the absorbing element. Theoretically, penetration of the beam into a medium continues indefinitely; however, in practical terms there is a specific distance at which the power density of the beam becomes reduced to a level where it no longer is capable of inducing interaction. This distance has been arbitrarily defined as the *extinction depth* of the laser beam. Extinction depths for various wavelengths and media are generally calculated at the distance where the intensity of the beam is reduced to 1% of its power density at the surface.

Therefore the optimal parameters for exposure of a given tissue required for ablation will be determined by: 1) the specific wavelength of absorption for that tissue; 2) the threshold power density required for ablation; and 3) exposure parameters that take into consideration the absorption characteristics and thermal relaxation time of the specific tissue.

Photomechanical and Photoelectrical Interactions

Photodisruption, photodisassociation, photoplasmolysis, and photoacoustic interactions are terms used to describe specific types of essentially nonthermal processes of laser-tissue interactions characterized by ultrashort pulses ($< 10^{-6}$ sec) of very high energy density. The high energy levels and rapid absorption that occur during photoablation by these processes result in rapid expansion or generation of shock waves that are capable of rupturing intermolecular and atomic bonds. Mechanical disruption or the breaking apart of matter by acoustic shock waves is accomplished by conversion of high intensity light (photon) energy to vibrational (kinetic) energy. Very high peak energy and ultrashort pulses are required to generate nonthermal photoablative interactions, therefore only pulsed lasers with very high photon energy and short wavelengths (< 319 nm) have this capability. Photodisruption occurs whenever the photon energy of the incident beam exceeds either the atomic or intermolecular bond energies of the target tissue.

The processes involved for photodisruption to occur can be divided into three interrelated mechanisms or phases: ionization, plasma formation, and shock wave generation. Ionization can occur in tissue at very high energy densities when the electric field strength of the beam becomes high enough to ionize atoms. The threshold value for the field strength necessary for ionization is determined by the level of the field strength, which binds the outer shell electron of an atom to its nucleus. Once ionization occurs, a hot electrically charged gas of free electrons and positive ions, or plasma, is formed. The plasma itself is maintained by absorption of energy from the incident beam reaching temperatures in excess of 15,000°C. As the temperature fluctuates within the electric field from the laser, electrons within the plasma begin to vibrate, creating a rapid expansion and contraction that leads to generation of shock waves that can be heard as a sharp popping sound. The pressures exerted by the acoustic shock wave on the target are responsible for the mechanical breaking apart or shattering of the target material observed during photoplasmolysis. Since it is a strong absorber of all wavelengths, the plasma acts as a shield preventing further penetration of the beam to the target tissue.

Only lasers that have high absorption in tissue and create extremely high power densities are able to produce the energy levels necessary to induce photoplasmolysis. Most biologic tissues readily absorb radiant energy within the ultraviolet spectrum. Lasers of this variety such as excimer have been shown to interact with dental hard tissue in a manner that results in minimal thermal effects (Stabholz et al, 1992; Neev et al, 1992). Other lasers with high peak energies and ultrashort pulse widths such as the Q-switched YAG lasers are also capable of inducing nonthermal photoablative interactions that may have potential applications to dental hard structures.

Clinical Manifestations of Laser-Tissue Interactions

Ablation and Incision

Removal of oral lesions by application of laser energy may easily be performed for surface, exophytic, and invasive lesions. The ablation of surface lesions by use of an unfocused beam of relatively large diameter (1 cm or greater) is easily accomplished through the effects of vaporization as previously described. Excision of exophytic or invasive lesions may also be performed with a focused beam of 1 mm or less to cut or incise tissue in a manner similar to that when a scalpel is used (Fig 3.11). The results of a histologic study conducted at Northwestern University Dental School indicate that laser wounds heal in a similar manner to that observed with more conventional surgical methods. In this study, laser wounds appeared to cause less collateral tissue damage than electrocautery, but healed slightly slower than scalpel wounds. Although one might argue in favor of scalpel vs laser due to this apparent delay in healing, laser surgery offers many other advantages over conventional methods, such as improved hemostasis and versatility of use, which warrant its application in oral soft tissue surgery.

The depth of penetration of the incision made by a focused laser beam or contact probe will vary with the power density used and the speed of movement of the beam across the tissue surface. These basic techniques may be mastered with some practice by most dental surgeons without difficulty.

Time-Dependent Tissue Effects

The amount of transfer of radiant light energy into thermal energy that occurs during absorption will necessarily be related to the power density of the incident radiation and the duration of the exposure. The extent of tissue damage therefore will be both power- and time-dependent. Additionally, the rate at which heat energy is dissipated within a given tissue type will also have an influence on the extent of thermal damage to surrounding tissue. This concept of thermal diffusion within tissue is fundamental to understanding the nature of the laser-tissue interaction that occurs within the various tissue types of the oral cavity.

Recognizing the differences in the TRT among tissue types is also essential to establish suitable exposure parameters for the various types of tissue encountered in the oral cavity. Values for TRT are tissue-specific and are related to the water content and vascularity of a particular tissue type. Variations in water content between fibrous noninflamed tissue and inflamed edematous tissue will require consideration when selecting laser parameters to avoid excessive heating and charring of tissues during surgical procedures. The significance of the TRT of tissue is that if tissues are allowed a period of cooling of approximately three times their TRT, accumulation of heat energy will be avoided and thermal diffusion from the exposure site can be minimized. Therefore, by controlling the diffusion of heat energy to surrounding tissue, the extent of collateral tissue damage can be managed effectively with the proper combination of power density and pulse duration for the desired procedure (Fisher, 1993; Miserendino et al, 1993).

Most surgical laser systems provide for the operation of the laser in either contin-

Fig 3.11 Comparison of wound healing for scalpel, carbon dioxide laser and electrocautery (hematoxylin & eosin; courtesy of Dr Paul Petrungaro). **(a)**, Scalpel incision of dog oral mucosa at 1 hour after treatment. **(b)**, Scalpel wound at 2 weeks showing complete epithelialization and connective tissue organization of the wound space (ws). Arrows show suture sites. **(c)**, CO_2 laser incision (in focus) of dog oral mucosa 1 hour after treatment. **(d)**, Laser wound at 2 weeks showing no histologic difference from the scalpel wound (fs indicates fibrin).

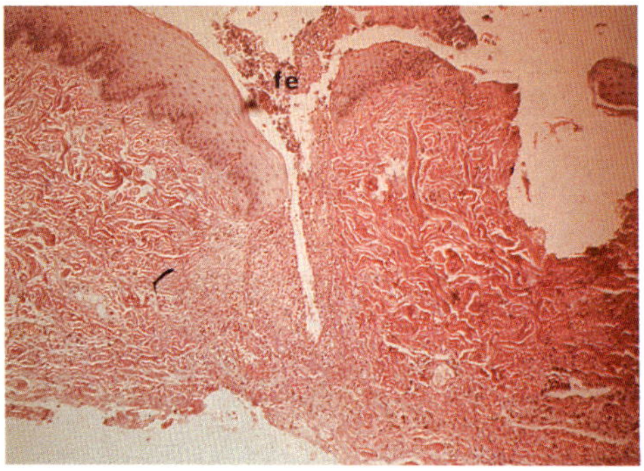

3.11a

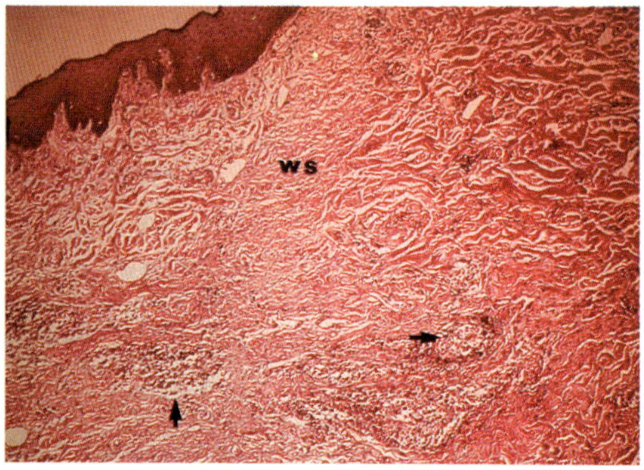

3.11b

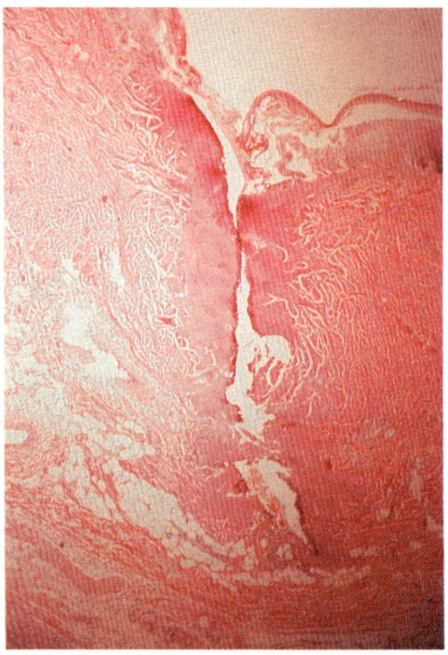

3.11c

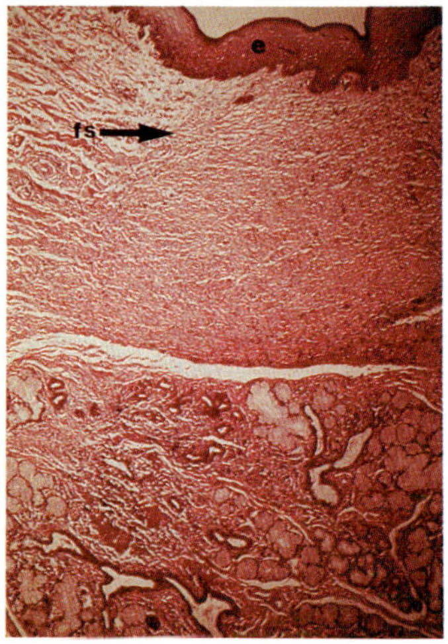

3.11d

uous or pulsed modes of delivery. In continuous mode, the laser beam is emitted as a constant stream of light energy as long as a control or foot pedal is depressed. Pulsed mode delivers the beam in bursts of energy at intervals and duration of exposure, which may be selected by the operator. The purpose of pulsing is to provide a brief cooling period for tissue to recover from the thermal stresses induced. By proper selection of the pulse width or duration of exposure, and the pulse repetition rate (PRR), it is possible to limit the extent of collateral tissue damage during surgical procedures. Surgical techniques for application of specific laser systems and procedures are presented in Chapter 9.

Hemostasis, Sterilization, and Tissue Welding

In addition to the basic techniques used for incision and ablation as previously described, lasers are capable of inducing other desirable effects that can be applied in soft tissue surgery. These include application of the coagulation effect afforded through protein denaturation and the sealing of small blood vessels and lymphatics for improved hemostasis; sterilization of wounds; and welding of tissues, all of which result from the thermal interaction of lasers with biologic tissues.

Hemostasis is a desirable characteristic of laser interaction with tissue. Coagulation of blood and tissue proteins is the primary mechanism by which hemostasis can occur. Irreversible damage to tissue in the form of coagulative or thermal necrosis of tissues inevitably accompanies the process of coagulation. Hemostasis is thus possible with many laser systems through the heating of blood elements, and by direct sealing of small blood vessels by desiccation and contraction of the vessel wall. Denaturation of serum and tissue proteins occurs at prolonged temperatures of 65°C to 70°C (Harris and Werkhaven, 1989). Absorption of different wavelengths by hemoglobin varies. Carbon dioxide lasers are reported to seal vessels of 0.5 mm or smaller. Neodymium:YAG and argon are more readily absorbed by hemoglobin with deeper tissue penetration and thereby display greater hemostatic capability, sealing vessels of 2- to 3-mm diameter (Castro, 1992).

The welding of soft tissue by laser irradiation has been suggested as a potential method to replace suturing in some surgical applications (Quigley et al, 1985; Garden et al, 1986). Tissue elements such as small blood vessels and tissue grafts may be joined together by an elevation of temperature from 70°C to 80°C. The process of tissue welding appears to be dependent on the denaturation of structural tissue proteins and may involve a limited amount of cellular necrosis over time. Collagen is the structural skeleton of all mammalian biologic tissues. At temperatures of 60°C or greater, the triple helix of collagen begins to unfold. Under mild heating of short duration, the collagen molecule may refold and intertwine with that of another tissue segment, thus joining the segments together. The partially reversible nature of collagen denaturation is the key to the process of tissue welding. Typically, argon, CO_2, and Nd:YAG lasers have been used by the medical surgical specialties to weld nerves, small blood vessels, and skin. Power densities from 50 to 250 W/cm^2 have been reported to produce favorable results, although initial tensile strength of the weld is relatively low (Buell and Schuller, 1983; Garden et al, 1986).

Sterilization or disinfection of tissue surfaces has been described as an additional benefit of laser use by a number of sources. When lasers are used to ablate tissue, the surface temperature is elevated to levels adequate to destroy microorganisms. The antibacterial effect of CO_2 laser use in soft tissue surgery has been well established (Pick et al, 1985). Noncontact laser surgery understandably will reduce the potential for contamination of the wound in addition to the effects attributed to the thermal destruction of bacteria, which occurs at relatively low power densities (Madden et al, 1970). The effectiveness of sterilization of dentin surfaces for potential application in endodontics (Hardee et al, 1990; Miserendino, 1988); periodontics (Pick and Miserendino, 1989); and restorative dentistry for the removal of caries (Miserendino et al, 1988; Stabholz et al, 1993) has been examined with positive results.

At present, the clinical benefits derived by sterilization of hard and soft oral tissues have been considered as ancillary effects of laser-tissue interaction. However, the potential use of laser energy for its specific therapeutic effects on dental caries, in vital pulp therapy (pulpectomy and pulpotomy), for wound healing, and for root surface and graft site preparation in periodontics and related surgical procedures will undoubtedly be forthcoming once a greater understanding of laser hard tissue interaction has been achieved.

Conclusions

The relationship between the interaction of radiant energy and its clinical manifestations on oral tissue has been described as being dependent on the three basic parameters of laser energy: *wavelength* specificity, which is determined by the inherent optical properties of tissue; *power density*, which influences the type of interaction, ie, photochemical, photoablative, photothermal, and photomechanical; and *time*, which limits the extent of the interaction. A thorough understanding of the complex interactions that occur when specific wavelengths of radiant energy interact with biologic tissue is prerequisite to the safe and effective application of lasers in clinical practice. These complexities may be more easily derived once the inherent characteristics of different laser systems, their modes of delivery, and the optical properties of oral soft and hard tissues are recognized. The effectiveness of dental laser therapy in clinical practice therefore will ultimately depend on selection of the proper wavelength and use of appropriate parameters necessary to produce the desired tissue response for the particular clinical circumstance. In this way, the laser dentist or surgeon may take full advantage of the unique features of lasers and may be assured of achieving predictable results.

References

Armon E, Laufer G. Analysis to determine the beam parameters which yield the most extensive cut with the least secondary damage. J Biomech Eng 1985; 107:286–290.

Barnes FS. Applications of lasers to biology and medicine. Proc IEEE 1975; 63:1269–1277.

Boehm R, Rich J, Webster J, Janke S. Thermal stress effects and surface cracking associated with laser use on human teeth. J Biomech Eng (Transactions of ASME) Nov 1977; 189–194.

Buell DR, Schuller DE. Comparison of tensile strength in CO_2 laser and scalpel skin incisions. Arch Otolaryngol 1983;109:465–467.

Castro DJ. The physical principles of lasers. In Apfelberg DB (ed): Atlas of Cutaneous Laser Surgery. New York: Raven Press;1992.

Carruth JA, McKenzie AL. The production of surgical laser lesions. In Carruth JA, McKenzie AL (eds): Medical Lasers: Science and Clinical Practice. Boston: Adam Hilger Ltd;1986:51–80.

Dederich DN. Laser tissue interaction. Alpha Omegan 1991;84:33–36.

Dederich DN. Laser/tissue interaction: what happens to laser light when it strikes tissue? JADA 1993; 124:57–61.

Fisher JC. Qualitative and quantitative tissue effects of light from important surgical lasers: Optimal surgical principles. In Wright VC, Fisher JC (eds): Laser Surgery in Gynecology. Philadelphia: WB Saunders Co;1993: 58–81.

Frank F. Laser light and tissue biophysical aspects of medical laser application. SPIE Lasers Med 1989; 1353:37–45.

Garden JM, Robinson JK, Taute PM. The low-output carbon dioxide laser for cutaneous wound closure of scalpel incisions: comparative tensile strength studies of the laser to suture and staple wound closure. Lasers Surg Med 1986;6:67–71.

Hardee M, Miserendino LJ, Kos W. Evaluation of intracanal Nd:YAG laser irradiation (abstract). J Endodontics 1990;16:194.

Harris DM, Werkhaven JA. Biophysics and applications of medical lasers. Adv Otolaryngol Head Neck Surg 1989;3:91–123.

Harris DM. Biomolecular mechanisms of laser biostimulation (editorial comment). J Clin Laser Med Surg 1991;9:277–280.

Levy G. A new laser for soft tissue and hard tissue applications. Alpha Omegan 1991;84:51–54.

Madden JE, Edlich RF, Custer JR, et al. Studies in the management of the contaminated wound, IV. Resistance to infection of surgical wounds made by knife, electrosurgery, and laser. Am J Surg 1970;119: 222–224.

Miserendino LJ. Sterilization of bacterially contaminated root apices by CO_2 laser irradiation (abstract). J Endodontics 1988;14:198.

Miserendino LJ, Pick RM, Kos W. In vitro sterilization of dental caries by CO_2 laser irradiation (abstract). Lasers Surg Med 1988;8:148.

Miserendino LJ, Neiburger EJ, Luebke N, Brantley W. Thermal effects of continuous wave CO_2 laser exposure on human teeth: an in vitro study. J Endodontics 1989;14:302–305.

Miserendino LJ, Abt E, Wigdor H, Miserendino CA. Evaluation of thermal cooling mechanisms for laser application to teeth. Lasers Surg Med 1993;13:83–88.

Neev J, Liaw LL, Raney DV, Fujishige JT, Ho PD, Berns MW. Selectivity, efficiency and surface characteristics of hard dental tissues ablated with ArF pulsed excimer lasers. Lasers Surg Med 1991;11:499–510.

Pick RM, Pecaro BC, Silberman CJ. The laser gingivectomy. J Periodontol 1985;56:492–494.

Pick RM, Miserendino LJ. Lasers in dentistry. J Clin Laser Med Surg 1989;7:33.

Quigley MR, Bailes JE, Kwaan HC, et al. Microvascular anastomosis using the milliwatt CO_2 laser. Lasers Surg Med 1985;5:357–365.

Rizoiu IM, Levy G. Efficiency of cooling mechanisms during the exposure of enamel to pulsed Nd:YAG laser beam: an in vitro study. Proceedings of Lasers in Orthopedic, Dental, and Veterinary Medicine II 1993; 188:212–220.

Stabholz A, Neev J, Kettering J, Torabinejad M. Effects of XeCl excimer laser on *Streptococcus mutans* (abstract no. 51). J Endodontics 1993;19:197.

Stabholz A, Neev J, Lih-Huei L, et al. Sealing of dentinal tubules by XeCl 308-nm excimer laser. J Endodontics 1993;19:267–271.

Chapter Four

Laser Effects on Dental Hard Tissues

Hans J. Koort and Matthias Frentzen

Only a few years after the discovery of the first ruby laser, investigations were performed to introduce laser technology into dentistry for "optical drilling" of teeth. Basic investigations on the effects of laser impacts on teeth were carried out by Goldman and Stern in the 1960s (Goldman et al, 1964; Stern and Sognnaes, 1964). Basic studies with Nd:YAG and CO_2 lasers followed in the 1970s. As a result of these investigations, unavoidable disadvantages such as damage to the dental pulp, carbonization of dentin, and crack formation in enamel were discussed as limitations in cavity preparation. Reviewing the early papers, Stern concluded in 1974 that laser technology may not replace the conventional drill unless heat-related structural changes and damage to the surrounding dental tissues could be reduced dramatically by new laser systems (Stern, 1974). Since then, further developments in laser technology have steadily been made. Today more than ten different laser types are used in dental research. A growing number of papers have been published during the past years, including those citing the advantages of laser applications in dental hard tissue treatment (Frentzen and Koort, 1990). A basic knowledge of laser effects is essential to decide whether laser applications really do offer new possibilities for advancement.

Lasers in Dental Hard Tissue Treatment

An increasing spectrum of laser types are currently used in dental research. These lasers emit electromagnetic energy from the infrared (10 μm) to the ultraviolet (200 nm) range (Table 4.1).

The number of commercially available dental laser systems is limited to some infrared lasers, namely CO_2, Nd:YAG, and Er:YAG lasers. In some European countries, the Er:YAG laser has just been introduced into the market for dental applications. To reduce unwanted side effects, water cooling systems are part of this mid-infrared laser. To facilitate handling in dentistry, fiber-guided delivery systems are preferable to mirror arms. While the manufacturing of fibers with good transmission for lasers in the range of 1 to 2 μm (Nd:YAG and Ho:YAG laser) is a standard, fibers for the 3-μm range

Table 4.1. Current Laser Types in Dental Hard Tissue Research

Laser	Wavelength (nm)	Pulsed/cw	Power/Energy	Delivery system
ArF excimer	193	Pulsed	> 300 mJ	Mirror system
KrF excimer	248	Pulsed	> 500 mJ	Mirror system
XeCl excimer	308	Pulsed	> 200 mJ	Fiber
XeF excimer	351	Pulsed	> 100 mJ	Fiber
Argon ion	488 + 512	cw	> 10 W	Fiber
KTP	532	Pulsed	> 50 mJ	Fiber
		cw	> 20 W	Fiber
Ruby	692	Pulsed	> 1,000 mJ	Mirror system
Nd:YAG	1,064	Pulsed	> 500 mJ	Fiber
		cw	> 50 W	Fiber
Ho:YAG	2,123	Pulsed	> 800 mJ	Fiber
Er:YSGG	2,790	Pulsed	> 600 mJ	Mirror system
Er:YAG	2,940	Pulsed	> 600 mJ	Mirror system
CO_2	10,600	Pulsed	> 300 mJ	Mirror system
		cw	> 100 W	Mirror system

(Er:YSGG and Er:YAG laser) and the 10-µm range (CO_2 laser) are still in the process of development. To enhance the flexibility of the delivery system, some CO_2 lasers are offered with hollow wave guide systems instead of mirror systems.

Models of Laser-Tissue Interaction

The interaction of laser light with living tissues is the interaction of photons with the atoms or molecules of the target. These interactions are followed by very complex reactions, and the involved mechanisms are not yet completely understood. In the field of mineralized tissues, the most thoroughly investigated interactions are the photothermal and thermomechanical interactions and the ablative photodecomposition (Müller et al, 1990; Koort and Frentzen, 1992a; Frentzen et al, 1992).

The biologic effects of laser light on dental tissues depend on a number of factors. To study the laser-tissue interaction, the properties of the laser radiation itself, such as wavelength, energy density, and pulse duration have to be considered. Furthermore, the effect of laser radiation on tissue depends on various properties of the irradiated material such as absorption, reflection, transmission, and scattering effects.

Optical Properties of Hard Tissues

In terms of the optical properties, enamel and dentin are thought to be optical systems with waveguiding, scattering, and absorbing elements (Altshuler et al, 1991; Zijp and Ten Bosch, 1991). Many effects caused by these optical elements are grossly unknown. Chapter 19 offers more details.

The absorption and transmission of laser light in human teeth is mainly dependent on the wavelength of the laser light (Koort and Frentzen, 1992a). Ultraviolet (UV) laser light is well absorbed. However

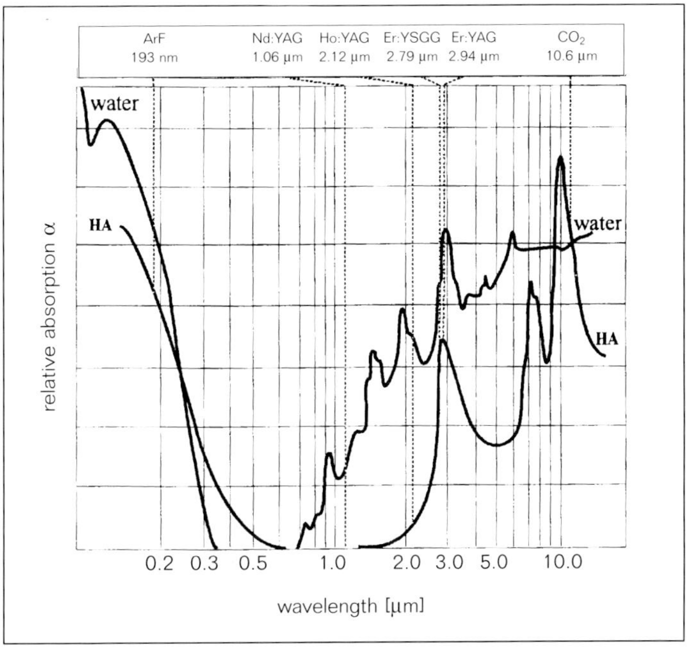

Fig 4.1 The absorption of laser light in water and hydroxyapatite (HA) in the spectral range from 200 nm to 10 µm.

in the mid-infrared spectrum, the absorption in water and in hydroxyapatite (HA) changes tremendously depending on the wavelength of the laser light (Fig 4.1). In water and in HA, there is a very low absorption at a wavelength of 2 µm in comparison to the high absorption of laser energy at 3 µm and 10 µm. At 1 µm, the absorption in water and in HA becomes about 10,000 times less than that at 3 µm (Hale and Query, 1973; Nagasawa, 1983; LeGeros, 1991).

The changing absorption effects can be observed, for example, by irradiating dentin slices of extracted human teeth with pulsed laser radiation of Nd:YAG, XeCl, and ArF excimer laser systems. The absorbed laser energy was found to be mainly dependent on the wavelengths of the laser light. With the ArF laser, the absorption was found to be very high. The transmitted energy decreases by 50% after a thickness of 20 µm. The whole energy was nearly absorbed after 100 µm (Fig 4.2). The absorption of the XeCl laser radiation at 50 µm thickness was 50%. After 200 µm, however, the radiation was still not completely absorbed. Due to a low absorption of the Nd:YAG laser radiation, the transmitted energy at 75 µm was 50% and 25% at a thickness of 3 mm (Koort and Frentzen, 1992b). In this study, a significant difference in transmission due to the orientation of dentin tubules could not be verified in contradiction to other findings with a He:Ne laser.

Investigations with lasers in the visible spectrum yielded the basis for an optical model of dental hard tissues (Altshuler et al, 1991; Zijp and Ten Bosch, 1991). The idea that dentin tubules may work as optical fibers transmitting high energy densities to pulpal tissues could explain unpredictable side effects when lasing dental tissues (Frentzen, 1992). These effects may also be the reason for the great deviation in the results of histologic studies and may be responsible for some laser-

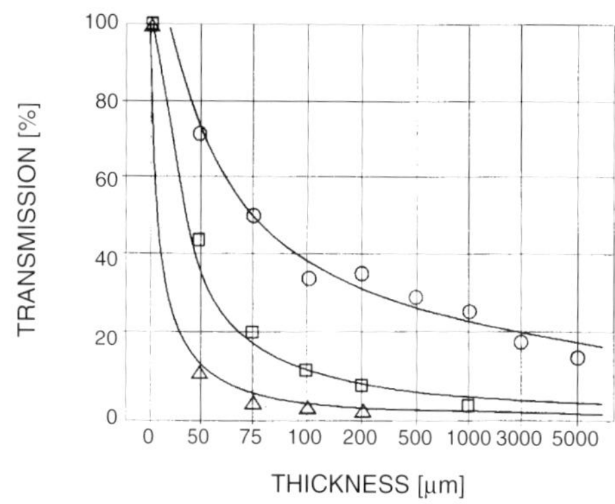

Fig 4.2 Measurement of transmitted pulsed laser light with different wavelengths through dentin sections. Δ = 193 nm wavelength (ArF laser); ❑ = 308 nm wavelength (XeCl laser); ❍ = 1.06 µm wavelength (Nd:YAG laser).

induced changes in the pulp. The absorption of laser energy in the superficial tissue layers can alter the optical properties of the affected tissue, causing a variation in the intensity of the penetration energy. To keep the intensity of light constant throughout a definite volume of tissue is not possible. Therefore laser effects are changing in dependence from the depth of penetration.

Thermal Effects

The best-known laser effect in dentistry is the thermal vaporization of tissue by absorbing infrared laser light. The laser energy is converted into thermal energy or heat that destroys the tissues. The laser beam couples to the tissue surface, and this absorption leads to a heating with denaturation at about 45°C to 60°C. Above 60°C coagulation and necrosis can be observed, accompanied by a desiccation of the tissue. At 100°C the water inside the tissue vaporizes. The absorption of the laser energy increases rapidly. Carbonization and later pyrolysis (> 300°C) with vaporization of the bulky tissue terminate the thermal laser-tissue interaction (Müller et al, 1990).

Mechanical Effects

High energetic and short pulsed laser light can lead to a fast heating of the dental tissues in a very small area. The formation of a plasma can be observed. The energy dissipates explosively in a volume expansion that may be accompanied by fast shock waves. These mechanical shock waves can lead to very high pressures so that adjacent tissue will be destroyed or damaged. The formation of mechanical shock waves can also be observed in nonlinear effects. Due to the short interaction time and the high energy density in a focus, the behavior of the irradiated tissue changes to nonlinear properties, inducing an optical breakdown in or above the tissue. This mechanism induces high and fast shock waves that lead to mechanical damage of the irradiated tissue (Table 4.2).

To study these photoacoustic effects in hard dental tissues, laser-induced shock waves can be measured with piezoelectric (PVDF) films. With the ArF excimer laser, energy densities of 2 J/cm^2 cause pressure amplitudes of 50 bar while energy densities of 20 J/cm^2 cause pressure am-

Table 4.2. Photomechanical Laser Interactions in Biologic Tissues

Mechanical Effects	Interaction
Photoablation	Fast thermal explosion Mechanical shock waves
Photodisruption	Nonlinear tissue behavior Optical breakdown Mechanical shock waves

plitudes of 1,000 bar (Bräucker et al, 1992).

To avoid microcracks in dental tissues, the maximum laser energy density of all pulsed laser systems must be kept below a certain threshold. Further basic investigations are necessary to determine the limitations of these threshold energies for the various laser systems.

Chemical Effects

The basis of the photochemical effect is the absorption of laser light without any thermal effect, which leads to an alteration in the chemical and physical properties of the irradiated tissues. Molecules can be dissociated directly with laser light of high photon energies. As an example, the ArF excimer laser has a photon energy of 6.4 eV. Only one photon is necessary to break one C=O double bond.

Thermally Induced Ablation of Dental Tissues

Volume effects can be observed as a result of heating tissues. The ablation effectiveness depends on the temperature of the solid-gaseous phase transition, the pulse duration of the laser radiation, and the energy density (Müller et al, 1990). In mineralized tissues, the ablation rate is low and accompanied by serious side effects. Variations of the thermally induced ablation are thermomechanical effects. In contrast to laser-induced thermal effects, mid-infrared lasers (Er:YAG and Er:YSGG) with varied absorption in water and HA can cause thermomechanical laser-tissue interactions (Zweig et al, 1988; Walsh et al, 1989). The local extensive heating of the water in mineralized tissues leads to microexplosions in the liquid phase. The resulting microfragments are removed by the high pressure caused by the steam. The thermal injury of the adjacent tissue could possibly be reduced, at least in hydrogenous tissues (Walsh and Deutsch, 1989; Walsh et al, 1989). The reduction of side effects in dental hard tissues may be achieved by a balanced absorption in water and HA. This is nearly fulfilled by using the Er:YAG laser at 2.94 µm: due to a high absorption in water and a good coupling to mineralized structures, only small zones of debris, necrosis, and carbonization can be found in dentin after laser irradiation with additional water cooling.

To reduce the side effects, especially in enamel, another erbium-doped laser is of interest. Because of the ratio of water to HA absorption, the Er:YSGG laser with 2.79-µm wavelength may be beneficial when used in dental tissue treatment. Compared to the Er:YAG laser at 2.94 µm, there is a stronger absorption in HA, which is the main mineral component in dental hard tissues. For that reason, the radiation might be less transmitted into enamel and dentin so that the extent of side effects might be reduced. Compared to the Er:YAG laser, the minor absorption in water might reduce heat effects caused by the steam phase (Sievers et al, 1992).

Ablative Decomposition

Laser decomposition by nanosecond pulsed lasers can remove soft and hard tissues with few side effects (Koort and Frentzen, 1992a; Frentzen et al, 1992). In this ablation process, the light energy is deposed in a very thin superficial tissue layer. The absorption of the laser radiation increases tremendously when a certain energy threshold is exceeded. The coupling of energy to the tissue is followed by nonthermal bond breaking (chemical effects) and/or by fast thermal expansions (mechanical effects) that lead to destruction of the tissue. Thermal-induced effects are significantly reduced. Serious photoacoustic side effects, however, are in discussion, especially with higher energy densities (Bräucker et al, 1992).

Ablation of Hydroxyapatite with Lasers

In the ablation of mineralized tissues with laser light, the characteristics of the inorganic matrix are of great importance. Therefore, highly pure hydroxyapatite ceramic (HAC) can be used as a test substrate for the inorganic part of bone and dental tissues (Frentzen et al, 1992). This material has been recently established in dentistry as a synthetic implant material. The chemical composition of HAC is similar to that of the minerals of bone and dental hard tissues. Specimens of sintered HAC blocks were irradiated with pulsed laser light of 193 nm (ArF), 248 nm (KrF), 308 nm (XeCl), 488 and 514 nm (Ar^+), 570 to 630 nm (Dye), 1.06 µm (Nd:YAG), 2.79 µm (Er:YSGG), and 10.6 µm (CO_2) to determine if it was possible to ablate HAC with these laser wavelengths.

Ablation of HAC was not possible with wavelengths in the infrared and visible spectral range (0.48 µm to 10.6 µm). Depending on the adjusted parameters, the material was destroyed after a shorter or longer time without signs of ablation. The ceramic burst into pieces. In contrast, ablation of the HAC surface without damage to the ceramic was only observed with use of lasers in the UV spectral range. With decreasing wavelengths (308 nm > 248 nm > 193 nm), the thermal side effects decreased while the ablation effects increased (Koort, 1991).

Efficiency of Laser Ablation

The mechanical drilling with burs is a well-known and accepted method for hard dental tissue preparation. Therefore any laser system has to be compared to this standard drilling method with respect to efficiency, side effects, and technical effort. A comparison of possible advantages and disadvantages of some laser systems that might be of interest for hard dental tissue treatment are shown in Table 4.3 (Müller et al, 1990).

To determine the advantages of lasers in dental hard tissue treatment, efficiency

Table 4.3. Advantages and Disadvantages of Different Laser Systems Used in Dental Hard Tissue Treatment*†

Characteristics	ArF (193 nm)	XeCl (308 nm)	Nd:YAG (1.06 µm)	Er:YAG (2.94 µm)	CO_2 (10.6 µm cw/pulsed)	TEA CO_2 (10.6 µm)
Fiber transmission	–	+	++	–	–/–	–
Ablation effectivity	+	–	– –	++	–/+	+
Thermal damage	++	+	–	(+)	– –/–	+
Pressure effects	+	nd	++	–	++/+	nd
Optical properties dependence	++	+	– –	nd	– –/– –	nd
Operating expenses	– –	–	+	+	++/+	–

*Modified from Müller, et al, 1990.

† + = Advantage; – = disadvantage; nd = not determined.

is an important factor to introduce this technology into therapy. Side effects, however, could be a limiting factor. Thus efficiency and side effects must be well balanced.

Histologic Results and Techniques

An important indicator for the control of side effects of laser radiation is histologic studies of dental hard tissues. The histologic results after conventional treatment of mineralized tissues are well known (Jarby and Dansgaard, 1959). The comparison of these results to those of laser-treated tissues will be a good standard.

To analyze structural changes in tissues, scanning electron microscopic (SEM) investigations and different light microscopic techniques are applied. Laser effects on the surface of mineralized tissues can be studied with SEM techniques or top-view light microscopy. A special problem of SEM techniques are artifacts caused by the preparation process. To study the depth effects, cross sections of the irradiated samples are necessary. Mineralized tissues are usually decalcified before preparing sections for histologic analysis. Because of this process, the laser-induced alterations in the mineralized components of the tissues cannot be observed, especially in dental hard tissues. To avoid these disadvantages, sawing and grinding techniques to cut undecalcified sections were developed. These methods are based on plastic embedding techniques with a penetrating UV-activated polymethylmethacrylate (PMMA) medium (Donath and Brenner, 1982). Vacuum chambers could be used to improve the penetration depth of the methylmethacrylate. The polymerization process should be prolonged to avoid artifacts caused by the polymerization shrinkage. High-power UV light sources should be used in the later polymerization steps to improve the polymerization rates in the deeper zones of mineralized dental tissues and the pulp chamber (Frentzen et al, 1990; Frentzen and Koort, 1992a). The staining of the prepared cross section can be performed with toluidine blue.

Continuous Wave and Pulsed CO_2 Lasers

When continuous wave (cw) or microsecond pulsed CO_2 lasers are used, structural changes and damage in dental hard tissues were reported: microcracks and zones of necrosis and carbonization are unavoidable. Steam and vapor can cause cracks in enamel and dentin. The extent and structure of effects and side effects are influenced by optical and other physical properties of the tissue. Because of drying effects, the microhardness of dentin increases (Brune, 1980; White et al, 1991). The organic matrix burns off. The laser radiation can fuse the apatite to a glazelike melt. The crystalline structure of HA changes (Kantola, 1973) (Fig 4.3). A transformation of apatite to tricalcium phosphate takes place. The rise of temperature can be so high that the pulp tissues will be destroyed. In the case of continuous wave lasers, the rise of ablation is mainly determined by the mean power and the interaction time. Pulsed CO_2 lasers are more effective than continuous wave CO_2 lasers in ablating mineralized tissues. In the case of pulsed lasers, the tissue ablation depends on the product of pulse energy, repetition rate (frequency), and treatment time. Because of a reduction of heat diffusion in dental tissues, the size of damage zones of pulsed lasers is smaller than the size of damage zones of continuous wave CO_2 lasers. The

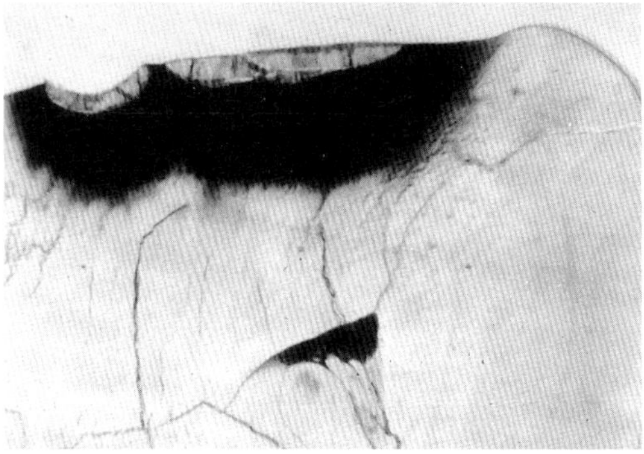

Fig 4.3 Undecalcified section of human enamel after continuous wave CO_2 laser radiation: glaze-like structure in the surface layer followed by zones of carbonization and thermally induced microcracks (magnification, × 20).

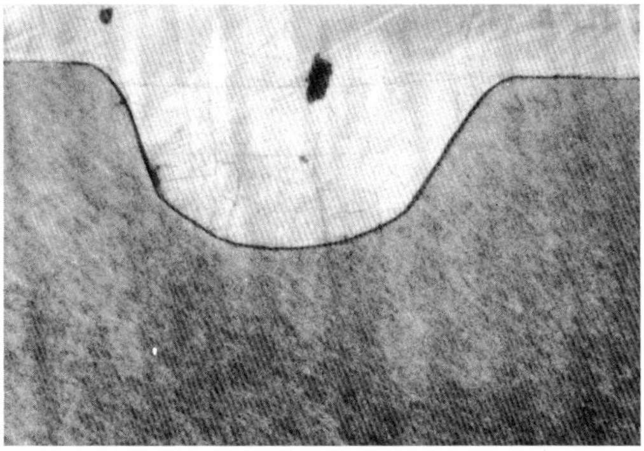

Fig 4.4 Undecalcified section of human dentin after TEA-CO_2 laser radiation: sharply defined cavity without carbonization and cracks (magnification, × 100).

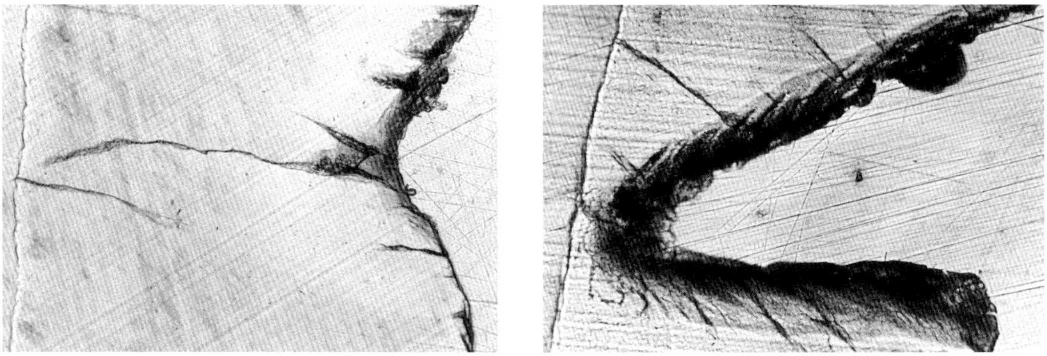

Fig 4.5 Undecalcified sections (× 100) of Er:YAG laser impact in enamel. Cracks and a wide zone of debris can be observed in both examples: **(a)**, with, and **(b)**, without water cooling.

extent of side effects seems to be highly influenced by the optical properties of the irradiated tissues.

TEA CO_2 Lasers

The effects of TEA CO_2 laser (100 nsec to 10 µsec) can be clearly distinguished from those of conventional CO_2 lasers. It is possible to create anatomic cavities with regular wall surfaces. The ablation rate of long pulsed TEA CO_2 lasers (10 µsec) are comparable to those of Er:YAG lasers (Melcer et al, 1992). The ablation rates are 23 µm/pulse in dentin and 14 µm/pulse in enamel, respectively (Melcer et al, 1992). The ablation efficiency decreases, shortening the pulse length. With the long pulsed TEA CO_2 laser, superficial melting on the surface appears. Thermal effects are significantly reduced compared to those with conventional CO_2 lasers.

In histologic investigations of nanosecond pulsed TEA CO_2 lasers, the gross view showed sharp defined cavities without zones of carbonization and cracks. Zones of debris, necrosis, or carbonization could not be observed in light microscopic

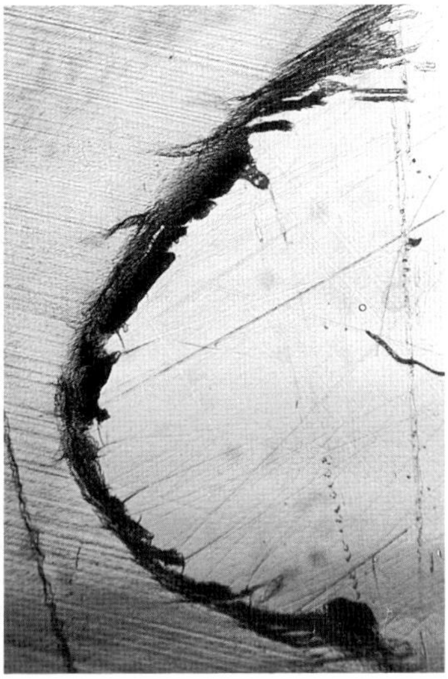

4.6a

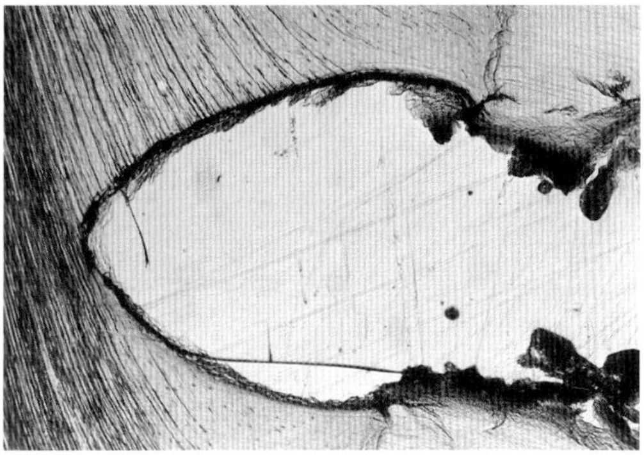

4.6b

Fig 4.6 **(a)**, Undecalcified sections of cavity enamel and dentin with the Er:YSGG laser. The side effects are less extensive compared to those with the Er:YAG laser. **(b)**, A cavity in enamel and dentin with wide debris in enamel and less damage below the enamel-dentin junction.

investigations. The surfaces of the cavities were comparable to those achieved with conventional preparation procedures (Koort and Frentzen, 1992c) (Fig 4.4). These histologic findings correspond with the results of Gertich et al (1991). However, the influence of laser-induced shock waves creating cracks cannot be excluded. Therefore further investigations are required to prove possible applications of TEA CO_2 lasers in dentistry.

Er:YAG Laser

Thermomechanical effects in mineralized tissues can be obtained with the Er:YAG laser. Recently a number of papers appeared about investigations with the Er:YAG laser (Keller and Hibst, 1989; Frentzen and Koort, 1992b), but there is still no common valuation about the possible benefit of this laser type.

In dentin, shallow cavities were surrounded by a zone of necrosis of 1- to 3-μm thickness when water cooling systems were used. In deeper cavities, areas of carbonization and microcracks were observed. Ablating enamel always cracked and deep zones of debris appeared (Frentzen and Koort, 1992b) (Fig 4.5). The extent of side effects did not correlate directly with the selected laser parameters. The location of carbonization and microcracks was not predictable.

Er:YSGG Laser

In the literature, there are only very few reports concerning the Er:YSGG laser with a wavelength of 2.79 μm. In preliminary histologic studies, the gross view showed well-defined cavities (Fig 4.6). In enamel, residual zones of debris and microcracks occurred in a range up to 140 μm. Adjacent to the irradiated area in dentin only very small zones of carbonization and necrosis were found (see Fig 4.6). In comparison to the interaction of the Er:YAG laser, the extent of the zone of side effects is distinctly smaller after Er:YSGG laser radiation (Sievers et al, 1992).

Ho:YAG and Tm:YAG Lasers

The ablation of dentin by pulsed Ho:YAG

Fig 4.7 Ho:YAG irradiated root surfaces (× 100). The cavity surfaces show small zones of intensive carbonization surrounded by a wide zone of thermal alterated dentin: **(a)**, without, and **(b)**, with water cooling. **(c)** and **(d)**, Tm:YAG irradiated root surfaces (× 100). The cavity surfaces show small zones of intensive carbonization surrounded by a wide zone of thermal alterated dentin: **(c)**, without, and **(d)** with water cooling. The histologic results of the Ho:YAG and the Tm:YAG laser only differ in the extent of the necrotic areas.

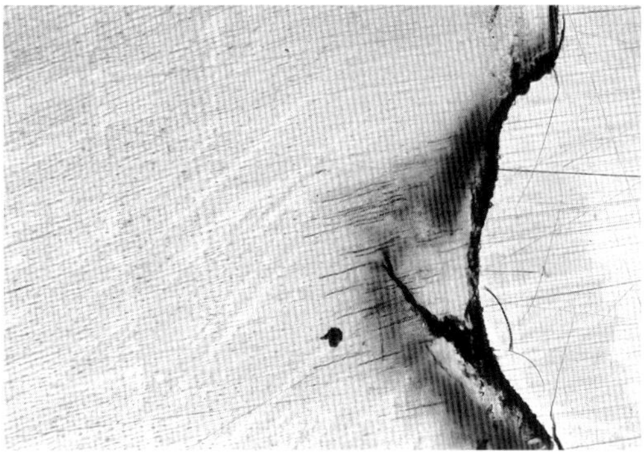

4.7a

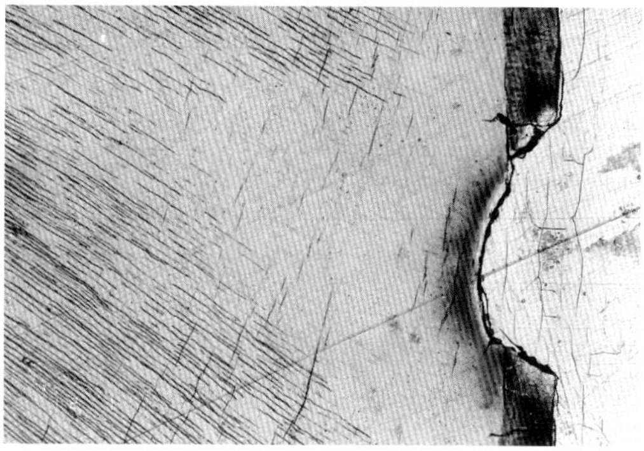

4.7b

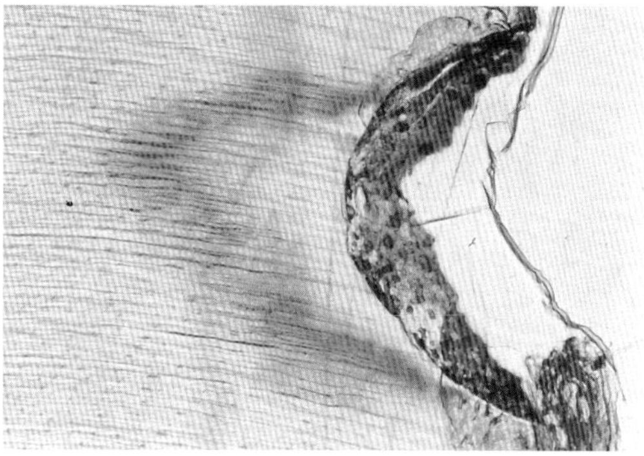

4.7c

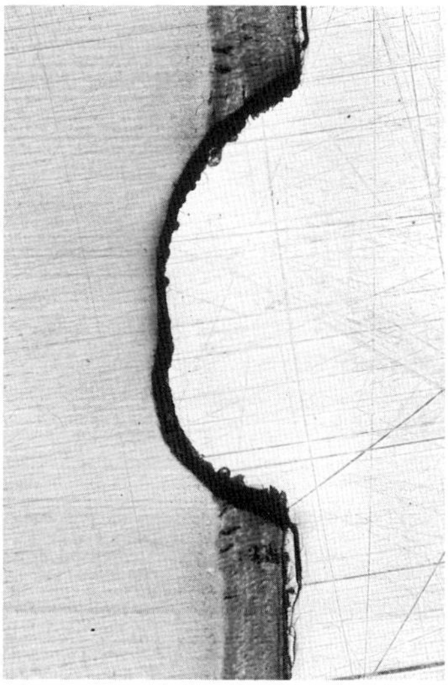

4.7d

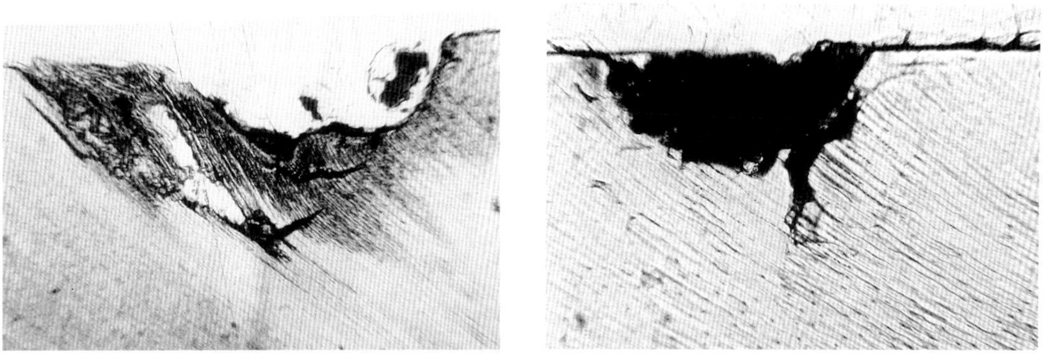

Fig 4.8 Undecalcified section of Nd:YAG laser prepared cavities in dentin (× 250). Zones of debris and carbonization are surrounded by an area of necrosis even when using low pulse energies: **(a)**,100 mJ, 15 Hz; **(b)**, 50 mJ, 15 Hz.

lasers (2.12 μm) and Tm:YAG lasers (2.09 μm) is very low. In preliminary investigations without cooling systems, the cavity surface shows a zone of intensive carbonization (Fig 4.7). Zones of necrosis and some microcracks can be observed below the carbonized surface (Fig 4.7). With additional water cooling systems, less carbonization can be observed. The cavity shows a dispersed surface. The extent of side effects was not predictable (Koort and Frentzen, 1992a–c).

Nd:YAG Laser

Many histologic studies describe the effects and side effects with use of Nd:YAG lasers in dental hard tissue treatment. The tissue removal of pulsed Nd:YAG laser radiation (1.06 μm, pulse duration 100 to 200 μsec) seems to be ineffective. The Nd:YAG laser radiation shows low absorption in water as well as in HA. Therefore the laser power diffuses deeply through the enamel and dentin and finally heats the pulp (Fig 4.8). In dentin, at the laser impact, zones of debris and carbonization are surrounded by an area of necrosis even when low pulse energies are used. Microcracks appear when energies above a threshold of 100 mJ/pulse are used (see Fig 4.8) (Koort and Frentzen, 1992a–c). The appearance and the extent of the side effects (areas of carbonization, necrosis, and microcracks) are not predictable.

Excimer Laser

In histologic investigations, no pathologic changes in the tissue layers adjacent to the dissected areas were found after the ablation of dental tissues with 193-nm ArF excimer lasers (Fig 4.9) (Frentzen et al, 1989). The cavity depth depends almost linearly on the number of laser pulses (Frentzen et al, 1992). The ablation depth per pulse in healthy enamel amounts to 0.15 μm and in healthy dentin to 0.20 μm in a 1-mm^2 focus area and with an energy density of about 10 J/cm^2 pulse. The ablation effects of dental hard tissues are predictable. Compared to conventional diamonds and burs, however, the effectiveness is low. Thermal side effects increase as photon energies of excimer lasers decrease (Frentzen et al, 1992). When, for example, XeCl excimer lasers (308 nm) are used to ablate dental tissues,

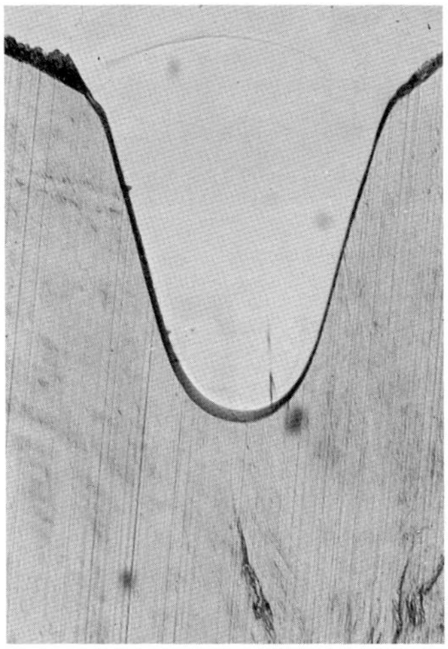

Fig 4.9 No pathologic changes in the tissue layers adjacent to the dissected areas could be found after the ablation of dental tissues with an ArF-excimer laser (in enamel, × 60).

thermal damage occurs in the subsurface layer of dentin and enamel (see Fig 4.9). Thermally induced microcracks appear.

Conclusions

The light microscopic observation of plastic-embedded, undecalcified histologic sections has advantages when the laser-tissue interaction in mineralized tissues is studied: enamel and zones of carbonization and debris are no longer etched away during the decalcification processes. Cracks can be clearly distinguished as laser-induced artifacts. Therefore these techniques should be introduced as a histologic standard method to discuss laser-tissue interactions in mineralized tissues.

The effects of the 193-nm ArF excimer laser radiation—no pathologic changes—can be explained by a nonthermal photoablative process. The radiation has a very high absorbency in only a very small layer of the tissue. In the focus, a plasma is formed that dissipates very fast in a small volume (diameter in µm) of the tissue layer. This could be explained with a fast thermal microexplosion leading to a mechanical destruction of the tissues. Because this process seems to be extremely effective and the involved area is very small, no residual energy is left to cause thermal injuries. Photochemical effects—nonthermal bond breaking by direct electron dissociation—are discussed to explain the effects of the UV laser ablation. The ablative decomposition of mineralized tissues with excimer lasers seems to be independent from the optical properties of the tissues.

Because of the longer wavelength of the XeCl excimer laser (308 nm), the histologic results indicate that the thermal effects increase. Supposed nonthermal photoablative effects as observed with the ArF excimer laser are superposed by thermal side effects.

Even when minimal energy densities are used, the Nd:YAG laser radiation causes wide zones of carbonization and necrosis (Fig 4.10). The reason is the lower absorption of the laser radiation in water than in HA. Because of the high transmission, the laser radiation is absorbed in the depth of the tissue, leading to volume effects that will damage the healthy tissue.

The penetration depth of the Ho:YAG and Tm:YAG laser radiation is less than in the case of the Nd:YAG laser because of a higher absorption (see Fig 4.10). The light energy is transformed into thermal energy mainly in a superficial tissue layer, leading to a strong zone of carbonization. Because of the very good absorption in water, as well as in HA, the laser energy of the CO_2 laser is well coupled to mineralized tissues. The main interaction of this infrared laser radiation in the continuous (cw) or chopped (ms) mode is a thermal interaction, comparable to the interaction

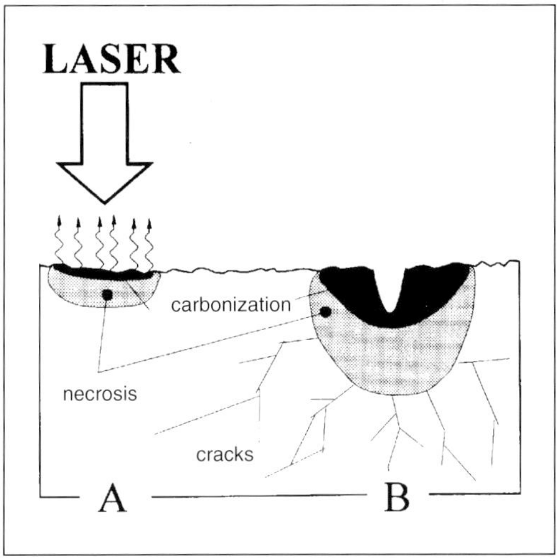

Fig 4.10 Thermal effects: The laser light will be absorbed and converts to thermal energy by stimulating the lattice vibrations of the tissue molecules (mainly water molecules). The lattice vibrations lead to a heating of the surrounding tissues, to a boiling of the water, and, after drying, to a rapid increase in the absorption followed by carbonization and tissue removal (A). Typically, serious damage of the adjacent tissue is found after treatment, manifested by massive zones of carbonization and necrosis as well as thermally induced cracks in hard dental tissues (B).

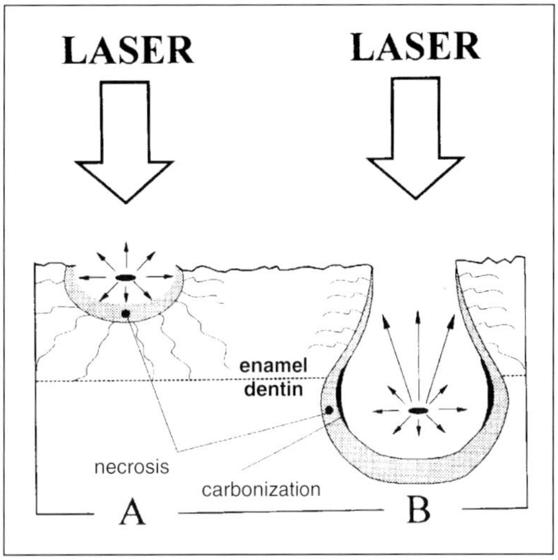

Fig 4.11 Thermomechanical effects: Due to the good absorption in water as well as in hydroxyapatite, an effective treatment of dental structures seems to be possible. The laser radiation leads to a fast heating of water inside the mineralized matrix followed by an explosive volume expansion. The material will be destroyed mechanically with little residual thermal damage. In enamel, cracks are always found (A). In dentin, no cracks but more thermal damage such as carbonization and necrosis are found (B). This seems to depend on the physical and chemical properties of the hard dental tissues.

described for the Ho:YAG and Tm:YAG lasers. The side effects in the depth of the tissue are limited compared to those with the Nd:YAG laser.

The tissue interaction of the TEA CO_2 laser radiation is similar to that of the excimer laser interaction. An ablative effect with little thermal injury is likely because of the high-energy densities in the focus of the short pulses (ns). Photoacoustic phenomena, however, could not be excluded. The radiation of the Er:YAG laser causes extensive damage in enamel. Only a few pulses lead to the unavoidable formation of cracks. Although the absorption in water as well as in HA is good, the zones of damage in dentin are smaller than those in enamel (Fig 4.11). This may be connected to the physical and chemical properties: dentin has a higher water content and can probably better absorb pressure waves created by the laser pulse.

With the exception of the ArF excimer laser and the TEA CO_2 laser, the effects of all laser systems investigated seem to be mainly dependent on unpredictable morphologic structures and physical and chemical properties of the dental hard tissues (Table 4.3). This may be the reason for a great deviation of histologic results.

The unpredictability of laser-induced effects in dental hard tissue treatment, however, is a serious problem and a limiting factor in clinical application.

References

Altshuler GB, Grisimov VN, Ermolaev, VS. Human tooth as an optical device. SPIE conference 1424: Lasers in Orthopedic, Dental, and Veterinary Medicine; 1991.

Bräucker G, Lubatschowski H, Koort HJ, et al. Laserinduzierte photoakustische Effekte im Dentin. Zahn Mund Kieferheilkd 1992;80:217–220.

Brune D. Interaction of pulsed carbon dioxide laser beams with teeth in vitro. Scand J Dent Res 1980; 88:301–305.

Donath K, Brenner G. A method for the study of undecalcified bones and teeth with attached soft tissues. J Oral Pathol 1982;11:318–326.

Frentzen M, Koort HJ, Kermani O, et al. Caries removal and conditioning of tooth surfaces for adhesive filling techniques by using a 193 nm excimer laser—preliminary results. In Yamamoto H, Atsumi K, Kusakari H (eds): Lasers in Dentistry. Amsterdam: Elsevier; 1989;235–240.

Frentzen M, Koort HJ. Lasers in dentistry: new possibilities with advancing laser technology? Int Dent J 1990;40:323–332.

Frentzen M, Koort HJ, Schulz B. Histological results after laser radiation using a new embedding technique for dental tissues. Innovative Tech Biol Med 1990;11: 105–112.

Frentzen M. Applications in restorative dentistry. "Let There Be Light—The Laser In Dentistry" London: Royal Society of Medicine; 1992.

Frentzen M, Koort HJ. Histological investigation of mid-infrared laser ablation of dental hard tissues. 3rd International Congress on Lasers in Dentistry; Salt Lake City, UT; 1992a.

Frentzen M, Koort HJ. The effect of Er:YAG laser radiation on enamel and dentin (abstract 450). J Dent Res 1992b;71:571.

Frentzen M, Koort HJ, Thiensiri I. Excimer lasers in dentistry: future possibilities with advanced technology. Quintessence Int 1992;23:117–133.

Gertich K, Krautschick G, Graehn G. Anwendung eines Mini-TEA-CO_2-Lasers in der Zahnheilkunde. Dtsh Stomatol 1991;41:446–450.

Goldman L, Hornby P, Mayer R, et al. Impact of the laser on dental caries. Nature 1964;203:417.

Hale GM, Querry MR. Optical constants of water in the 200 nm to 200 μm wavelength region. Appl Opt 1973;12:555–563.

Jarby S, Dansgaard W. The thermal effect of different operations on teeth. Odontol Tidskr 1959;67:208–240.

Kantola S. Laser induced effects on tooth structure. VII. X-ray diffraction study of dentine exposed to a CO_2 laser. Acta Odontol Scand 1973;31:381–386.

Keller U, Hibst R. Experimental studies of the application of the Er:YAG laser on dental hard substances. II. Light microscopic and SEM investigations. Lasers Surg Med 1989;9:345–351.

Koort HJ. Processing of bioceramic implants with excimer laser. In Jacques SL, Katzir A (eds): Laser-Tissue Interaction II. SPIE Proc 1991;1427:173–180.

Koort HJ, Frentzen M. YAG-lasers in restorative dentistry. A histological investigation. In Anderson RR, Katzir A (eds): Laser Surgery. Advanced Characterization, Therapeutics and Systems III. SPIE Proc 1992a; 1643:403–411.

Koort HJ, Frentzen M. Absorption of laser radiation in dentin. 3rd International Congress on Lasers in Dentistry; Salt Lake City, UT; 1992b.

Koort HJ, Frentzen M. The effect of TEA-CO_2-laser on dentin. 3rd International Congress on Lasers in Dentistry, Salt Lake City, UT; 1992c.

LeGeros RZ. Calcium Phosphates in Oral Biology and Medicine. Basel-München-Paris: Karger; 1991.

Melcer J, Helias G, Farcy JC, et al. Ablation of mineralized dental tissues by the long pulsed TEA CO_2 laser. 3rd International Congress on Lasers in Dentistry; Salt Lake City, UT; 1992.

Melcer J, Farcy JC, Hellas G, et al. Preparation of cavities using a TEA CO_2 laser. 3rd International Congress on Lasers in Dentistry, Salt Lake City, UT; 1992.

Müller G, Scholz C, Ertl T, et al. Biophysics of laser tissue ablation in bone and dental treatment. Innovative Tech Biol Med 1990;11:1–22.

Nagasawa A. Research and development of laser in dental and oral surgery. In Atsumi K (ed): New Frontiers in Laser Medicine and Surgery. Amsterdam-Oxford: Elsevier;1983;233–241.

Sievers M, Koort HJ, Altshuler G, et al. The ablation of dental hard tissue by Er:YSGG-laser. 3rd International Congress on Lasers in Dentistry; Salt Lake City, UT; 1992.

Stern RH, Sognnaes RF. Laser beam effects on dental hard tissues. J Dent Res 1964;43:873–876.

Stern RH. Dentistry and the laser. In Wolbarsht ML (ed): Laser Applications in Medicine and Biology, vol II. New York-London: Plenum Press;1974:361–387.

Walsh JT, Deutsch TF. Er:YAG laser ablation of tissue: measurement of ablation rates. Lasers Surg Med 1989;9:327–337.

Walsh JT, Flotte TJ, Deutsch TF. Er:YAG laser ablation of tissue: effect of pulse duration and tissue type on thermal damage. Lasers Surg Med 1989;9:314–326.

White JM, Goodis HE, Wong WS. Nd:YAG laser treatment effects on microhardness of dentin (abstract 351). J Dent Res 1991;70:309.

Zijp JR, Ten Bosch JJ. Angular dependence of HeNe-laser light scattering by bovine and human dentine. Arch Oral Biol 1991;36:283–289.

Zweig AD, Frenz M, Romano V, et al. A comparative study of laser tissue interaction at 2.94 μm and 10.6 μm. Appl Phys Bull 1988;47:259–265.

Chapter Five

Laser Effects on the Dental Pulp

Charles Arcoria and Leo J. Miserendino

Within the oral cavity, the proximity of soft tissue to vital calcified tissues has precipitated a persistent problem regarding tissue viability. Coupled with this obstacle, the nature of soft/hard tissue density types has made it exceedingly difficult to accurately characterize laser-tissue interactions of specific wavelengths. In essence, the predicament has been one of too much data in the form of specific parameters (power density, beam transmissive mode, time of pulse duration, wavelength, etc). To accurately characterize the tissue effects of lasers, these essential features perhaps need to be embedded in a mathematical formula or model that will help the researcher and clinician determine an appropriate and safe clinical response. The pulp tissue characteristics and attributes in response to externally applied trauma have historically used three forms of evaluation: 1) histologic analysis; 2) radiographic or clinical observations; and, most recently 3) laser doppler flowmeter measurement.

The histologic descriptions have dominated the literature and therefore consume the emphasis of the pulp biology discussion. Radiographic/clinical observation has been inconsistent and lacks standardization because of the degree of difficulty in the assessment of clinical judgments. In the future, it is anticipated that a noninvasive technique, eg, possibly utilizing doppler flowmeters, can become both accurate and standardized (Friedman et al, 1991). As a corollary, histologic observation can then be used to confirm the flowmeter determinations.

The pulpal effects of existing laser wavelengths used in dentistry (10,600 nm; 9,320 nm; 2,900 nm; 2,100 nm; 1,064 nm; 693 nm; 514.5 nm; 488 nm; 308 nm; and 193 nm) have been well documented in the scientific literature. In particular, effects on the odontoblasts and the erythrocytic matrix have received special attention. Most studies have focused on the interaction between the specific wavelength and tissue in addition to the resultant heat response. Because the vast majority of these wavelengths have the capacity to convert light energy to thermal energy, it is important to understand that pulpal heat convection has been a significant problem.

Collectively, many dental laser studies have been based on the nature of the

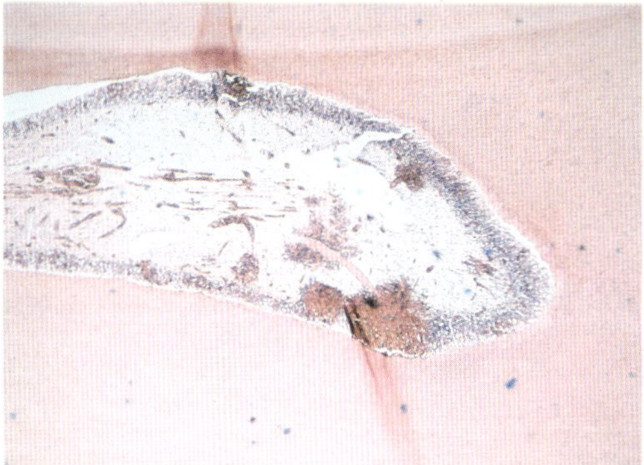

Fig 5.1 Disruption of odontoblastic layer and focal hemorrhage in dog pulp resulting from Nd:YAG laser irradiation of enamel surface (hematoxylin and eosin). (From J Clin Laser Med Surg 1993; 11(2): 83–85. Reprinted with permission.)

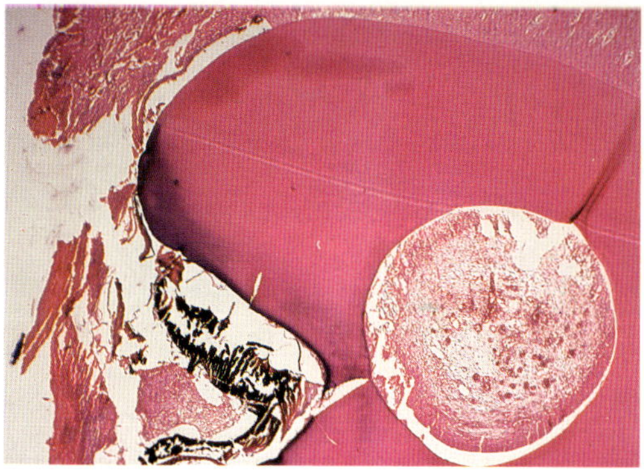

Fig 5.2 Carbonization of dentin and necrosis of dog pulp resulting from carbon dioxide laser pulse (15 W, 0.5 sec, 1-mm focal spot). **(a)**, × 25; **(b)**, hematoxylin and eosin, × 100. (Courtesy of Dr. Shawn Noorvash.)

laser-tissue interaction involving absorptive qualities of tissue and their relationship with the infrared (IR) spectra. Wavelengths greater than approximately 390 nm have been shown to possess inherent heat-producing characteristics. In particular, carbon dioxide lasers, when ablating pulp tissue, can produce a significant amount of heat. Neodymium:YAG lasers also have the potential for inducing heat production depending on the overall interaction with the tissue with darkened pigmentation.

If one surmises that, because of the potential for transmission through enamel and dentin into the pulp, ablation can occur with an Nd:YAG laser, the 1,064-nm wavelength may have somewhat limited indications at higher power levels (Fig 5.1). Research, on the other hand, has demonstrated that carbon dioxide lasers produce a different type of response, but no less damaging effect on pulpal tissue (Fig 5.2).

When examining dental pulp in a histologic manner after laser ablation, the presence of odontoblastic nuclei is extremely important. Recent histologic evidence suggests that a normal odontoblastic layer, stroma, and viable epithelial root sheath can be retained (Figs 5.3 and 5.4) following laser radiation provided damage threshold energy densities are not exceeded (Abt et al, 1992). If pulp temperatures are raised beyond the 5°C level, research has shown that the odontoblastic layer may not be present (Fig 5.5). Moreover, odontoblastic alignment may also be acutely disrupted, displaying a vertical or layering type of structure. Characteristics of the dentinogenesis process related to root development, predentin and reparative dentin formation, dentinal bridge presence, and remaining dentin thickness typically reflect the overall trauma that has been induced in the odontoblasts via either the response to heat production or from the interaction between light energy and the cellular substance. Although the latter mechanism is poorly understood, it may account for the possibility of cell damage in pulp specimens that have not exhibited a significant rise in temperature.

The carbon dioxide laser can induce predentin, reparative dentin, and dentinal bridging responses while exhibiting a measurable amount of remaining dentin thick-

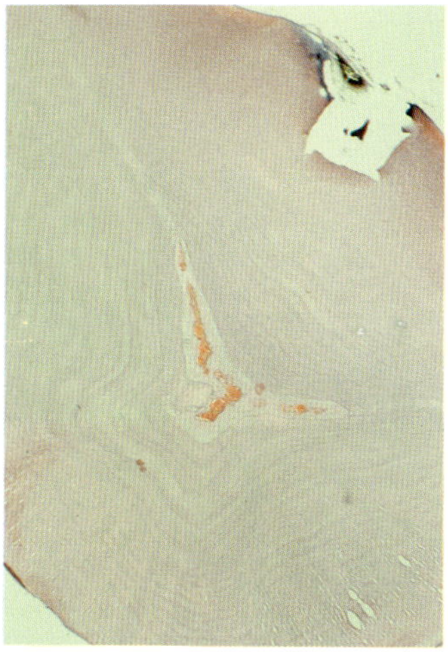

Fig 5.3 Nd:YAG laser cutting of dentin (hematoxylin and eosin cross section) at the level of the cementoenamel junction. (Courtesy of Elliot Abt.)

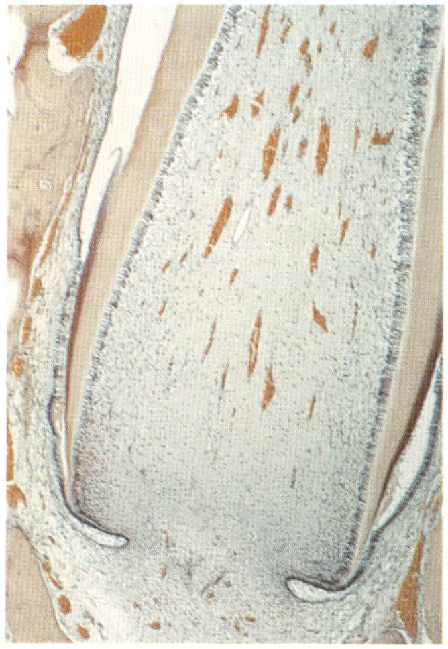

Fig 5.4 Periapical region of Nd:YAG irradiated rabbit tooth at 30 days after treatment. Note absence of inflammatory cell infiltrate and normal-appearing root development (hematoxylin and eosin). (Courtesy of Elliott Abt.)

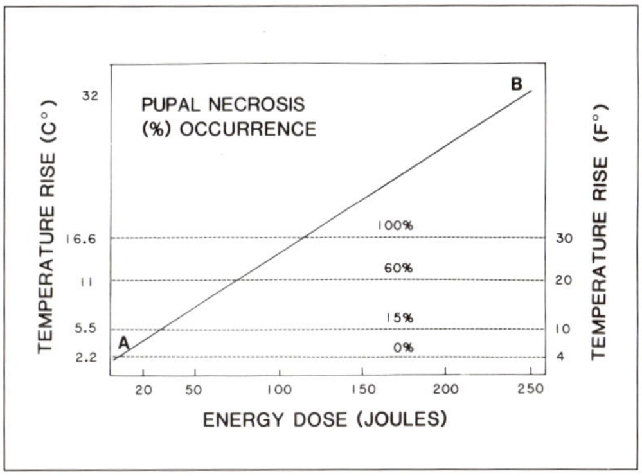

Fig 5.5 Relationship of pulp temperature elevation to pulp necrosis. (From J Endodent 1989; 15:302–305. Reprinted with permission.)

ness. The Nd:YAG wavelength can also produce these phenomena, but in a radically different fashion. Researchers have postulated that the mechanism occurs primarily as a function of the laser-tissue interaction and the IR spectra. The 488- and 514.5-nm wavelengths, when they penetrate calcified tissues, can also produce all of these reactions. As a consequence, the interaction of any laser-induced trauma can theoretically stimulate the dentinogenesis process.

The consistency and composition of the intracellular tissue is another factor influencing cell viability. If heat is intensive and exists for an extended time, the consistency of the intracellular ground substance may not be preserved. This is a function of the interaction both at the surface where first contact of the beam is evident and also very deep, where a specific wavelength can penetrate profoundly into the tissue. Accordingly, the application of excessive energy densities has been shown to result in significant damage to pulp tissue and, in particular, to odontoblasts. The threshold response for pulp reaction appears to lie at energy densities somewhat less than 60 J/cm^2.

With the aforementioned in mind, it is apparent that there is a window of survivability with any dental laser system irrespective of wavelength. This is dependent on the parameters within the system, specifically power, pulsing nature, beam duration, pulse width, and spot size. Unfortunately, from a clinical perspective, this window of tissue viability is extremely narrow and may not produce a desirable clinical response on bone, enamel, dentin, or caries (ie, cavitation).

Laser-Tissue Interactions of Pulp

Although the destructive effects of laser beams on pulpal tissue have been delineated for several years (Goldman et al, 1965; Kinersly et al, 1965; Nelson et al, 1987; Zakariasen et al, 1990), safe windows regarding hard-tissue use are slowly achieving acceptance. Historically, the use of a continuous wave apparatus had been shown to generate significant thermal tissue damage in the oral cavity (see Fig 5.5) extensively disseminating into surrounding tissues (Lobene et al, 1968; Launay et al, 1987; Miserendino et al, 1989; Jeffrey et al, 1990).

Characteristically, pulpal tissue cannot survive in an environment of elevated temperatures for protracted periods when tooth structure is irradiated with lasers (Adrian et al, 1971; Melcer et al, 1987; Renneboog-Squilbin et al, 1989; Arcoria et al, 1991). With the advent of superpulsed laser systems, a potential decrease in soft tissue necrosis became possible because heat was given sufficient time to dissipate from the site of irradiation as a result of the rapid interruption of the beam (Franquin and Salomon, 1986; Lanzafame et al 1988; Walsh et al, 1988). Although the use of a discontinuous beam has produced a more workable tissue-management system, the thermal effects have not completely abated in excess of 60 J/cm^2 (Taylor et al, 1965; Lobene et al, 1968; Brune, 1980). As a result, infrared and/or visible light mediums utilizing a pulsed mode have also exhibited pulpal damage indigenous to a wavelength with a measurement larger than 390 nm (Adrian, 1977).

The development of thermal reduction mechanisms intended to reduce heat transfer from the enamel or dentinal surface may answer some of the inherent problems experienced during laser treatment (Miserendino et al, 1993). Pulsing has been used during soft tissue laser ablation as an effective mechanism for reducing the extent of collateral tissue damage. This principle however has been shown to be less effective when laser exposures involve dental hard tissues, which perhaps can be attributed to differences in the thermal diffusion rate and relaxation time between the hard calcified and soft oral tissues. The extent of these differences may therefore preclude the use of pulsing alone as an effective means of temperature control when lasers are to be applied to enamel and dentin of teeth with vital pulps (Table 5.1).

The use of a combination of air-and-water spray before, during, or immediately after laser irradiation to enamel and dentin may be a more effective method for temperature control and reduction of heat transfer to the pulp and other vital structures surrounding the teeth. Precooling by air-and-water spray prior to lasing may be

Table 5.1 Temperature Change*

Group	10 J	20 J	30 J	40 J	50 J
No cooling	1.85	3.65	5.10	5.12	5.56
Air	1.95	2.75	3.00	3.65	4.06
Air/water	3.95	3.3	3.06	3.10	2.19
Pulsed 10 ms	1.64	3.88	5.12	5.50	7.06
Pulsed 50 ms	2.69	4.56	4.75	5.56	6.75
Drill and air	3.10	< 0.1	< 0.1	4.65	< 0.1

*|Tmax| Mean Values

used with laser systems with wavelengths such as carbon dioxide, holmium, and erbium, which are more readily absorbed by water. Neodymium:YAG, which has little absorption in water, may be effectively cooled with simultaneous air-and-water spray. Lasers with limited transmission through enamel and dentin may also be effectively cooled with application of an air-and-water spray immediately after lasing. The application of an air-and-water spray has been found to provide adequate heat protection to the pulp equivalent to that of the common dental drill (Miserendino et al, 1993; Abt et al, 1992). The use of other methods of delivery, pulse configuration, or wavelengths such as excimer, which exhibit less thermal interaction with enamel and dentin, are other possible mechanisms for preserving pulp vitality during laser treatment of teeth.

Obviously, unabated or uncontrolled laser irradiation of oral structures can cause pulpal inflammation with any type of laser (Stern et al, 1972; Adrian, 1977; Launay et al, 1987). This undesirable side effect can vary primarily with power and energy density and secondarily with the type of laser used. Little information is available regarding intracellular response of dental pulp to several types of lasers. Continuous wave CO_2 lasers can produce varying degrees of pulpal necrosis (Miserendino et al, 1989), but at low power or in a pulsed mode, new dentin formation may ensue (Melcer et al, 1987). Since animal studies have demonstrated that laser irradiation of oral tissues induced increases in pulpal warming (Adrian, 1977; Serebro et al, 1987), this is likely the reason for cell death. Intermittent formation of new dentin, with concomitant pulp vitality, is a normal response of the pulp to external insult. Unfortunately, significant heat escalation within the pulp precludes this sustained formation.

Continuous wave and pulsed devices with single laser sources produce consistent, characteristic effects on the tissues, particularly when using a CO_2 medium (Walsh et al, 1988). In previous studies involving tissue outside the oral cavity, the results of combining or sequentially using the Nd:YAG beam, despite its inherent penetration potential, with CO_2 or argon have been inconsistent. From the general inferences noted throughout the literature, the interaction of the differing wavelengths in tissue may sometimes favor new dentin formation over odontoblastic degeneration, depending on relative power levels.

In a comparison of the histologic response of the dental pulp to dentin ablation by various wavelengths of laser in dog teeth, Wigdor and others (Wigdor et al, 1993) suggest that Er:YAG may display a lower thermal effect than the other lasers tested. They conclude that other important factors, such as the selection of optimal parameters for efficient ablation, need to be identified before lasers may be used to replace the dental drill for removal of enamel and dentin in clinical practice (Figs 5.6 and 5.7).

Laser Effects on Enamel

Typical processes for describing the ablation effect of lasers on enamel have been donated from other research specialties. The modalities used for measuring enamel surface morphology characteristics have included: 1) profilometric recordings with a surftester; 2) scanning electron microscopic examination; 3) digital image processing of photomicrographs; 4) customized software programs for developing fractal dimension equations characterizing surface morphology; 5) elemental analysis of the physicochemical alterations on the surface; and 6) three-dimensional topo-

Fig 5.6 Er:YAG laser cavity preparation in dentin (hematoxylin and eosin). (From JADA 1993; 124:65–70. Reprinted with permission.)

Fig 5.7 Carbon dioxide laser cavity preparation in dog tooth (hematoxylin and eosin). (From JADA 1993;124:65–70. Reprinted with permission.)

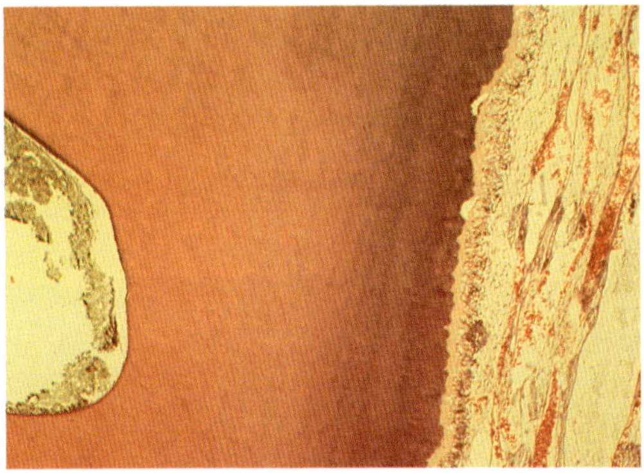

5.6

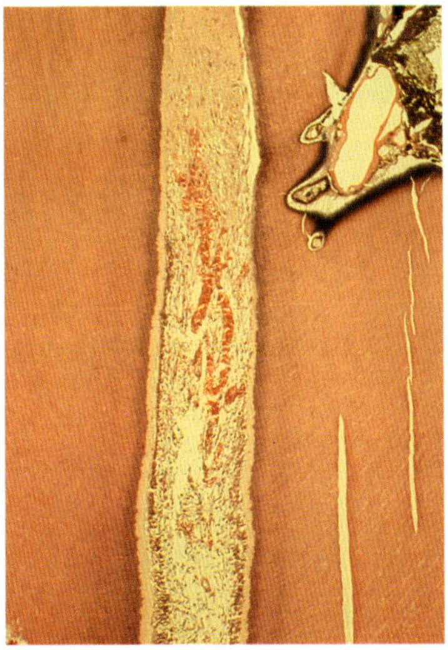

5.7

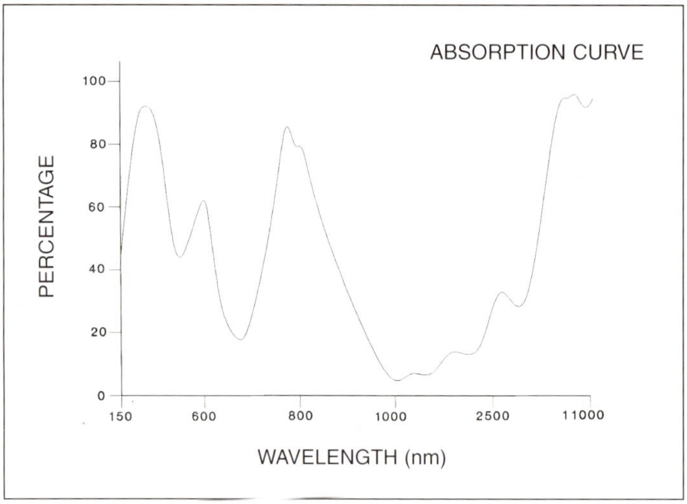

Fig 5.8 Absorption spectrum for enamel from 150 to 11,000 nm.

graphic reconstruction of enamel. All of these modalities have been used to accurately assess the capacity of specific wavelengths to interact with hydroxyapatite and induce permanent, and hopefully desirable, calcified tissue changes.

The nature of the hard tissue response of laser light has always been a primary function of the IR spectral wavelength absorption factors. Absorption spectra for enamel (Fig 5.8) denote the lack of consistency across the spectra regarding absorption characteristics of enamel. Carbon dioxide wavelengths at 9,320 nm and 9,900 nm have been shown to be the most highly absorbed of any wavelength into hydroxyapatite. Conversely, 1,064 nm and other near-infrared wavelengths possess minimal absorbance characteristics with enamel. Absorbance peaks also occur at

200 nm, 600 nm, and 700 nm. As such, the effect on enamel can be described in a variety of fashions depending on the specific wavelength. Table 5.2 lists the respective wavelengths, their corresponding enamel surface characteristics after laser ablation, the potential clinical applications, and the research studies that have produced this body of evidence.

Parameter factors and wavelength specificity relate to the degree of change that can be induced into enamel. Understandably, enamel changes are a function of parameter variance and, as such, can be controlled by the operator. For instance, varying the pulse width, pulse mode, and spot size can produce significant changes in enamel surface morphology. Studies have demonstrated that the variance is proportional to the degree and time of laser exposure. Moreover, the specific wavelength also contributes to the quality of the surface appearance.

Researchers have used etching as a precondition for significant subsurface cavitation by either measuring the ablation rate and evaluating the efficiency of single vs multiple wavelength systems. For instance, the coaxial CO_2/Nd:YAG beam (10,600 and 1,064 nm) induces significantly different surface changes than those with either CO_2 or Nd:YAG independently. Interestingly, the characteristic surface changes are representative of the

Table 5.2 Enamel Surface Response to Laser Ablation

Medium	Wavelength (nm)	Enamel Characteristics	Potential Clinical Applications
CO_2[*]	10,600	Surface fusion, roughness, etching, partially fused crystallites, charred, cracking	Resin bonding, enamel etching, caries reduction, fusing apatite, cavitation
CO_2/Nd:YAG[†]	1,064/10,600	Terraced surface, rough, fused crystallites, charred, cracking	Resin bonding, enamel etching, caries reduction, fusing apatite, cavitation
CO_2[¥]	9,320	Etched, partially fused crystallites, reduction in demineralization, charred, cracking	Resin bonding, enamel etching, caries reduction, fusing apatite, cavitation
Er:YAG[§]	2,900	Etched, cavitated, scaly or flaky rough surface	Cavitation, enamel etching
Nd:YAG[‖]	1,064	Unless photoabsorptive is placed, reflection of beam is seen	Decay removal, etching with placement of dye
Ruby[¶]	693	Cratering, irregular cavitation surface, charred	No known applications
Argon[#]	514/488	Reflection of beam produces minimal effect on surface	Resin polymerization only
ArF[**]	193	Slight etching, smooth, lacking in charring, planed enamel prisms	Cavitation, enamel etching

[*]Ferreira et al, 1989; Kuroda and Fowler, 1984; Liberman et al, 1984; Walsh et al, 1991.
[†]Arcoria et al, 1991.
[¥]Featherstone and Nelson, 1987; Nelson et al, 1986; Nelson et al, 1987.
[§]Hibst and Keller, 1989; Keller and Hibst, 1989.
[‖]Dederich, 1991; Von Lenz et al, 1976; White et al, 1992.
[¶]Gordon, 1967.
[#]Kelsey et al, 1989; Launay et al, 1987.
[**]Arcoria et al, 1992; Frentzen et al, 1992.

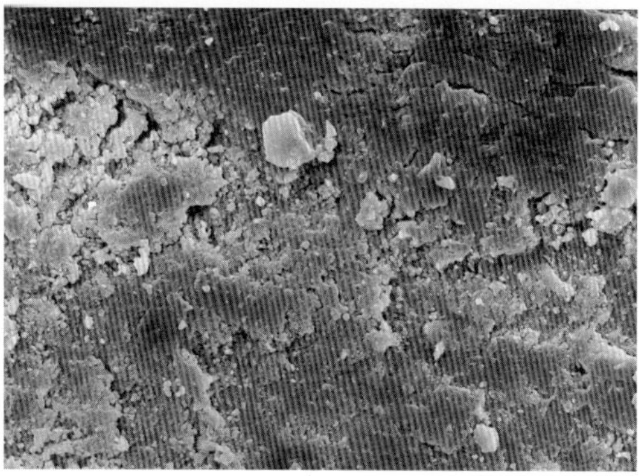

Fig 5.9 Coaxial Nd:YAG and CO_2 laser-etched enamel surface.

CO_2 laser because of the deep, etching changes. Also, the degree of subsurface cavitation by the coaxial laser is more profound than with either independent beam (Fig 5.9).

The argon and Nd:YAG beams possess significant reflecting properties, with the latter beam also having penetration potential. As a result, these wavelengths, devoid of photoabsorptive dye placement, produce a superheated and beaded enamel structure, not particularly desirable for an etched enamel surface. Effective etching of enamel with use of photosensitizers (dyes) has been demonstrated (unpublished data). The surface characteristics of the laser-etched surface compared to that of acid-etched enamel display a more uniformly roughened appearance (Figs 5.10 and 5.11). The CO_2 beam, known for its efficient absorption into enamel, also produces a superheated enamel surface similar to the previous ablations.

In essence, the morphologic appearance of the enamel with the argon, Nd:YAG, and CO_2 lasers represents recrystallized or resolidified hydroxyapatite and enamel prismatic structure. However, the coaxial CO_2/Nd:YAG laser can induce a surface roughness value similar to the acid-etched surface. Because of the nature of these specific coaxial wavelengths and their tandem effects in tissue (Arcoria et al, 1991), the terracing of enamel is quite profound, albeit significantly different from that with the use of either beam independently.

Of principal interest in enamel ablation studies is the fact that acid-etched samples appear markedly different than laser ablations, with the possible exception of the CO_2/Nd:YAG and ArF irradiation. The combined nature of the CO_2 and Nd:YAG beams produces a synergistic effect that is measurably different from the independent use of the two beams. The surface morphologic appearance exhibits a highly roughened or terraced topography, similar to a chipping or slight fracturing of the enamel prisms. Furthermore, ArF excimer ablations are qualitatively different from all other ablations. Understandably, the 193-nm ultraviolet wavelength possesses inherent differences relating to overall calcified tissue effects as compared to those with visible light and infrared wavelengths (Srinivasan, 1986). For instance, the capacity of excimer lasers to dissociate the peptide bonds of organic molecules without inducing substantial temperature elevation in tissue (Srinivasan, 1986; Srinivasan and Leigh, 1982; Lustmann et al, 1991) is significant regarding the lack of surface fissuring and carbonization. Moreover, the clinical enamel surface, using the ArF excimer displays a slightly roughened appearance devoid of heat-induced alterations.

Previous studies have demonstrated the potential of an assortment of visible and infrared wavelength lasers to induce surface fissuring and carbonization above the 50 to 60 J/cm^2 energy density threshold (Featherstone and Nelson, 1987; Arcoria et al, 1991; Boran et al, 1991). Similarly, the visible light systems have displayed surface cracking representative

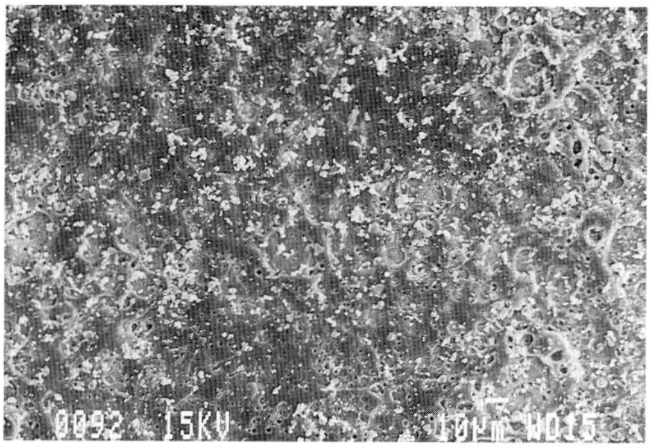

Fig 5.10 Scanning electron micrograph of Nd:YAG laser-etched enamel surface. (Courtesy of TD Myers.)

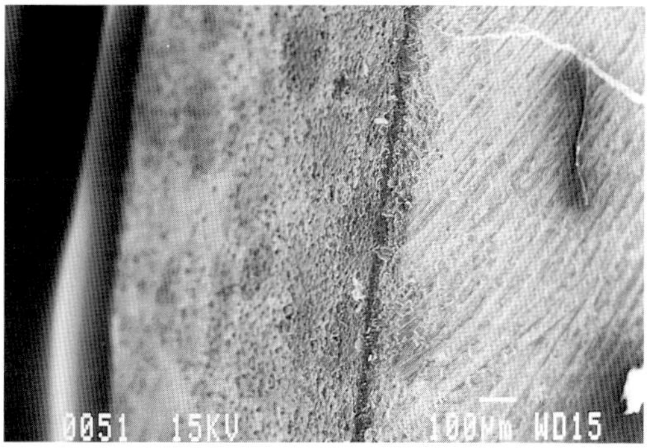

Fig 5.11 Scanning electron micrograph cross-sectional view of Nd:YAG laser-etched enamel surface. (Courtesy of TD Myers.)

of a superheated, then rapidly cooled enamel surface, undergoing a severe dimensional change; thus, the reason for the heat-induced enamel morphologic appearance.

The mapping of enamel surface contour after laser ablations vs acid etching is important for several reasons. First, a prediction regarding the degree of restorative material mechanical bond strength and subsequent correlation of these values with the attachment of the material to tooth structure is needed. Second, the use of a profilometer to precisely measure the degree of surface roughness without the need for additional quantitative analyses has been previously used (Ferreira et al, 1989; Arcoria et al, 1991), but may not generate a comprehensive picture of the surface. Third, qualitative analyses of scanning electron micoscopic (SEM) photographs have adequately described the breadth of surface roughness alterations, but lacked the capacity to express the contour in a mathematical equation. Thus, a qualitative analysis (SEM), in combination with the use of a profilometer, cannot accurately compare the differences between similar wavelength ablations (ie, Nd:YAG continuous wave vs Q-switched)

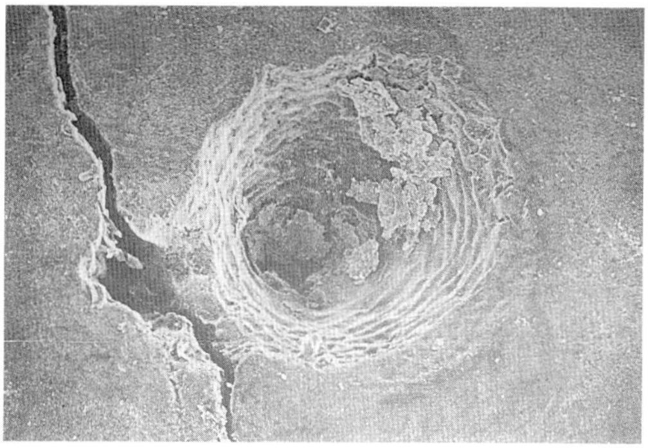

Fig 5.12 Scanning electron micrograph of laser crater produced by Q-switched Nd:YAG laser in enamel. Notice induced thermal fracture (left). (Courtesy of D Harris, 1987.)

in a quantitative fashion (Fig 5.12). Therefore, in the future, the use of a more quantifiable method, probably digital texture analyses with computer scanning imagery, should be investigated to assess the enamel surface morphology. Subsequently, a correlation of these values with the in vitro restorative material bond strength is indicated.

Calcified tissue responses are largely dependent on wavelength specificity (Featherstone and Nelson, 1987). The portion of the electromagnetic spectrum

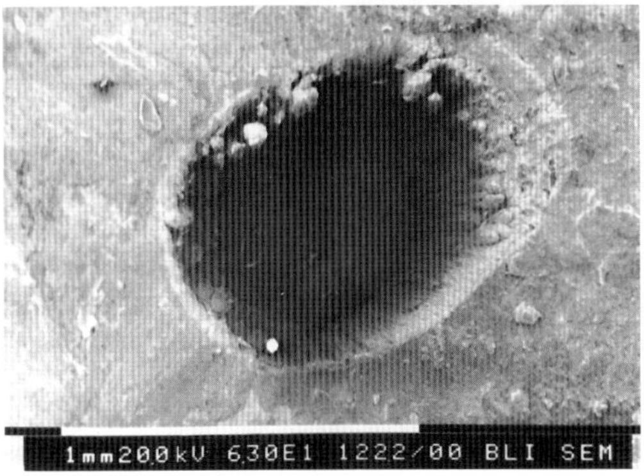

Fig 5.13 Scanning electron micrograph of laser crater produced by excimer laser. (Courtesy of Dr Joseph Neev.)

occupied by the CO_2 laser, 9,000 to 11,000 nm, respectively, exhibits the most efficient pathway of absorption into enamel (Featherstone and Nelson, 1989). High energy densities (in excess of 100 J/cm^2) have produced the desired ablative effects (Gordon, 1967; Lobene et al, 1968; Kuroda and Fowler, 1984; Ferreira et al, 1989; Walsh and Perham, 1991). Typically, the ablated surface has been measured with a profilometer (Arcoria et al, 1991), in addition to determining crater depth (Walsh and Deutsch, 1988; Ferreira et al, 1989). Lased enamel surface characterizations have also encountered a fused enamel appearance (Stern et al, 1972; Featherstone and Nelson, 1987; Featherstone and Nelson, 1989; Walsh and Perham, 1991; Slayton and Wefel, 1991) and an increased calcium/phosphorus content as compared to unlased enamel (Kantola, 1972; Kuroda and Fowler, 1984; Nelson et al, 1986, 1987; Kempler et al, 1991). Furthermore, the inhibition of enamel subsurface demineralization (Yamamoto and Ooya, 1974; Kuroda and Fowler, 1984; Boran et al, 1991) has resulted in a degree of acid resistance after laser usage, which may be beneficial for the prevention or inhibition of dental caries (Stern and Sognnaes, 1972; Yamamoto and Sato, 1980; Shirasuka et al, 1991; Yu et al, 1991).

Tissue responses encompass an interaction between laser wavelengths and tissues, leading to localized heat convection into surrounding structures (Hillenkamp, 1989). Also, the induction of nonlinear absorption and plasma formation, resulting in vaporization and explosive tissue removal, becomes likely (Walsh and Deutsch, 1988). Furthermore, inadequate characterization of laser-tissue interaction has occurred because of the incomparable nature of different laser systems. The heterogeneous nature of tissue types makes it difficult to detect penetration depths and the totality of ablations (Walsh and Deutsch, 1988; Hillenkamp, 1989).

Characterizations of enamel and dentin alterations have been performed with nontraditional laser models (Arcoria et al, 1991). Irradiation with a coaxial infrared beam produced different cavitations from other types of ablations (Arcoria et al, 1991). Moreover, ultraviolet mediums, such as ArF excimer lasers (193 nm), have induced a nonthermal ablation in calcified tissue, suggestive of photodissociation of organic molecular bonds (Srinivasan and Leigh, 1982; Srinivasan, 1986; Lustmann et al, 1991). The wavelength is specific with regard to dissociating the bonds of molecular structures at a high enough intensity before heat transfer to the remaining molecular entity can occur (Linsker et al, 1984; Srinivasan, 1986; Frentzen and Koort, 1990). Thus, a disintegrating effect on calcified tissue occurs (Fig 5.13) without surface charring or temperature elevation (Keyes et al, 1985). Consequently, the excimer laser possesses the potential to ablate tooth structure without the deleterious effects on pulpal structure and function. A more complete description of excimer laser interaction with dental hard tissue is presented in Chapter 19.

References

Abt E, Miserendino LJ, Levy GC. Histologic effects of Nd:YAG and Er:YAG on dentin, pulp, and bone (abstract). Proceedings of Third International Congress on Lasers in Dentistry. International Society for Lasers in Dentistry Meeting; Salt Lake City, UT; Aug 1992.

Adrian JC. Pulp effects of neodymium laser. Oral Surg Oral Med Oral Pathol 1977;44:301–305.

Adrian JC, Bernier JL, Sprague WG. Laser and the dental pulp. Am Dent Assoc 1971;83:113–117.

Arcoria CJ, Steele RE, Wagner MJ, Judy MM, Matthews JL, Hults DF. Enamel surface roughness and dental pulp response to coaxial carbon dioxide-neodymium:YAG laser irradiation. J Dent 1991; 19:85–91.

Bahcall JK, Miserendino LJ, Howard P, Walia H. Preliminary investigation of the histopathologic reaction of pulpal tissue from Nd:YAG laser treatment on enamel of dog teeth. J Clin Laser Med Surg 1993;11:83–86.

Boran TL, Zakariasen KL, Peters J. The effects of CO_2 laser radiation on smooth surface enamel in vitro (abstract). J Dent Res 1991;70:1819.

Brune D. Interaction of pulsed carbon dioxide laser beams with teeth in vitro. Scand Dent Res 1980;88: 301–305.

Featherstone JDB, Nelson DGA. Laser effects on dental hard tissues. Adv Dent Res 1987;1:21–26.

Featherstone JDB, Nelson DGA. Recent uses of electron microscopy in the study of physico-chemical processes affecting the reactivity of synthetic and biological apatites. Scan Microsc 1989;3:815–828.

Ferreira JM, Palamara J, Phakey PP, Rachinger WA, Orams HJ. Effects of continuous-wave CO_2 laser on the ultrastructure of human dental enamel. Arch Oral Biol 1989;34:551–562.

Franquin JC, Salomon JP. Pulp-dentin reactions after CO_2 laser treatment of dentine. J Biol Buccale 1986;14:53–64.

Frentzen M, Koort HJ. Lasers in dentistry: new possibilities with advancing laser technology? Int Dent J 1990;40:323–332.

Goldman L, Gray JA, Goldman J. Effect of laser beam impacts on teeth. J Am Dent Assoc 1965;70:601–606.

Gordon TE. Single-surface cutting of normal tooth with ruby laser. J Am Dent Assoc 1967;74:398–402.

Hillenkamp F. Laser radiation tissue interaction. Health Phys 1989;56:613–616.

Jeffrey IWM, Lawrenson B, Saunders EM. Dentinal temperature transients caused by exposure to CO_2 laser irradiation and possible pulpal damage. J Dent 1990;18:31–36.

Kantola S. Laser-induced effects on tooth structure: V. Electron probe microanalysis and polarized light microscopy of dental enamel. Acta Odontol Scand 1972;30:475–484.

Keyes T, Clarke RH, Isner JM. Theory of photoablation and its implications for laser phototherapy. J Phys Chem 1985;89:4194–4196.

Kinersly T, Jarabak JP, Phatak NM, DeMent J. Laser effects on tissue and materials related to dentistry. J Am Dent Assoc 1965;70:593–600.

Kuroda S, Fowler BO. Compositional, structural, and phase changes in in vitro laser-irradiated human tooth enamel. Calcif Tissue Int 1984;36:361–369.

Lanzafame RJ, Naim JO, Rogers DW, Hinshaw JR. Comparison of continuous-wave, chop-wave, and super pulse laser wounds. Lasers Surg Med 1988;8:119–124.

Launay Y, Mordan S, Cornil A, Brunetaud JM, Moschetto Y. Thermal effects of lasers on dental tissues. Lasers Surg Med 1987;7:473–477.

Liberman R, Segal TH, Nordenberg D, Serebro LI. Adhesion of composite materials to enamel: comparison between the use of acid and lasing as pretreatment. Lasers Surg Med 1984;4:323–327.

Linsker R, Srinivasan R, Wynne JJ, Torres A, Geronemus RG. Far-ultraviolet laser ablation of atherosclerotic lesions. Lasers Surg Med 1984;4:201–206.

Lobene RR, Bhussry BR, Fine S. Interaction of carbon dioxide laser radiation with enamel and dentin. J Dent Res 1968;47:311–317.

Lustmann J, Ulmansky M, Fuxbrunner A, Lewis A. 193 nm excimer laser ablation of bone. Lasers Surg Med 1991;11:51–57.

Melcer J, Chaumette MT, Melcer F. Dental pulp exposed to the CO_2 laser beam. Lasers Surg Med 1987; 7:347–352.

Miserendino LJ, Neiburger EJ, Walia H. Thermal effects of continuous wave CO_2 laser exposure on human teeth: an in vitro study. J Endodontics 1989;15: 302–305.

Miserendino LJ, Abt E, Wigdor H, Miserendino CA. Evaluation of thermal cooling mechanisms for laser application to teeth. Lasers Surg Med 1993;13:83–88.

Nelson DGA, Jongebloed WL, Featherstone JDB. Laser irradiation of human dental enamel and dentine. NZ Dent J 1986;82:74–77.

Nelson DGA, Shariati M, Glena R, Shields CP, Featherstone JDB. Effect of pulsed low energy infrared laser irradiation on artificial caries-like lesion formation. Caries Res 1987;20:289–299.

Nelson DGA, Wefel JS, Jongebloed WL, Featherstone JDB. Morphology, histology and crystallography of human dental enamel treated with pulsed low energy infrared laser radiation. Caries Res 1987;21:411–426.

Renneboog-Squilbin C, Nammour S, Coomans D, Barel A, Carleer M, Dourov N. Measurement of pulp temperature increase to externally applied heat (argon laser, hot water, drilling). J Biol Buccale 1989;17:179–186.

Shirasuka T, Kodaka T, Debari K, Matsumoto K. Acid resistance on human dental enamel by laser irradiation and fluoride treatment (abstract). J Dent Res 1991; 70:679.

Serebro L, Segal T, Nordenberg D, Gorfil C, Bar-Lev M. Examination of tooth pulp following laser beam irradiation. Lasers Surg Med 1987;7:236–239.

Slayton RS, Wefel JS. Effects of laser irradiation on occlusal surfaces of human molars (abstract). J Dent Res 1991;70:1818.

Srinivasan R. Ablation of polymers and biological tissue by ultraviolet lasers. Science 1986;234:559–565.

Srinivasan R, Leigh WJ. Ablative photodecomposition: action of far-ultraviolet (193 nm) laser radiation on poly (ethylene terephthalate) films. J Am Chem Soc 1982; 104:6784–6785.

Stern RH, Sognnaes RF, Goodman F. Laser effect on in vitro enamel permeability and solubility. J Am Dent Assoc 1966;73:838–843.

Stern RH, Sognnaes RF. Laser inhibition of dental caries suggested by first tests in vivo. J Am Dent Assoc 1972;85:1087–1090.

Stern RH, Vahl J, Sognnaes RF. Lased enamel: ultrastructural observations of pulsed carbon dioxide laser effects. J Dent Res 1972;51:455–460.

Taylor R, Shklar G, Roeber F. The effects of laser radiation on teeth, dental pulp, and oral mucosa of experimental animals. Oral Surg Oral Med Oral Pathol 1965;19:786–795.

Walsh JT, Deutsch TF. Pulsed CO_2 laser tissue ablation: measurement of the ablation rate. Lasers Med Surg 1988;8:264–275.

Walsh JT, Flotte TJ, Anderson RR, Deutsch T. Pulsed CO_2 laser tissue ablation: effect of tissue type and pulse duration on thermal damage. Lasers Surg Med 1988;8:108–118.

Walsh LJ, Perham SJ. Enamel fusion using a carbon dioxide laser: a technique for sealing pits and fissures. Clin Prev Dent 1991;13:16–20.

Wigdor H, Abt E, Ashrafi S, Walsh JT. The effect of lasers on dental hard tissues. J Am Dent Assoc 1993;124:65–70.

Yamamoto H, Ooya K. Potential of yttrium-aluminum-garnet laser in caries prevention. J Oral Pathol 1974;3:7–15.

Yamamoto H, Sato K. Prevention of dental caries by acousto-optically Q-switched Nd:YAG laser irradiation. J Dent Res 1980;59:137.

Yu D, Hsu J, Higuchi WI, Powell GL, Fox JL. Temperature profiles during laser irradiation of human enamel (abstract). J Dent Res 1991;70:683.

Zakariasen KL, Boran T, MacDonald R. The emerging role for lasers in endodontics and other areas of dentistry. Alpha Omega Sci 1990;83:65–67.

Part II

Practical Considerations for Lasers in Dentistry

Chapter Six

Laser Safety in Dental Practice

Leo Miserendino, Robert M. Pick, and Richard Blankenau

Laser safety is an issue limited not only to the performance of treatment within the dental operatory, but one that also encompasses the interrelationship among health-care providers, educational institutions, government, and the commercial sector (Miserendino et al, 1992). The safe and appropriate use of lasers in the field of dentistry requires the conscious and cooperative efforts of all of the aforementioned groups to be effective (Abt et al, 1993). The responsibility for the safe application of lasers in dentistry therefore is one that is shared by all those concerned: dentist, educator, manufacturer, and scientist. Each has a role, from design and development to practical application.

Prior to any clinical or research application of lasers, clinicians and researchers should participate in a formal comprehensive laser training program administered by qualified and experienced instructors to ensure their safety, and the safety of the staff and patients. Laser safety training should be considered an essential component of basic laser instruction and a prerequisite to any application within the dental clinic or research facility. The importance of this premise cannot be overemphasized. Given the proper training and with appropriate precautions, lasers may be used safely for the mutual benefit of both the patient and the dental health-care practitioner.

Dentistry is unique within the health-care industry in that most dentists work as solo practitioners in private office settings. For the most part, their use of lasers is not monitored. In contrast, within the medical community, laser use is more strictly controlled by institutional review boards, credentialing, and hospital surgical privilege committees (Harris et al, 1992; Miserendino et al, 1993). Furthermore, the level of training and experience of the dental staff is generally far less than that of the laser surgical nurse or hospital laser safety officer (Harris et al, 1993).

The subject of dental laser safety is broad in scope, including not only an awareness of the potential risks and hazards related to how lasers are used, but also a recognition of existing standards of care and a thorough understanding of safety control measures. This chapter reviews several of the safety standards and regulatory agencies that pertain to the dental use of lasers; specific educational requirements related to laser safety in the dental office setting; identification of biologic hazards that may be encountered; and proposed laser safety control measures that may be applied by the dental practitioner.

Regulations, Safety Standards, and Guidelines

Safety regulations and standards may be classified as either voluntary or mandatory, and as governing either manufacturers or users of lasers. In many countries, voluntary standards have been established to guide the laser user and manufacturer based on the standard developed by the Technical Committee no. 76 (TC-76) of the International Electrotechnical Commission (IEC) initially released as IEC publication 825 in 1984 and revised 1990 (IEC, 1990). One such version has been adopted by the European Organization for Electrotechnical Standardization and serves as the European Norm (EN 60825). Industrial laser safety standards are currently being developed by the European Organization for Standardization (CEN) and the International Standards Organization (ISO).

Within the United States, the Center for Devices and Radiological Health (CDRH) of the Food and Drug Administration (FDA) is the regulatory agency that governs the manufacture and sale of all laser devices used in the United States. The CDRH sets forth the standards governing the manufacture of lasers in the Code of Federal Regulations (CFR) Title 21: Food and Drugs; chapter 1, Food and Drug Administration; subchapter J, Radiological Health; part 1040, Performance Standards for Light Emitting Products (U.S. Department of Health and Human Services, 1985). This standard categorizes all laser devices into one of four classes based on their total energy output and wavelength (Table 6.1). The surgical lasers currently used in dentistry generally fall into the class IV category, which is considered the most hazardous group of lasers. Additionally it mandates that manufacturers of lasers fix warning labels, sets limits on collateral radiation emitted, and generally imposes specific performance requirements for lasers such as protective enclosures, safety interlocking mechanisms, and emission indicators.

Prior to 1976 there were no published standards or regulations governing the clinical use of lasers. That year Congress passed the Medical Device Amendments to the U.S. Food, Drug, and Cosmetic Act giving jurisdiction over all medical devices, including laser products, to the Food and Drug Administration of the Department of Health and Human Services. The FDA regulates the manufacture, promotion, and

Table 6.1. Laser Hazard Classification According to ANSI and OHSA Standards

Class	Description
I	Low-powered lasers that are safe to view
IIa	Low-powered visible lasers that are hazardous only when viewed directly for longer than 1,000 sec
II	Low-powered visible lasers that are hazardous when viewed for longer than 0.25 sec
IIIa	Medium-powered lasers or systems that are normally not hazardous if viewed for less than 0.25 sec without magnifying optics
IIIb	Medium-powered lasers (0.5 W maximum) that can be hazardous if viewed directly
IV	High-powered lasers (> 0.5 W) that produce ocular, skin, and fire hazards

sale of lasers for specific applications, thus indirectly controlling their clinical use. Independently, the Laser Institute of America, which serves as secretariat for the American National Standards Institute (ANSI), has developed both general and clinical standards that currently serve as voluntary guidelines for the safe use of lasers in dentistry and medicine. General safety recommendations for the use of lasers have been published as ANSI Z-136.1 (ANSI, 1993), and for the safe use of lasers in health-care facilities as ANSI Z-136.3 (ANSI, 1988). Although voluntary, for legal purposes, these standards may be considered as the standard of care for dentistry and medicine (Griffith, 1989).

Specific recommendations relevant to dentistry are listed within Appendix B12 of the ANSI Z-136.3 document, which is currently under revision. The present standard contains discussions on hazards related to reflection from dental instruments, fire, combustion of general anesthetic gases, eye injury, tissue damage, and smoke inhalation. Appendix III contains general recommendations concerning standards of practice that have been adopted from those developed by the American Society for Laser Medicine and Surgery. Appendix III also describes the educational and certification requirements for the use of lasers in medicine and surgery, while leaving the responsibility for granting of privileges to the hospital governing board. Among the most important information contained in the ANSI standard is: the classification of specific hazards and control measures related to the clinical use of lasers; the designation of responsibility for laser safety in health-care facilities, including private offices, to the laser safety officer (LSO); and specific administrative procedures for ensuring safe application of lasers in the clinical setting.

In addition to the ANSI standard, detailed guidelines have been published by the Occupational Safety and Health Administration (OSHA) of the United States Department of Labor. The OSHA "Guidelines for Laser Safety and Hazard Assessment" (U.S. Department of Labor, 1991) are mandatory and enforceable under strict penalty by federal and state agencies throughout the United States. Contained in the OSHA guidelines, which are based heavily on the ANSI Z-136.1 document, are requirements for hazard evaluation; hazard control measures; personal protective equipment; training of personnel; and reporting of incidents involving laser accidents. The purpose of the OSHA guideline is to ensure the safety of employees who work in areas where lasers are used or who may be accidentally exposed to laser radiation. The OSHA regulations pertain to any dental employee, ie, dentist, dental hygienist, or dental assistant. The safety of patients being treated by lasers, however, is not considered within the scope of the OSHA regulations.

Other state and local governmental agencies, and professional societies may impose additional restrictions on the use of lasers within dental practice. The question of who may use lasers, and how they may be applied in dentistry, has come to the attention of the profession recently (McCann, 1992). Several state dental licensing boards and agencies have enacted legislation to limit the use of lasers to date (Table 6.2). Certainly other restrictions will follow once there is more widespread use of lasers in dentistry.

Hazard Classification and Identification

According to the CDRH and ANSI system of classification, class IV lasers are defined as those devices that pose a biologic

Table 6.2. Regulation of Laser Use by State*

State	Governing Agency
Alaska	Department of Environmental Conservation
Arizona	Radiation Regulation Agency
Arkansas	Division of Radiation Control and Emergency Management
Florida	Department of Health and Rehabilitation Services
Georgia	Department of Public Health
Illinois	Department of Nuclear Safety
Massachusetts	Department of Public Health
Montana	Department of Health and Environmental Services
New York	Department of Labor
Texas	Department of Health
Washington	Department of Labor and Industry

*These are the only states that regulate lasers.

hazard from either direct or diffuse reflection. Generally any laser capable of emitting power greater than 500-mW continuous wave output belongs in this class. The types of hazards that may be encountered within the clinical practice of dentistry may be grouped as follows: (1) ocular injury; (2) tissue damage; (3) respiratory hazards; (4) fire and explosion; and (5) electrical shock.

Ocular Hazards

Potential injury to the eye can occur either by direct emission from the laser or by reflection from a specular (mirrorlike) surface. Dental instruments have been capable of producing reflections that may result in tissue damage to both operator and patient (Neiburger and Miserendino, 1988). The use of carbonized or nonreflective instruments has been recommended during laser treatment by some authorities (Sosis, 1990). Several structures of the eye may be injured as a result of laser emissions. The site of injury is directly dependent on the preferential absorption of various wavelengths by specific structures of the eye (Fig 6.1).

The primary ocular injury that may result from a laser accident is a retinal or corneal burn. Retinal injury is possible with emissions in the visible (VIS, 400 to 780 nm) and near-infrared (NIR, 780 to 1,400 nm) spectral regions. Direct (intrabeam) and specular reflections of relatively low intensity are capable of causing retinal damage because of the focusing effect of the lens and cornea.

For purposes of calculation of potential retinal injury at wavelengths from 400 nm to 1,400 nm, an effective limiting aperture of 7 mm is used as an estimate of the diameter of the dilated pupil. Incident radiation passing through the pupil may be increased up to 100,000 times at the retina due to the focusing action of the eye (Laser Institute of America, 1993). For example, if an individual stared directly into the laser beam (Fig 6.2), an incident beam of 1 W/cm^2 power density would be resolved to a small spot on the retinal surface with a power density of 100,000 W/cm^2. Such a concentrated exposure at this site could conceivably render the person legally blind. Approximately 95% of the incident radiation entering the eye is absorbed by pigmented epithelium of the retina and choroid layer. Irreversible retinal burns resulting in permanent blindness can occur by conversion of incident radiation to heat energy within a fraction of a second. Thermal damage to the macula is most likely to occur as a result of direct intrabeam viewing or by specular reflection from a class IV laser where the laser beam acts as a point source. Diffuse reflections or extended exposures of lower intensity can produce retinal injuries of a larger spot size than intrabeam viewing and are only

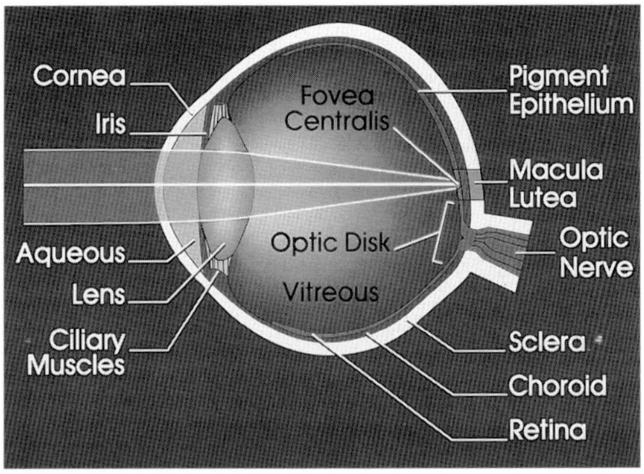

Fig 6.1 Potential sites of ocular injury. (Modified from Sliney DH [ed]: Laser Safety Guide, ed 9. Orlando, FL: Laser Institute of America, 1993.)

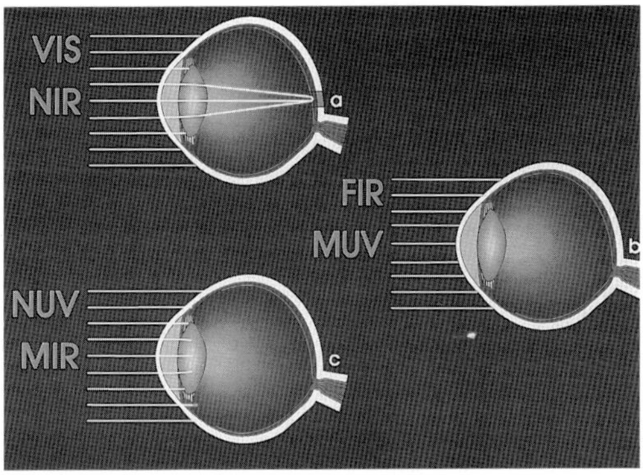

Fig 6.2 Sites of potential ocular injury based on absorption of specific wavelengths: *(a)* visible (VIS) and near infrared (NIR); *(b)* far-infrared (FIR), and mid-ultraviolet (MUV); *(c)* mid-infrared (MIR), and near ultraviolet (NUV) radiation. (Modified from Sliney DH [ed]: Laser Safety Guide, ed 9. Orlando, FL: Laser Institute of America, 1993).

considered a hazard with class IV lasers. In these situations, the degree of retinal damage could be extensive since larger image sizes (greater than 100 μm) and exposures of long duration (greater than 10 seconds) require more time for diffusion of thermal energy.

Most laser safety exposure limits are based on the premise that potential injury to the retina is dependent on thermal damage mechanisms since early data suggest a linear relationship between damage thresholds and exposure duration for single pulses greater than 10 μsec. Pulsed exposures of less than 20-μsec duration display a reduction of the damage threshold. Repetitive pulses appear to produce an additive effect that does not correlate with a strictly linear thermal damage relationship. Although the exact mechanism for this phenomenon is not yet well understood, it is conceivable that nonthermal mechanisms may be responsible.

The CDRH allows a cumulative radiant exposure limit of 3.85 mJ, which is based on the assumption of a linear biologic effect for continuous wave exposures from 10 to 10^4 seconds. The ANSI standard requires an adjustment of the maximum permissible exposure (MPE) for multiple pulsed laser emissions with pulse repetition rates from 1 to 15 kHz. The correction factor for pulsed emissions is calculated according to the following formula:

$$MPE_{\text{multiple pulse}} = [N^{1/4}] \times MPE_{\text{single pulse}}$$

where N = total number of pulses. The maximum permissible exposure limits for several common types of surgical lasers are in Table 6.3 and adopted from ANSI Z-136.3 for comparison. The MPEs listed for various exposure durations represent the different limits for acute (short-term) to delayed (long-term) biologic effects. For further information refer to "Safe Use Of Lasers," ANSI Z-136.1.

Other potential ocular injuries from various wavelengths may occur (Fig 6.2). Damage to the sclera or corneal surfaces can occur from exposure to radiant energy within the far ultraviolet (FUV < 300 nm) and far infrared (FIR > 7,000 nm) spectral

Table 6.3. Ocular Exposure Limits (in seconds) for Common Lasers Based on ANSI and OSHA Standards*

Laser Type	Wavelength (μm)	Maximum Permissible Exposure Limits (MPE) (W/cm^2)			
		0.25 sec	10 sec	600 sec	3×10^4 sec
CO_2	10.6	—	1×10^{-1}	—	1×10^{-2}
Nd:YAG (cw)	1.064	—	5.1×10^{-3}	—	1.6×10^{-3}
Nd:YAG (Q-switched)	1.064	—	1.7×10^{-6}		2.3×10^{-6}
HeNe	0.633	2.5×10^{-3}	—	2.93×10^{-4}	1.76×10^{-5}
Argon	0.514	2.5×10^{-3}	—	1.67×10^{-5}	1.0×10^{-6}
Excimer (XeCl)	0.308	—	—	—	1.3×10^{-6}
Excimer (XeFl)	0.351	—	—	—	3.33×10^{-6}
Excimer (ArFl)	0.193	—	—	—	1.0×10^{-7}
Holmium	1.9–2.2	—	1.0×10^{-1}	—	1×10^{-2}
Diodes (GaAs)	0.840	—	1.9×10^{-3}	—	6.1×10^{-4}

Note: To convert MPE values in W/cm^2 (power density) to J/cm^2 (energy density), multiply by the exposure time in seconds.
*Data compiled from ANSI Z–136.1, ANSI Z–136.3, and OSHA guidelines.

ranges. Cataracts are most likely to result from radiant exposure from wavelengths within the 300 to 400 nm (near ultraviolet) region by absorption of the lens and cornea as well as potential injury to the sclera or aqueous humor.

Tissue Hazards

Laser-induced damage to skin and other nontarget tissue can result from the thermal interaction of radiant energy with tissue proteins as described in Chapter 3. Temperature elevations of 21°C above normal body temperature (37°C) can produce cell destruction by denaturation of cellular enzymes and structural proteins, which interrupts basic metabolic processes. Additionally, exposures of 1 sec or greater duration can interfere with vascular perfusion and thus compound the problems associated with thermal diffusion of heat energy within tissues. Histologically, the thermal effect of absorbed radiant energy is manifested as thermal coagulation necrosis for wavelengths above 400 nm. Short exposures producing temperature elevations less than 30°C, however, may be within physiologic limits of recovery.

Other nonthermal tissue interactions are thought to induce injury through photochemical and photoacoustic mechanisms. These types of interactions are most likely to occur with single or repetitive pulses of very short duration (less than 10 μsec). Nonthermal interaction has been associated with radiant exposures within the ultraviolet spectrum such as those with excimer lasers. Although there have been no reports of laser-induced carcinogenesis to date, the potential for mutagenic changes, possibly by the direct alteration of cellular DNA through breaking of molecular bonds, has been questioned (Goldman, 1991; U.S. Department of Labor, 1991).

The terms *photodisruption* and *photoplasmolysis* have been applied to describe the type of tissue interactions that may occur as a consequence of high intensity irradiation with ultrashort laser pulses in the nanosecond and picosecond range. As previously mentioned, the damage mechanism for repetitively pulsed laser-induced tissue damage appears to be the result of the cumulative effects of radiant exposure and not entirely thermal in nature.

In general, laser-induced tissue injury is primarily dependent on the extent of absorption of the incident radiation by tissue. At present, there is insufficient information related to the absorption coefficients for many tissues found in the oral cavity, particularly oral hard tissue. It is important therefore to recognize what factors may strongly influence the extent of laser-tissue interaction. These include: (1) the relative amount of absorption, transmission, and scatter of the particular wavelength; (2) the pulse duration and pulse repetition rate; (3) the level of radiant exposure (energy density or exposure dose); and (4) the relative degree of vascularity of the tissue.

Of clinical significance is the potential damage to deeper tissue from penetration of specific wavelengths such as the continuous wave Nd:YAG. Though not commonly used in dentistry, this configuration is effective in general surgery when coagulation of deeper structures and destruction of pigmented tissues is the desired surgical effect. However, with prolonged exposures of low power density from this type of laser, excess thermal necrosis that may not be apparent at the tissue surface can occur. When surface cutting or ablation of soft tissues within the oral cavity is the objective, then application of the carbon dioxide or pulsed YAG lasers may be a better choice, provided the appropriate parameters are used.

During ablation of oral tissue with the carbon dioxide laser a carbonized layer of tissue residue, or char layer, forms on the surface as the more volatile and liquid components within tissue are vaporized. This carbon material is a strong absorber of most wavelengths of laser light. As such it acts as a heat sink that transfers thermal energy to surrounding tissues. The extent of collateral damage is therefore greatly influenced by the presence of this char layer. Further lasing will only increase the zone of collateral thermal damage to adjacent tissue. Mechanical removal of the char or escar is necessary to allow continuation of tissue ablation (see laser wipe down in Chapter 9).

Other factors that may influence the nature of interaction, aside from those differences attributed to wavelength or mode of delivery (continuous vs pulsed) are related to delivery instrumentation. For example, a noncontact Nd:YAG laser delivery system will produce a very different effect than that of a contact tip laser scalpel or bare fiber delivery system. Generally there will be greater penetration into deeper structures with the noncontact system vs the others mentioned. A more detailed explanation of the clinical significance of laser delivery systems and related instrumentation is presented in Chapter 8.

Environmental Hazards

Another class of hazards involves the potential inhalation of airborne biohazardous materials that may be released as a result of the surgical application of lasers. These secondary hazards belong to a group of potential laser hazards sometimes referred to as nonbeam hazards since they do not pertain to injuries resulting from direct exposure to the laser beam. Inhaled airborne contaminants can be emitted in the form of smoke or plume generated through the thermal interaction of surgical lasers with tissue or through the accidental escape of toxic chemicals and gases from the laser itself. While most surgical lasers used in dentistry are capable of smoke generation to some extent, toxic gases and chemicals are a more common hazard in dental research facilities and laboratories. Excimer lasers, for example, contain inert gases (argon, krypton, or xenon) mixed with toxic gases such as fluorine or hydrogen chloride as the active medium. Toxic dyes and solvents are used in other types of laser systems for photodynamic therapy. Chapter 18 presents the subject of photodynamic therapy in greater detail.

The generation of smoke or laser plume during surgery can be a hazard to operating personnel and patients. Inhalation of toxic or infectious matter in the form of aerosols and particles has been found to be potentially damaging to the respiratory system following both long-term and short-term exposure (Kirschner and Unger, 1984).

During ablation or incision of oral soft tissue, cellular products are vaporized due to the rapid heating of the liquid components in the tissue. In the process, extremely small fragments of carbonized, partially carbonized, and relatively intact tissue elements are violently projected into the area, creating airborne contaminants that are observed clinically as smoke or what is commonly called the laser plume. Inhalation of particulate matter of this type has been identified as hazardous to patients and operating room personnel (Baggish et al, 1991). Ablation of infected tissue poses an even greater hazard due to the possible presence within the plume of viable intact infectious agents including HIV (Baggish et al, 1991; Garden et al, 1988; Sawchuck et al, 1989; Shapsky et al, 1980).

The generation of smoke during laser surgery occurs as the result of dehydration of tissue and heating of the residual solid matter to temperatures sufficient for combustion. In this process, oxygen, which is present in ambient air, combines with tissue elements to form a variety of by-products, many of which are biohazardous. A partial list of chemical compounds that have been recovered from laser plume are listed in Table 6.4 (Koksa and Eugene, 1989; Koksa and Bendetto, 1992).

Standard surgical masks are able to filter out particles down to 5 μm in size. Particles from laser plume however may be as small as 0.3 μm in diameter. Evacuation of laser plume is therefore necessary to reduce the level of airborne contaminants to acceptable levels. The effectiveness of dental high-volume evacuators may be adequate for this purpose, although there have been no controlled studies to substantiate this premise to date. Surgical smoke evacuation equipment is commonly

Table 6.4. Some Chemicals Found in Laser Plume After Soft Tissue Vaporization

Laser Plume Chemicals	
Water	Carbon dioxide
Formaldehyde	Benzene
Acrolein	Methane
Cyanates	Acetone
Cyclohexane	Toluene
Fatty acid esters	Alkanes
Xylene	Acetaldehyde

used in the operating theater for control of particulate emissions during laser surgery (Fig 6.3). Most of these devices filter out and recirculate the air by collection of the plume through a nozzle connected to the filtration apparatus. Research has indicated that the distance of the nozzle opening and volume of filtration are critical factors in the effectiveness of filtration (Smith et al, 1990). Based on these findings, it is recommended that the collection nozzle should be placed no more than 2 inches from the surgical site and the rate of evacuation should be above 40 ft^3/min.

The extent of plume generation during laser surgery is dependent on the absorption of various wavelengths by the target tissue. The greatest producers of smoke are the carbon dioxide and erbium lasers followed by Nd:YAG laser. Plume generation is possible whenever thermal interaction occurs. Carbon dioxide and Er:YAG have high coefficients of absorption because of the high water content of oral tissue. Nd:YAG is more highly absorbed by pigmented tissue elements.

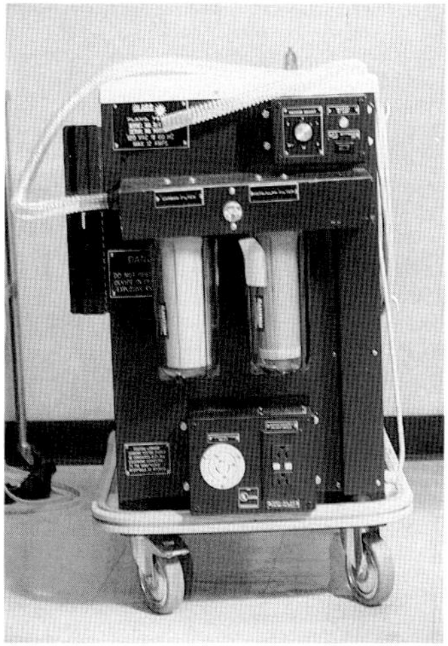

Fig 6.3 Surgical laser smoke evacuator for removal of airborne contaminants (laser plume) generated during laser surgery.

Combustion Hazards

In the presence of flammable materials, the laser may pose other significant hazards. Flammable solids, liquids, and gases used within the surgical setting can be easily ignited if exposed to the laser beam. Of particular concern is the potential combustion of flammable gases and endotracheal tubes used during general anesthesia due to their proximity during head and neck procedures. Toxic fumes released as a result of the combustion of flammable materials present an additional hazard as previously discussed. The use of flame-resistant materials and other precautions therefore is recommended. A partial list of flammable substances commonly found in the dental operatory and operating room is presented in Table 6.5.

Table 6.5. Flammable Materials Found in Dental Treatment Areas

Solids	Liquids	Gases
Clothing	Ethanol	Oxygen
Paper products	Acetone	Nitrous oxide*
Plastics	Methylmethacrylate	General anesthetics
Waxes and resins	Solvents	Aromatic vapors

*Generally classified as nonflammable, but will support combustion. Not recommended for use in laser airway surgery (Sosis, 1990).

Electrical Hazards

Because class IV surgical lasers often use very high currents and high voltage power supplies, there are several associated hazards that may be potentially lethal. Electrical hazards of lasers can be grouped as electrical shock hazards, electric fire hazards, or explosion hazards. Safe manufacturing practices for the most part offer adequate protection from these hazards in dental laser systems. Considerable effort has been made by biomedical and electrical engineers in the design and manufacture of safe laser systems. Insulated circuitry, shielding, grounding, and housing of high-voltage electrical components provide adequate protection under most circumstances from electrical injury. However, within the surgical setting, the laser may be exposed to conductive liquids that may contribute to an electrical hazard. Installation and servicing of laser equipment should always be performed by qualified personnel according to established safety standards. The clinician should never attempt to repair or remove safety panels from the laser since a number of fatalities by electrocution have been reported during servicing of the laser's electrical system (Sliney and Trokel, 1993).

Laser Hazard Control Measures

According to the OSHA guidelines for laser safety and hazard assessment (OSHA, 1991) and the ANSI standard Z-136.3 for the safe use of lasers in health-care facilities, control measures are required to reduce the possibility of unwanted exposure of patients and personnel to laser radiation within the dental and medical clinical setting. Four categories of control measures have been identified in the standards that have relevance within the dental laser environment (Table 6.6). These include: (1) engineering controls; (2) personal protective equipment; (3) administrative and procedural controls; and (4) environmental controls. Additionally, both documents identify or designate responsibility for implementation of these four categories of control measures to the LSO.

Role of the Laser Safety Officer

The LSO has been identified as the individual having administrative control over all measures that are to be implemented for the safe operation of lasers within industry and health-care facilities. The responsibilities of the LSO include: hazard identification and assessment within the operative setting; determination of the potential hazard zone otherwise termed the nominal hazard zone (NHZ); establishing the stan-

Table 6.6. Summary of Laser Safety Control Measures Recommended by ANSI Z–136.3

Engineering controls	Personal protective equipment
Protective housing	Eyewear
Interlocks	Optical density
Beam enclosures	Transmission
Shutters	Identification
Service panels	Visibility
Equipment labels	Comfort and fit
Warning systems	Clothing
Key switch	Screens and curtains
Administrative controls	Special controls
Laser safety officer (LSO)	Fire and explosion
Standard operating procedures	Repair and maintenance
Output limitations	Fiber optic delivery systems
Training and education	
Maintenance and alignment	
Warning signs	
Protective devices	
Medical surveillance	
Incident reporting	

dard operating procedure (SOP) for operation of the laser within the facility; ensuring proper laser safety training for all persons working within the environment; approving use of protective equipment; specifying use of warning signs and labels; and implementing medical surveillance and accident report programs. In hospitals and laser clinics, the LSO is also actively involved in the assurance of safe practices and policies through cooperation with hospital credentialing and laser use committees.

Within the dental profession, the designation of a specialized individual, the dental LSO, may be required to fulfill the responsibilities of the LSO due to certain unique features of dental practice (Miserendino et al, 1993). The specific educational and training requirements for the LSO are listed in the OSHA document. These include knowledge of: (1) the operational characteristics of the laser; (2) the bioeffects and potential hazards of the laser; (3) requirements of applicable laser safety standards including the ANSI and OSHA regulations; and (4) practical safety control measures for lasers. In the absence of a qualified LSO in the private office setting where lasers are used, the laser dentist may assume all the previously mentioned responsibilities or delegate them to another qualified individual. The need for the LSO or dental equivalent, however, is mandated in the OSHA regulations.

Specific Recommendations

All dental lasers that are classified as class IV lasers should be considered potentially hazardous to anyone present during the time of their operation. It is strongly advised that any safety precautions delineated by the manufacturer in the operator's manual be strictly followed as well as all general laser safety precautions listed within the ANSI and OSHA standards. When used properly, lasers are a very safe and effective dental tool, provided that adequate safety measures also are followed.

Training Requirements

Prior to any clinical or research application of a laser, the intended operator of any laser system must have a thorough knowledge of the operation and safety requirements of the specific laser system and should have received hands-on instruction related to its practical application. A variety of laser safety training courses have been developed by the Laser Institute of America and other laser centers to suit the needs of the laser clinician, scientist, engineer, LSO, service technician, and industrial worker. Current estimates conservatively project that by the mid 1990s, more than 1 million persons will be directly involved with the application of lasers in relation to their employment (U.S. Department of Labor, 1991).

Specific educational guidelines describing the curricula for dental laser training courses are listed in Chapter 7 for consideration. Four levels of education have been established within these guidelines, ranging from general informational courses to instructor-level training courses. The guidelines outline the recommended course content for the various levels of laser training for the dental profession. To date, a number of national and international dental laser associations and dental schools have adopted these guidelines for laser proficiency training and dental continuing education courses. Development of the educational guidelines through the cooperative efforts of technical experts within the dental profession and industry

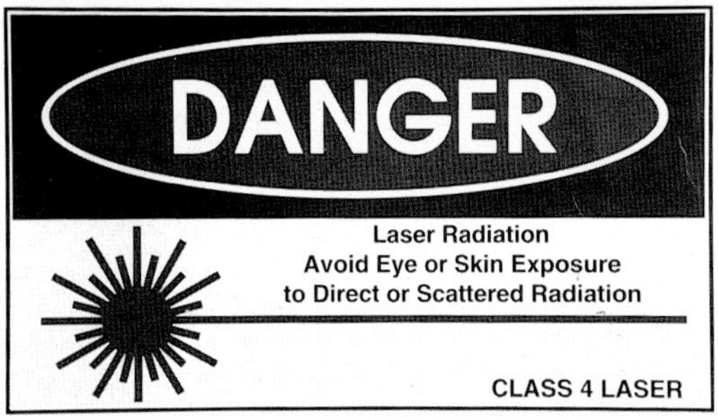

Fig 6.4 Laser safety warning signs as presented in ANSI and OSHA guidelines.

represents a giant step forward in the evolution of laser dentistry.

All staff or other personnel present within the laser operating environment should be well-versed in the general safety practices applicable to laser operation. The scope of laser safety training for dental assistants and staff should include a complete understanding of the concepts and requirements of a safe laser operating environment, identification of potential hazards that may be encountered in the dental practice setting, awareness of laser safety devices and personal protective equipment available, knowledge of safe operating procedures to be used during operation and maintenance of the laser, and mechanisms for reporting accidental laser beam exposures.

Environmental Control Measures

Evaluation of environmental hazards involves an assessment of three primary aspects of the laser treatment area that should be considered to establish adequate control measures for the particular application. These include: (1) the physical environment in which the laser is used; (2) the potential for injury attributed to direct exposure from the laser beam output and delivery mechanism; and (3) the level of training and knowledge of laser safety of the persons who may use or be exposed to the laser beam. Secondary considerations may include potential exposure to airborne contaminants, fire, and electrical and explosion hazards within the vicinity of the laser.

Laser Treatment Controlled Area

Defined within the ANSI Z-136.3 and OSHA standards is the concept of the nominal hazard zone (NHZ), which is described as the space or area in which the level of direct, reflected, or scattered radiation exceeds the MPE for a given laser system. Calculation of the NHZ for specific laser systems involves considerations such as: (1) power output of the laser; (2) beam diameter and divergence; (3) pulse repetition rate (PRR); (4) wavelength of emission; and (5) exposure duration. The purpose of the NHZ evaluation is to define the region where control measures are required. In general dental practice however, this region may be defined as or confined to the dental treatment room, providing that access is restricted to operating personnel. This would require enclosed entrances and doorways with properly marked warning signs.

Preferably, laser use should be confined to controlled areas with restricted access. Since many dental operatories have open doorways and pass-through floor plans, the use of protective laser curtains should be considered to prevent accidental exposure to passersby. Fail-safe mechanisms that prohibit the laser from firing when doors are opened are also useful to prevent accidental exposure to persons entering the operating room during laser procedures.

All entrances to the operating theater

must be clearly marked with a removable sign that contains the words "DANGER" and "LASER RADIATION: Avoid Eye or Skin Exposure to Direct or Scattered Radiation." Removable signs have been proven to be more effective in alerting people to the presence of danger because they can be posted and removed and are not as likely to be taken for granted as a fixed sign would be (Fig 6.4).

Since laser emissions travel in a straight line until obstructed or reflected, care should be taken regarding the type of material beyond or behind the intended target. This is necessary to protect tissue other than that intended for treatment and surgical personnel from accidental exposure to the treatment beam. Highly reflective instruments and surfaces should be avoided to prevent reflection of the laser beam onto nontarget tissues.

Fire and Electrical Control Measures

To avoid an electrical hazard during the operation of the laser unit, the floor of the theater must be kept dry to avoid having the operator standing in a pooled liquid. Additionally, the control panel and its electrical power unit should be protected from splashing that can sometimes emanate from working in a wet field environment.

Because laser energy generates heat, care must be taken to avoid the use of flammable or explosive liquids or gases in the operating room. In addition to heat, combustible materials may also be ignited by exposure to the focused laser beam. As a result, the presence of combustible materials, either in the field of operation or in the operating theater, is discouraged. This care must be extended to the choice of any cleansing solutions applied to either the patient or the instruments. Vapors from certain solutions (ie, alcohol and ether) can be ignited either by heat or by direct contact with the laser beam. If the presence of a potentially hazardous material is necessary, a certain measure of protection can be gained, in some cases, by wetting or moistening these items or by draping them with nonflammable materials. Flammable materials such as surgical drapes and gauze sponges may be soaked in sterile saline to reduce the potential of burning by accidental exposure to the laser beam.

Personal Protective Equipment

Eye Protection

Light produced by all class IV lasers by definition presents a potential hazard for ocular damage by either direct viewing or reflection of the beam. Therefore, all people within the NHZ must wear adequate eye protection, including the patient. This can be provided by either safety goggles or screening devices; however, the means selected must be designed specifically for use with the particular wavelength of laser radiation.

When selecting appropriate protective eyewear several factors should be considered: (1) wavelength of laser emission; (2) maximum permissible exposure limits; (3) degradation of the absorbing media or filter; (4) optical density of the eyewear; (5) radiant exposure limits; (6) need for corrective lenses; (7) multiple wavelength requirements; (8) restriction of peripheral vision; and (9) comfort and fit.

Optical density (OD) is one of the most important factors to consider when choosing laser eye protection. Optical density is the parameter that specifies the degree of attenuation of the incident radiation for a given optical material. Laser protective eyewear filters are specified according to their OD, which is determined by a mathe-

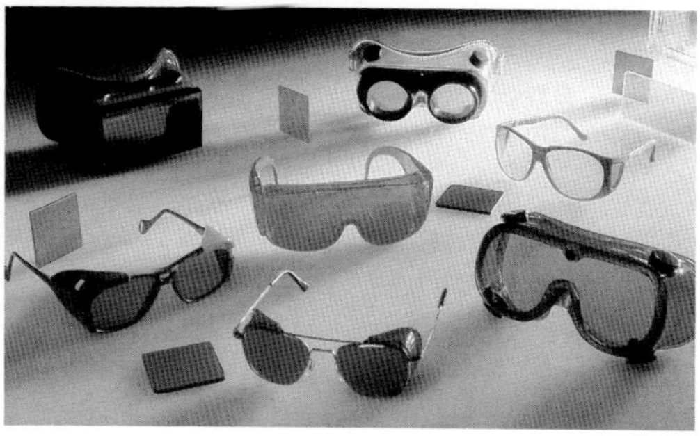

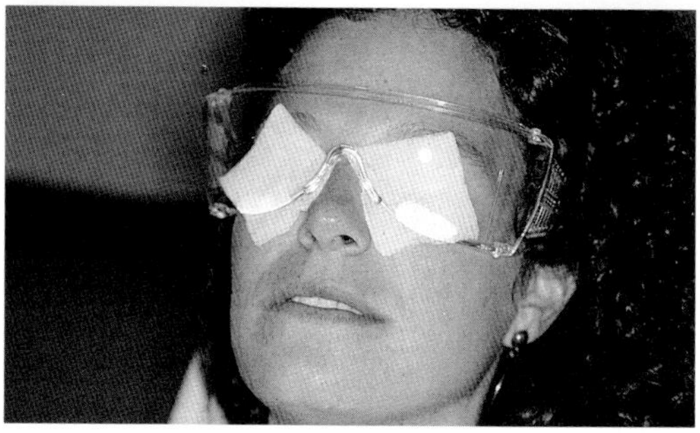

Fig 6.5 (a), Various designs of laser safety glasses and goggles. (Courtesy of Laser-R Shield Inc, Albuquerque, NM.) **(b)**, Laser safety goggles and saline-soaked gauze pads placed over patient's eyes during CO_2 laser surgery.

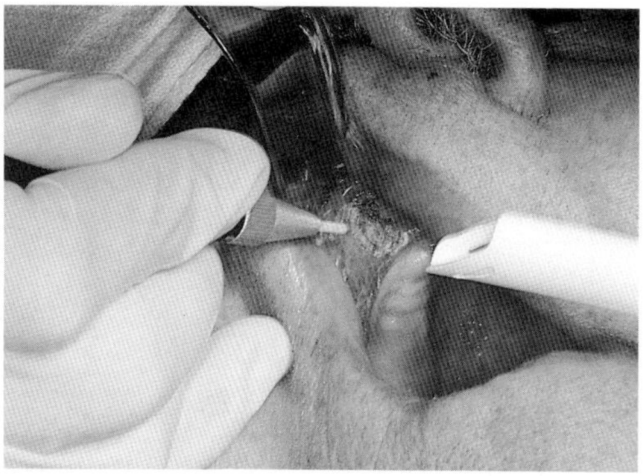

Fig 6.6 Dental high volume evacuator removal of laser plume.

matical formula that takes into account the wavelength, power, and diameter of the beam. For pulsed lasers, consideration is also given to the pulse duration and repetition rate. The purpose of the calculation of OD is to determine the minimum level of attenuation needed to reduce the beam exposure to the eye to relatively safe levels. Laser protective eyewear is intended to provide a level of protection that may occur from brief accidental exposures and should not be used to stare directly into the beam. Several varieties of protective viewing devices are currently available to suit the needs of virtually any situation (Fig 6.5). Laser protective eyewear should also be clearly labeled or coded to indicate the wavelength and optical density attenuated and should be inspected regularly for degradation of the filter by cracks and pitting.

Control of Airborne Contaminants

The laser plume, which is the smoke or vapor emitted from the site of surgery during exposure to laser energy, is a special concern. This plume should be regarded as potentially hazardous both in terms of particulate matter and infectivity. Although it is highly unlikely that viable tumor cells occur in the laser plume, it has been reported that intact viral DNA can be liberated into the air with the vapor created during carbon dioxide laser treatment of verrucae. Additionally, the exposure to carbon dioxide laser smoke has been demonstrated to have harmful effects on the respiratory system in animal models (Tomita et al, 1981).

Airborne contaminants may be controlled by ventilation, evacuation, or other methods of respiratory protection. Laser surgery within the oral cavity or near respiratory passages requires sufficient evacuation of the plume for patient protection (Fig 6.6). Airborne contaminants should be removed as near as possible from the point or origin by evacuation and ventila-

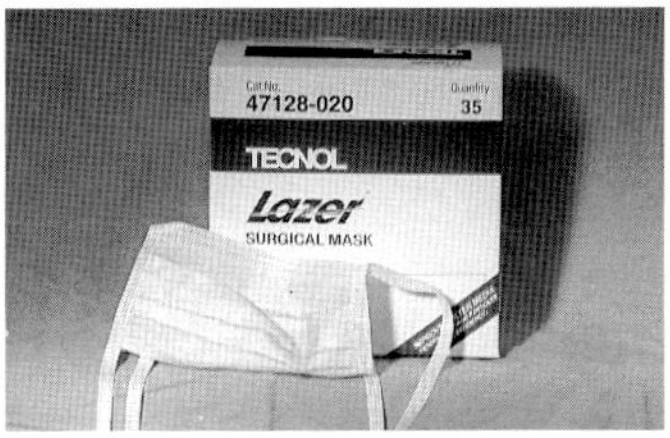

Fig 6.7 Laser filtration masks: Lazer Surgical Mask filters to 0.1 μm at 98% efficiency. (Courtesy of Technol Inc, Fort Worth, TX.)

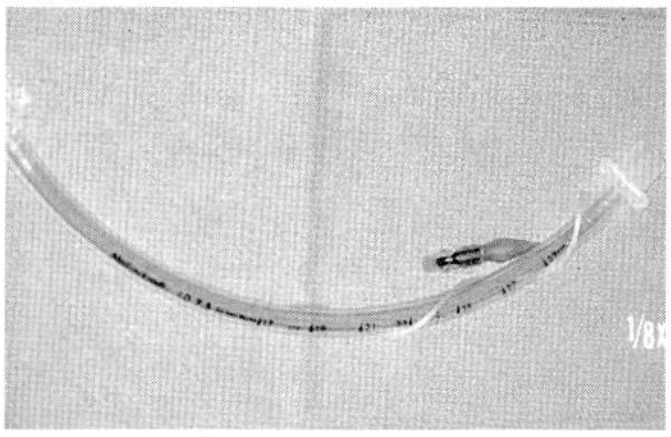

Fig 6.8 Flammable PVC endotracheal tube.

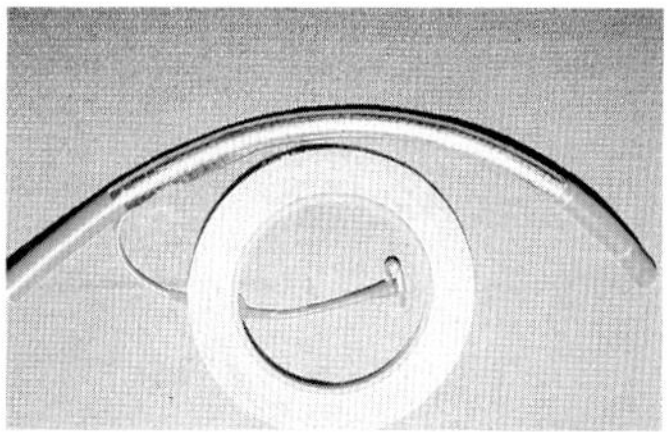

Fig 6.9 Endotracheal tube wrapped with aluminum tape to prevent perforation by the laser beam.

tion to the outside if possible, or by recirculating air filtration systems. Adequate suction in the surgical field must be maintained at all times, especially when treating pathologic conditions that are suspected of being viral in origin to limit the possibility of spreading that virus via the laser plume. Accordingly, the evacuation system should be able to remove particles as small as 0.3 μm with at least an 80% efficiency. The filter of the evacuation system should be changed regularly in accordance with the manufacturer's instructions to maintain a full air flow and to prevent the possible accumulation of infectious material. Surgical staff should wear masks that remove particles as small as 0.3 μm (Fig 6.7). Conventional surgical masks are not adequate. Eyewear or face shields and caps and gowns that protect against spatter and laser light should be worn for the protection of operating room personnel.

Administrative and Procedural Controls

When using a laser within the private office setting or hospital operating theater, special precautions need to be observed if general anesthesia is administered. Laser surgery in and around the oral cavity presents the potential risk of exposure of the nasotracheal or endotrachael tube to the laser beam; therefore, special anesthesia techniques are required. In place of the standard polyvinyl chloride (PVC) intubation tube, a red rubber or Silastic tube should be used (Fig 6.8). For further protection, the tube can be wrapped with ⅓- to ½-inch aluminum tape (Fig 6.9). In this way, if the beam strikes the tube it will be reflected and not penetrate or ignite it. Polyvinyl chloride tubes should be avoided because they produce toxic breakdown products and create extensive tissue destruction associated with combustion of the PVC material (Davis and Simpson, 1983; Hermens et al, 1983; Ossoff et al, 1983; Sosis, 1990).

Other safe operating practices involve the protection of nontarget tissue during laser surgery in the mouth. Highly reflective instruments and those with mirrored surfaces should be avoided since they may cause damage to nontarget tissue. Damage to dental structures can also occur when lasers are used improperly. Appropriate power settings and time frames are essential to reduce the risks of undesirable laser effects on teeth and supporting structures. Special precautions have been recommended for the protection of teeth when the CO_2 laser is used on surrounding soft tissue (Pick et al, 1985; Neiburger and Miserendino, 1988). Tooth protection is needed when using lasers at

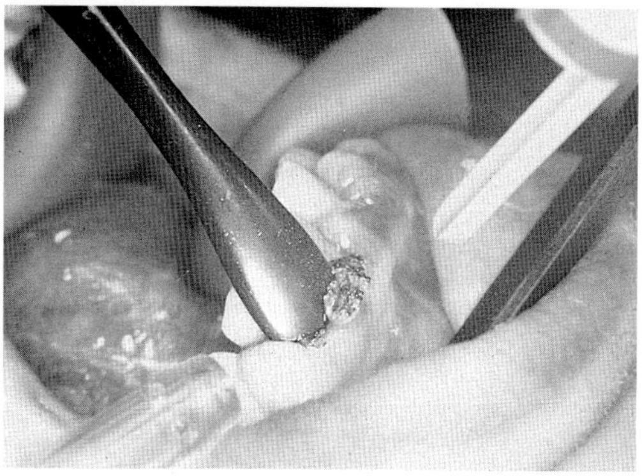

Fig 6.10 Blackened (anodized) instrument used as a shield to prevent damage to tooth enamel.

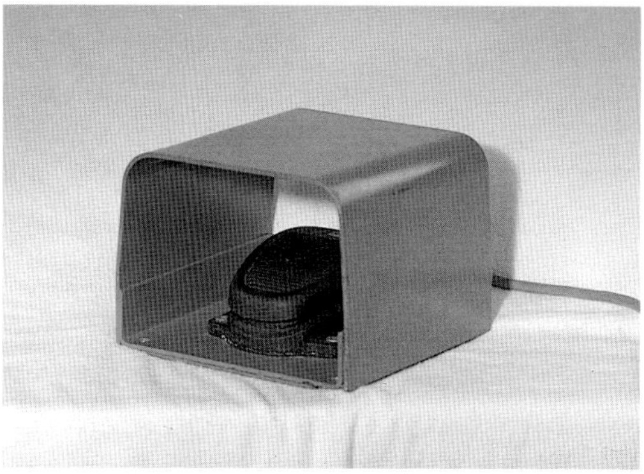

Fig 6.11 Foot pedal control switch with protective hood to prevent accidental depression by surgical staff.

high power settings and whenever the beam is directed at angles other than those parallel to tooth surfaces. Shielding may be used as an effective method to avoid inadvertent contact of the beam with tooth enamel or root surfaces. A no. 7 wax spatula or the small end of a Prichard periosteal elevator can be inserted into the gingival sulcus to serve as an effective shield when lasing soft tissue near teeth (Fig 6.10).

Neodymium:YAG, argon, holmium, and erbium:YAG lasers are also capable of destructive effects to teeth at high power levels. Holmium and erbium:YAG lasers have been shown to ablate tooth hard structures and therefore should be used cautiously when in proximity to teeth. At lower settings and when applied properly, however, all of the previously mentioned lasers may be used effectively without unwanted tissue damage.

Proper knowledge of the specific laser in use and its tissue effects is essential for the operator. With adequate knowledge and appropriate power and time settings, the clinician may be assured of achieving the desired result. For most applications it may be advisable to use low power and time settings initially before progressing to higher and faster times. One should never use power settings that result in uncontrollable tissue effects. Experience ultimately will dictate the speed at which procedures may be performed safely irrespective of the instrument that is used. When lasers are not actually being used for treatment or if long pauses occur between use, the unit should be placed in the standby mode to prevent inadvertent firing of the laser beam. Once placed in the open or fire mode, the operator should always be aware of the location of the foot pedal to avoid accidental firing of the laser by anyone in its vicinity. Most manufacturers provide a cover or metal hood (Fig 6.11) to help prevent accidental activation of the laser beam. The foot switch should be cleaned and inspected each day prior to use. In the highly unlikely event that it should become stuck in a position with the laser operating, it is recommended that someone stationed near the laser console during surgery be familiar with procedures necessary to deactivate the laser.

In addition to the safety recommendations previously described, it is advisable for surgical staff as well as the private practitioner to develop standard operating procedures and adhere to a written laser safety policy for their laser facility to ensure a safe operating environment for themselves and their patients. These topics are covered in greater detail in the ANSI and OSHA guidelines. Most laser accidents and injuries can be prevented if appropriate control measures are recognized and implemented.

References

Abt E, Miserendino LJ, Pick RM, Harris D, Wigdor H. Credentialing for the safe and effective use of lasers in dental practice. Lasers Surg Med 1993;5:19.

American National Standard for Safe Use of Lasers in Health Care Facilities (ANSI Z-136.3–1988). Orlando, FL: Laser Institute of America;1988.

American National Standard for the Safe Use of Lasers (ANSI Z-136.1–rev. 1993). Orlando, FL: Laser Institute of America;1993.

Baggish MS, Poiesz B, Jorot D, Williamson P, Refai A. Presence of immunodeficiency virus DNA in laser smoke. Laser Surg Med 1991;11:197–203.

Davis RK, Simpson GT. Safety with the carbon dioxide laser. Otolaryngol Clin North Am 1983;16:801–814.

Garden JM, O'Banion K, Sheintz L, Bakus A, Reichman M, Sundberg J. Papilloma virus in the vapor of carbon-dioxide-laser-treated verrucae. JAMA 1988;259: 1119–1202.

Goldman L. Laser techniques in various medical specialties. In Laser Non-surgical Medicine. Lancaster, PA: Technomic Publishing Co; 1991;223–230.

Griffith JL. ANSI guidelines strongly influence policies, procedures. Clin Laser Mon 1989;7:49–51.

Harris DM, Miserendino LJ, Abt E, Wigdor H, Pick RM. Education, training and certification for the use of lasers in the dental profession. Presented at the International Laser Safety Conference; Cincinnati, OH; Dec 4, 1992.

Harris D, Miserendino LJ, Wigdor H, Abt E, Pick RM. Laser training and experience in the dental profession. Lasers Surg Med 1993;5:19.

Hermens JM, Bennett MJ, Hirshman CA. Anesthesia for laser surgery. Anesth Analg 1983;62:218–229.

IEC 825. Radiation safety of laser products, equipment classification, requirements and user's guide with amendments 1, 1990. Geneva, Switzerland: International Electrotechnical Committee.

Kirschner RA, Unger M. Laser surgery. Surg Clin North Am. Philadelphia: WB Saunders; 1984;64:851–859.

Koksa JM, Eugene J. Chemical composition of laser-tissue interaction smoke plume. J Laser Appl 1989; 1:59–63.

Koksa JM, Bendetto MD. Probing plume protection problems in the health care environment. J Laser Appl 1992;4:39–43.

McCann D. States look at who may use lasers. ADA News 1992;23:1–6.

Miserendino LJ, Abt E, Harris D, Pick RM, Wigdor H. Recommendations for safe and appropriate use of lasers in dentistry. J Laser Appl 1992;4:16–17.

Miserendino LJ, Harris D, Abt E, Wigdor H, Pick RM. Laser safety in the dental profession. Lasers Surg Med 1993;5:18.

Neiburger EJ, Miserendino LJ. Laser reflectance hazard in the dental operatory. J Oral Surg 1988;66:659–661.

Ossoff RH, Eisenman TS, et al. Comparison of tracheal damage from laser-ignited endotracheal fires. Ann Otol Rhinol 1983;92:333–336.

Pick RM, Silberman CJ. The laser gingivectomy. The use of the CO_2 laser for removal of phenytoin hyperplasia. J Periodontol 1985;546:492–496.

Sawchuck WS, Weber PJ, Lowey DR, et al. Infectious papillomavirus in the vapor of warts treated with carbon dioxide laser or electrocoagulation: detection and protection. J Am Dermatol 1989;21:41–49.

Shapsky SM. Removal of rhinophyma with the carbon dioxide laser. Arch Otolaryngol 1980;106:257–259.

Sliney DH (ed). Laser Safety Guide, ed 9. Orlando, FL: Laser Institute of America;7–10.

Sliney DH, Trokel SL. Medical Lasers and Their Safe Use. New York: Springer-Verlag;1993:98–100.

Smith J, Topmiller J, Schulman S. Factors affecting emission collection by surgical smoke evacuators. Laser Surg Med 1990;10:224–233.

Sosis MB. Operating room safety during laser surgery. Proc Int Laser Safety Conf ISLC Nov 1990; section 6–9.

Tomita Y, Mihashi S, Nagata K, et al. Mutagenecity of smoke condensates induced by CO_2 laser irradiation and electrocauterization. Mutat Res 1981;89:145–149.

U.S. Department of Health and Human Services. Performance Standard for Laser Products. Code of Federal Regulations, 1985, title 21, subchapter J, part 1040.

U.S. Department of Labor. OSHA Instruction Publication 8–1.7. Directorate of Technical Support, Aug 5, 1991.

Chapter Seven

Regulation, Standards, and Education for Lasers in Dentistry

Harvey Wigdor and Leo J. Miserendino

This chapter reviews the present regulations that effect laser use in dentistry and the existing standards that have been developed to ensure safe and effective laser use in the health professions. It also reviews and identifies the educational standards and guidelines that either currently exist or are being developed for dentistry. Three agencies exert either indirect regulatory control over the use of lasers in dentistry or have developed safety standards or guidelines that directly regulate or control how lasers are applied in dental practice: the Food and Drug Administration (FDA); the Occupational Health and Safety Administration (OSHA); and the American National Standards Institute (ANSI). The Laser Institute of America is another organization that serves as secretariat for the ANSI, exerts influence over the dental use of lasers through its development and approval of the two American National Standards, ANSI Z-136.1 and Z-136.3, which specify the laser safety standards governing both operators of lasers and patients treated with lasers (ANSI, 1988, 1993). There are a number of other professional societies and associations devoted to laser use that have either published or are presently developing educational, certifying, or credentialing programs, or standards of practice for both the medical and dental professions. Included among these are the Academy of Laser Dentistry, the International Society of Laser Dentistry, the American Board of Laser Surgery, and the American Society for Lasers in Surgery and Medicine.

Medical Devices and the FDA

The FDA has developed a system that has only recently been applied to dentistry to evaluate new technologies used to treat patients in the United States. Lasers for dentistry are being scrutinized by the FDA and come under the purview of the Center for Devices and Radiological Health (CDRH). The CDRH, formed in 1982, develops and implements national programs to protect the public health in the fields of medical devices and radiological health (CDRH, 1989). The intent of these programs is: to assure the safety, effectiveness, and proper labeling of medical devices; to control unnecessary human exposure to potentially hazardous ionizing and nonionizing radiation; and to ensure the safe, efficacious use of such radiation (FDA, 1990).

The medical device amendments were formally initiated in 1976 and were intended to guide the medical device industry. Section 201(h) of the Federal Food, Drug, and Cosmetic Act defines "device" as an instrument, apparatus, implement, machine, contrivance, implant, in-vitro reagent, or other similar or related article, including any component part, or accessory that is: (1) recognized in the national formulary, or the United States pharmacopoeia, or any supplement to them; (2) intended for use in the diagnosis of disease or other condition, or in the cure, mitigation, treatment, or prevention of disease, in man or other animals; or (3) intended to affect the structure or any function of the body, of man or other animal, and which does not achieve its primary intended purposes through chemical action within or on the body of man or other animals and which is not dependent on being metabolized for the achievement of its principal intended purposes (FDA, 1990).

The act and amendments are intended to affect manufacturers and other persons marketing medical devices and do not directly regulate practitioners. The three components of the act that have an indirect effect on dentistry are the 510K provision, the investigational device exemptions (IDE), and the pre-market approval application (PMA).

There is a progression of events that may ultimately lead to the marketing clearance of a new device by the FDA. This progression begins with the determination of whether or not a new device is substantially equivalent to any device that was either on the market before May 28, 1976, or equivalent to one that is currently being legally sold in the U. S. market. This distinction and date is important for the FDA. The amendments became law on this date and gave the FDA the jurisdiction over devices used to treat patients. If there was a product being used prior to this date that produces an effect similar to that of a new product, then a marketing clearance can be given by the FDA under the 510K provision.

Based on this premise, manufacturers who wish to be given 510K clearance by the FDA only need to show that their device, by application, is substantially equivalent to a device that was in existence before May 28, 1976. These devices are "grandfathered" because of their equivalency. Under the safe medical device act of 1990, devices may receive a 510K marketing clearance if found to be substantially equivalent to other legally marketed devices.

With one exception, the only marketing clearance given to all the dental lasers, to date, is for oral soft tissue surgery. These clearances come under the 510K section, which states that these lasers affect oral tissues in a similar way to lasers that were in use for other tissues before May 28, 1976, or other lasers that are currently on the U. S. market. The equivalency did not have to be specifically in oral soft tissue. Any soft tissue laser surgery can be used to establish equivalency for 510K clearance purposes. The only non–soft tissue application for the oral cavity cleared by the FDA is for composite curing with the argon laser. Since CO_2 lasers were used for surgery on oral tissues and other tissues prior to the 1976 date, manufacturers of dental lasers needed only to prove substantial equivalency to these lasers to market them for oral soft-tissue surgery. The application for pre-market notification [510(K)] just needs to prove equivalency and does not require the extensive research necessary to prove safety and efficacy for a new device.

Hard Tissue Applications of Lasers

When there is a desire to use a dental laser for a new intended use such as hard tissue surgery, a PMA is required. Since there were no lasers that had clearance for surgery on dental hard tissue prior to May 28, 1976, any laser manufacturer that wishes to market their laser for hard dental tissues must apply for a PMA. The FDA has suggested that the PMA application must include multicenter research, first evaluating the effect of the specific laser on dental hard tissue in vitro. Only after a sufficient amount of basic research has been completed can the manufacturer apply for an IDE. The intent of this basic research must address the question of safety and the potential for harm to the patient. The IDE allows for a designated group of clinicians to treat patients in a very limited scope. An IDE is only granted after proving to the FDA that the intended treatment method is safe for the patients being treated. An IDE must be granted before a new device receives clearance from the FDA that will allow it to be used in human trials and shipped in interstate commerce. The transition from the laboratory to the clinic where the device will be used on human subjects is not very well-defined, and it is left to the FDA to determine whether or not sufficient basic research has been performed to allow clinical studies to begin (CDRH, 1989).

This brings up some issues that are of great interest to any laser company that wishes to bring a new technology to the marketplace. One of these issues relates to what occurs if a laser company funds the research necessary to take a laser through the IDE, which eventually leads to a PMA, and this laser company can sell their laser only for the procedures cleared by the PMA. The question that arises is can a laser manufacturer with a similar laser apply for a clearance based on this equivalency clearance? If this were the case, no laser manufacturer would be willing to fund the research necessary to receive PMA clearance. The FDA states that each laser manufacturer must provide multicenter research for their PMA device, no matter how similar it is to existing cleared lasers. This means that if a manufacturer develops, for example, an Er:YAG laser for hard tissue surgery, no other manufacturer can market their laser for the same application without providing the same research done by the cleared manufacturer, even though it is the exact same laser wavelength and delivery system. This provision is meant to protect the manufacturers who are willing to fund the research necessary for hard tissue clearance or new intended use. The PMA requirements apply to the first four units that have the same wavelength and parameters of treatment. A device that is brought to the market after the first four PMAs have been granted is eligible to apply for clearance under substantial equivalence.

An important part of the FDA monitoring policy is that any manufacturer that develops a device must maintain an inventory of incidents or accidents that occur with that product. Through this inventory and reports from practitioners who use the product, the FDA can determine if the device has the potential for causing harm to patients. Once aware of any potential problems that may arise from the use of a product (drug or device), the FDA may either issue warnings to practitioners to prevent other injuries or occurrences, or it may withdraw the product from the marketplace. The reporting of unwanted or undesirable effects to the FDA is an important responsibility of practitioners.

OSHA Guidelines and ANSI Standards

There are two agencies that have an interest in the safe and effective use of lasers on the American public: the American National Standards Institute (ANSI) and the Occupational Safety and Health Administration (OSHA) of the United States Department of Labor. The OSHA guidelines and ANSI standards serve as the primary documents that regulate the use of lasers in both industry and health care. The OSHA guidelines for laser safety and hazard assessment (U. S. Department of Labor, 1991) are mandatory and enforceable under strict penalty by federal and state agencies throughout the United States. The ANSI standards are strictly voluntary in nature, serving only as guidelines. The ANSI is not a part of the federal government, as one might expect, but is an independent organization that serves to develop national standards for various industries (including health care) in the United States.

The ANSI Z-136.3 Standard

The ANSI has approved the Z-136.3 standard for the safe use of lasers in health-care facilities, with the LIA as secretariat, which recommends both basic laser safety parameters and for specific applications (ANSI, 1993). The basic standard provides guidance for the safe use of lasers and laser systems for diagnostic and therapeutic uses in health-care facilities. It is intended for use by all persons associated with the installation, operation, maintenance, and service of health-care laser systems (HCLS). This standard covers engineering, procedural, and administrative controls necessary for the safety of patients and health-care professionals. These controls are based on evaluation of potential hazards from laser radiation; unique problems related to operating rooms, outpatient clinics, private medical and dental offices; and exposure risks to patient and professional staff. Included are engineering and administrative controls, personal protective equipment, and laser safety training. The specific standards for safe use of lasers in general and specifically in dentistry are available through the LIA. The dental standards are included in Appendix IV for reference. These standards are continually being updated, so as new lasers and applications are added in dentistry, updated standards will be developed.

OSHA Guidelines

OSHA has established safety guidelines with the ANSI Z-136.3 standards as a guide (OSHA, 1991). The objectives of the guidelines are to provide a general overview of lasers, laser uses, laser hazards and hazard analysis that are required to provide appropriate background for understanding the applicable industry standards and regulatory requirements. The two documents listed ANSI Z-136.3 and OSHA that would give the dental practitioner all the relevant information and regulations on the safe and effective use of lasers in dentistry. A more extensive description of the OSHA guidelines is presented in Chapter 6.

The intent of these previously mentioned regulations, from both the FDA and OSHA, is to protect both the patient and staff (doctor, assistant, nurse). These regulations have at their core the basic research that has been done with lasers since their development in the early 1960s. Understanding the effects of lasers on tissue, especially dental hard tissues, has to be a prerequisite before additional standards can be developed. As dentists, we must understand the parameters we must work within to protect our patients. To develop these parameters, basic research is required. Since the field of lasers in dentistry is exploding with new information, laser users must keep abreast of this new information. Only when these components, ie, research, education, and continued education, are realized can all of the above come together for the goal of safe and effective use of lasers in dentistry.

Laser Education and Training Programs

Laser education and training in dentistry have evolved out of necessity. As laser technology improved and became available to dentists, innovative clinical and research applications for lasers were developed by pioneering individuals in the field of dentistry. Early dental researchers and clinicians acquired their technical skills and knowledge of lasers either through practical experience or from laser courses offered at hospitals, laser centers, or other institutions such as the Laser Institute of America or Wenske Laser Center (Harris et al, 1992). Initially, laser education and training were borrowed from the medical surgical specialties and industry. As the specific needs and requirements of dentistry became apparent and the use of lasers in dentistry became more widespread, the desire for structured dental laser education became an important issue (McCann, 1992). Once armed with this powerful tool, clinicians began to search for the sources of information and experience required to safely use lasers in clinical dental practice. To date, there are few dental schools that include any form of structured dental laser training programs either at the undergraduate or graduate levels. The ultimate goal of dental education within any field or discipline must center around the delivery of safe and effective patient care (Miserendino et al, 1993). Therefore at this time, structured programs for dental laser education are prerequisite to any clinical application in the practice of dentistry.

Current sources of training for laser users include: (1) dental residency training programs; (2) hospital based credentialing and training courses; (3) continuing dental education programs offered at dental schools; (4) short courses and workshops offered through meetings of professional dental associations and societies; and (5) preceptorships or supervised observation by dental laser experts sponsored by manufacturers of dental laser systems. A limited number of universities and hospitals currently offer surgical laser training as part of residencies or advanced training programs for the surgical specialties of oral and maxillofacial surgery and periodontics, while others have introduced continuing education courses on a more limited scale. Because of the increasing interest and popularity of lasers within the profession, many educational programs and training seminars have been presented in conjunction with national, state, and regional meetings of dental societies and professional associations such as the American Dental Association, the Academy of General Dentistry, and the Academy of Laser Dentistry. These types of programs are intended to provide various levels of laser instructional and informational courses to the general practitioner. More recently, an increasing number of elective undergraduate level courses are being offered or developed at several dental educational institutions to familiarize the future dental professional with the potential advantages of laser application. Undoubtedly, as the use of lasers in dentistry increases, it is likely that laser education and training will become a more integral part of the regular dental-school curricula.

Because of the scarcity or absence of formal laser training, most dentists who currently use lasers have been trained through manufacturer-sponsored courses; preceptorships; or hospital, professional association, or university-based training seminars. Understandably, the extent and level of knowledge and experience among those groups vary considerably. Much of the variation in education and clinical experience to date can be attributed to the logical differences in course content related to specific features of various laser systems and wavelengths. Other differences may also be imposed by the level of training and educational skills of the instructors of laser courses and the physical limitations of the facilities at which they were trained. The important factor to recognize at this time is that laser education in dentistry can no longer be administered effectively without the development of a more formally structured process and without consideration of certain essential elements (Miserendino et al, 1992).

Essential Elements of Laser Training Programs

Elements of laser training programs include: (1) course content (didactic component); (2) hands-on experience (practical component); (3) evaluation of competency or clinical proficiency (certification or credentialing); (4) instructor competency (educational skills); and (5) advanced training and continuing educational needs (updating). Specific educational and training requirements for laser users (dental practitioners) will also vary from that needed for proper training of dental auxiliaries and other support staff.

Four levels of safety training programs required for the various types of health-care personnel involved with laser use are described in the ANSI Z-136.3 guidelines in Appendix IV. Listed in the ANSI document are the essential elements of the specific training requirements for physicians and laser technical support staff (D1); health-care support staff (D2); the laser safety officer (D3) (Table); and medical laser service personnel (D4). Pertinent to dental practitioners and chairside auxiliaries are the requirements described in Table D1. These include two categories of knowledge, the first consisting of an understanding of the bioeffects and hazards

Table. Sample LSO Laser Training Requirements*

Operational Characteristics of the Laser
Operation of laser
The laser "language" (definitions)
Review of laser application(s)
Bioeffects and Potential Hazards of the Laser
Eye and skin hazards of direct and reflected beams
Laser exposure criteria (MPEs, AELs)
Hazard assessment methods (ODs, NHZs)
Non-beam hazards: electrical hazards; fire hazards; hazards of laser-produced fumes and articles . . . etc.
Other associated hazards
Requirements of Laser Safety Standards
Specific company laser regulations
The ANSI Z-136.1 Standard "For Safe Use of Lasers"
The U.S. Federal Laser Product Performance Standard
OSHA laser regulations
Regional (state) and local regulations, if applicable
International Laser Regulations (as applicable)
Practical Controls for Lasers
Reducing beam hazards
Laser eye protection: types and proper selection
Methods of electrical safety
Methods for fume removal
Methods to reduce fire hazards
Standard operating procedures (SOP) for laser use

*From OSHA Instruction, PNB 8-1.7, August 5, 1991, Directorate of Technical Support.

of lasers; and second, a knowledge of the requirements of laser safety standards and practical controls for lasers in the medical environment.

Standards of Practice

Suggested standards of practice for the use of lasers by clinicians have been published by the American Society for Lasers in Medicine and Surgery (ASLMS). These have also been incorporated into the ANSI Z-136.3 as Appendix IV (ANSI Z-136.3, 1988). Within the ASLMS proposed standard are general recommendations for the training of physicians and surgeons who use lasers. These recommendations describe training requirements and standards of practice beyond the scope of course work included in basic laser science and safety courses. According to the ASLMS recommendations, laser training courses should include: (1) basic laser physics; (2) laser tissue interaction; and (3) hands-on experience and discussions relevant to the particular clinical specialty field. Additionally, course time for the didactic component is specified to be a minimum of 8 to 10 hours; with observation and hands-on experience in actual clinical applications, appropriate to the specific training procedures, the minimum is 6 to 8 hours. Practitioners are also directed to perform only those procedures for which they have been formally trained or certified and which they are capable of accomplishing by conventional methods.

Educational Requirements for Dental Auxiliaries and Staff

Additional training requirements for dental office personnel employees are specified in the OSHA guidelines (U. S. Department of Labor, 1991). The OSHA guidelines are not intended to ensure the proficiency of laser use in health-care facilities, but instead focus on the safety training of health-care workers to provide a safe workplace for those employees who either work with or work around lasers.

Detailed in the OSHA guidelines are the training requirements for four classes of health-care personnel based on the class of laser that is used as defined in the OSHA and ANSI documents (see Chapter 6). Generally, dental lasers capable of continuous output greater than 500 mW are classified as class IV lasers. According to the OSHA guidelines, training for class IV personnel should provide an understanding of and familiarity with practical and safe laser techniques; safe operational procedures; safety equipment and devices; personal protective equipment, hazard identification and avoidance, environmental control measures, and the requirements of a medical surveillance program. Training should be tailored for each level of employee and according to the specific type of laser system, ie, wavelength or delivery system used, with updating when appropriate. Records should also be maintained to document the dates and times of formal training programs, laser accident or incident occurrences, and medical surveillance. Medical surveillance describes the periodic monitoring of injuries or damage (principally ocular) that could potentially result from long-term exposure to radiant energy.

The responsibility for implementing and administering the laser safety program, which includes ensuring the education and training of all personnel at the specific health-care facility, is the laser safety officer (LSO). Additional educational and training requirements are specified in the OSHA guidelines, which also apply to private offices, clinics, and other health-care facilities, including dental offices (Abt et al, 1993). The OSHA guidelines further mandate that an LSO must be appointed for each facility. The training requirements for the LSO as listed in the OSHA guidelines can be found in the Table.

Curriculum Guidelines for Dental Laser Education

Although dentistry is included in the ANSI document, the educational requirements and respective courses previously described pertain to all health-care workers involved with the use of lasers and were not specifically developed for or intended for the dental profession. On January 22, 1993, the research and education committee of the Academy of Laser Dentistry elected to formally adopt curriculum guidelines previously formulated by a group of technical experts, clinicians, and dental educators for the purpose of developing an educational standard for the profession.

On July 25 and 26, 1992, curriculum guidelines for dental laser education were drafted at a workshop held at the University of California, San Francisco, for the development of standards for dental laser education and laser instructor certification. Within these guidelines, four levels of education are defined for dental practitioners. Outlined for each level of training are the recommended course contents, which range from the introductory course level to instructor-level training courses. Specific educational guidelines describing the curricula for dental laser training courses are listed in Appendix IV for reference. To date, a number of national and international dental laser associations, including the Academy of Laser Dentistry, the International Society of Laser Dentistry, and a number of dental schools have adopted these guidelines as a basis for their laser training and continuing education courses.

Course Content. A typical laser course intended to provide education that is sufficient to prepare an individual for laser use in clinical practice will necessarily be extensive. Similarly, courses designed to prepare dental auxiliaries and staff will also be quite involved. Both levels of training will necessitate each of the essential components required for a clinical training program as described earlier (Harris et al, 1993). These components can be summarized briefly as didactic, practical experience, and testing.

The didactic component of any laser course should include a discussion of the basic sciences or principles of physics and optics that pertain to lasers. All aspects of clinical laser safety, hazard identification, and control methods should also been covered. Prior to any description of surgical techniques relevant to the procedures to be performed, an adequate understanding of the biologic effects of each laser type (wavelength) and specific types of tissue interactions that may occur should be provided. Once these basic principles of lasers and their effects on tissues are understood, one is prepared to learn and master the surgical techniques necessary to perform clinical procedures safely and effectively. Practical experience is required for the performance of specific procedures and will provide the clinician or auxiliary with the opportunity to develop the hand-eye coordination skills essential to achieve a mastery of the surgical techniques necessary for laser treatment.

Because of variations among lasers attributable to wavelength of emission, instrumentation, and methods of delivery, the tissue effects of various laser systems, even those of the same wavelength, will vary greatly. It is advisable then that laser training should be designed to provide system-specific information and that training in one wavelength or system should not be considered equivalent to that with others.

Clinical experience in the actual treatment of patients should also be separate from dental laser courses and training programs. It is advisable that prior to the practical treatment of patients, workshops or preceptorships that allow observation of a number of cases be attended. It is also desirable that a variety of cases be practiced under supervision before the learning clinician attempts treatment alone. The practical component of laser training courses should also include information related to appropriate follow-up care, management of potential complications, standard operating procedure, and safety methods specific to the procedures to be learned. Indications for treatment, as well as alternatives, advantages, and disadvantages of laser use and diagnosis should also be covered. In general, at least 50% of the course time should be devoted to practical experience. The novice should attempt only relatively simple procedures with the newly learned techniques until he or she has gained sufficient experience to perform more challenging cases.

Credentialing and Certification

Often when credentialing and certification are mentioned in dental circles, groups of individuals become alarmed or incensed. Curiously, this situation does not frequently arise within the medical profession. Certification in dentistry usually implies specialization, which is not necessarily true in medicine. Credentialing and certification in the medical field describe a recognition of training obtained for purposes of exercising certain surgical privileges at hospitals (Abt et al, 1993). Physicians and surgeons certified for training in specific procedures are thereby approved by hospital boards or surgical privilege committees to exercise or practice those procedures. This is what is meant by certification and credentialing in this chapter. To further clarify this potentially controversial subject, we, who have been involved with literally thousands of dental laser users for several years, have not encountered a single individual who has ever mentioned or favored the idea of establishing laser use as a specialty field in dentistry.

At present, there is no recognized certifying board within the practice of medicine or dentistry related to the use of lasers. The American Board of Laser Surgery (Milwaukee, WI) is one organization that certifies clinicians, including dentists, in laser use. The certification process involves examination to determine a level of knowledge related to laser use specific to the area of practice, but it is not universally accepted by hospitals or other institutions. Each hospital surgical privilege committee or equivalent body establishes its own criteria for granting privileges.

The Academy of Laser Dentistry (ALD) also offers certification (certificates of completion) for the three levels of dental laser training courses offered either through the organization itself or from dental schools and other institutions with equivalent courses based on the Educational and Curriculum Guidelines described earlier. The certification process of the Academy of Laser Dentistry is similar to the various levels of membership status of the Academy of General Dentistry, although the titles of Mastership or Fellowship are not applied. Certification and courses offered through ALD are wavelength- and system-specific.

Acknowledgment

Special thanks to Neal Ogden from the Center for Devices and Radiological Health of the Food and Drug Administration for help in reviewing the manuscript.

References

Abt E, Miserendino LJ, Pick RM, Harris D, Wigdor H. Credentialing for the safe and effective use of lasers in dental practice. Lasers Surg Med 1993;5:19.

American National Standard for Safe Use of Lasers in Health Care Facilities (ANSI Z-136.3–1988). Orlando, FL: Laser Institute of America; 1988.

American National Standard for the Safe Use of Lasers (ANSI Z-136.1–rev. 1993). Orlando FL: Laser Institute of America; 1993.

CDRH. Investigational Device Exemptions: Regulatory Requirements for Medical Devices. Rockville, MD: U. S. Department of Health and Human Services, DHHS Publication No 89-4159, 1989.

FDA. Everything You Always Wanted to Know About the Medical Device Amendments . . . and Weren't Afraid to Ask, ed 3. Rockville, MD: U. S. Department of Health and Human Services, Public Health Service, Food and Drug Administration, Center for Device and Radiological Health, DHHS Publication No 90-4173; 1990.

Harris DM, Miserendino LJ, Abt E, Wigdor H, Pick RM. Education, training and certification for the use of lasers in the dental profession. Presented at the International Laser Safety Conference; Cincinnati, OH: Dec 4, 1992.

Harris D, Miserendino LJ, Wigdor H, Abt E, Pick RM. Laser training and experience in the dental profession. Lasers Surg Med 1993;5:19.

McCann D. States look at who may use lasers. ADA News 1992;23:1–6.

Miserendino LJ, Abt E, Harris D, Pick RM, Wigdor H. Recommendations for safe and appropriate use of lasers in dentistry. J Laser Appl 1992;4:16–17.

Miserendino LJ, Harris D, Abt E, Wigdor H, Pick RM. Laser safety in the dental profession. Lasers Surg Med 1993;5:18.

OSHA: Guidelines for Laser Safety and Hazard Assessment. U. S. Department of Labor OSHA Instruction Publication 8-1.7. Directorate of Technical Support, August 5, 1991.

Chapter Eight

Surgical Technique

V. Kim Kutsch and Robert M. Pick

Dental lasers fall into two basic categories: there are those that work solely in the noncontact mode, either focused or defocused, such as CO_2 lasers, and those that work either in the contact or noncontact modes, the contact mode being focused and the noncontact mode being defocused. This group includes the lasers delivered by fiberoptics such as argon, Ho:YAG, and Nd:YAG.

Noncontact Lasers

The discussion of noncontact lasers will address carbon dioxide lasers and overall surgical technique. Carbon dioxide lasers can be divided into those CO_2 lasers that work by articulated arm technology, those that operate via hollow waveguide technology, and those that operate by hand-held technology.

Most CO_2 lasers applicable in medicine can also be used effectively in dentistry. Carbon dioxide lasers work primarily in a noncontact mode. They can also be used in either a focused or a defocused mode. The focused mode is when the laser beam hits the tissue at its focal point or smallest diameter. This diameter is dependent on the size of the lens used. Most CO_2 laser systems today have a lens that can focus the beam down to spot sizes ranging from 0.1 mm to 0.35 mm or larger. This focused mode can also be referred to as a cut mode. For example, the cut mode is used when performing biopsies.

The other method of using the laser is the defocused mode. By defocusing the laser beam or moving the focal spot away from the tissue plane, the beam size that hits the tissue has a greater diameter, thus causing a wider area of tissue to be vaporized (Figs 8.1 and 8.2a). By defocusing the beam, however, laser intensity or power density is reduced. A defocused beam, for example, is used when performing frenectomies, or for the removal of inflammatory papillary hyperplasia. Because all optical fibers have a high absorptive index for CO_2 laser light, true fiberoptic delivery cannot be used. Instead, some CO_2 lasers use articulating arms (Fig 8.3) with properly aligned mirrors at knuckle joints and then a handpiece with a specific lens is used to create the desired spot size in the focused mode. Because of their some-

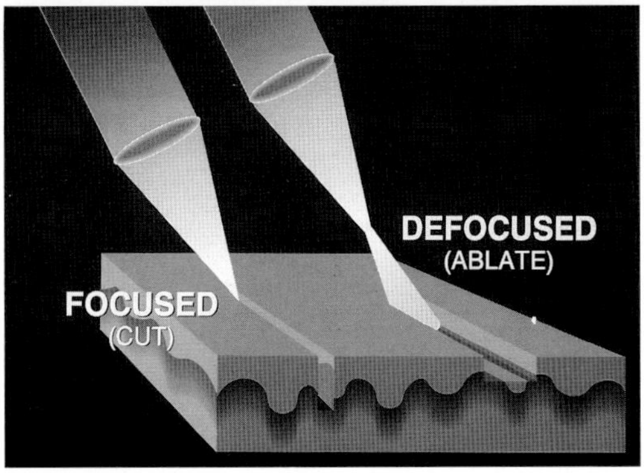

Fig 8. 1 Focused and defocused modes of delivery. With the defocused mode, there is a wider zone of tissue removal but a shallower depth of penetration as compared to the focused mode.

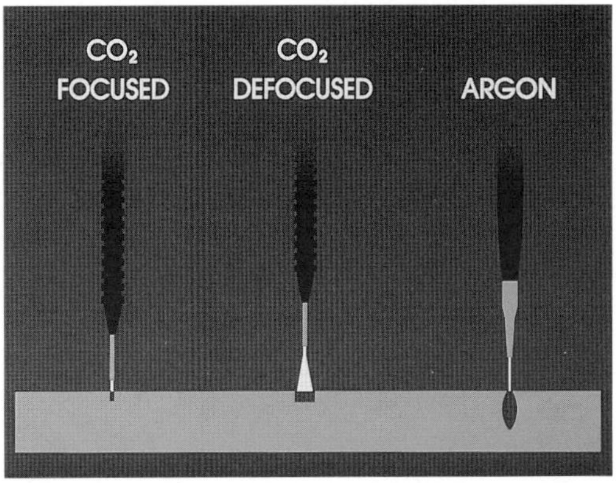

8.2a

Fig 8.2 Various types of dental lasers and surgical delivery modes. **(a)**, CO_2 laser in focused and defocused modes and argon laser in contact modes. **(b)**, Ho:YAG laser in the pulsed, contact mode and continuous wave (cw) Nd:YAG laser in both contact and noncontact modes. With the continuous wave mode, there is greater depth of penetration. **(c)**, Pulsed Nd:YAG laser used with coated tips or an air-and-water spray to control depth of penetration.

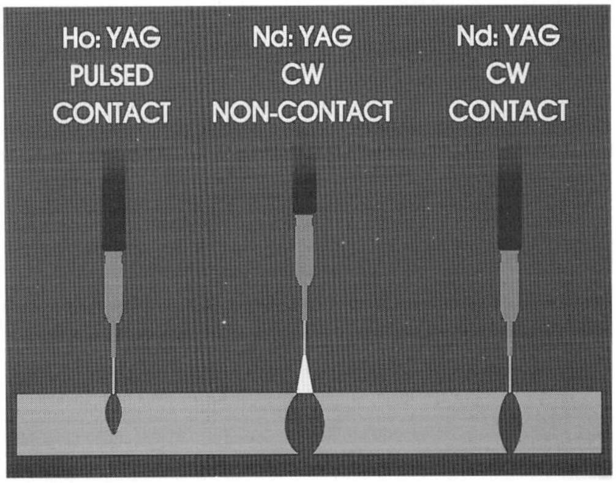

8.2b

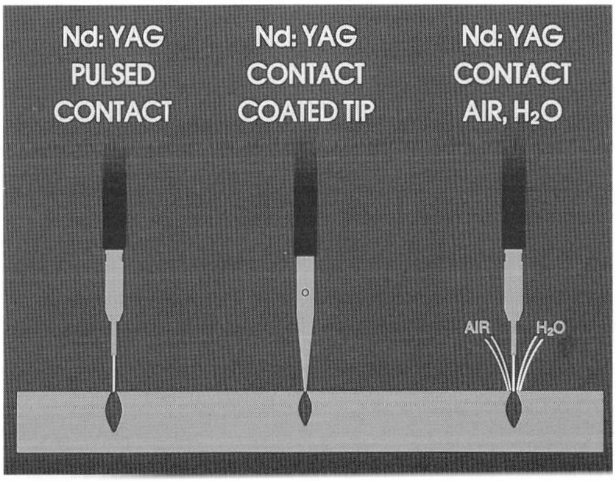

8.2c

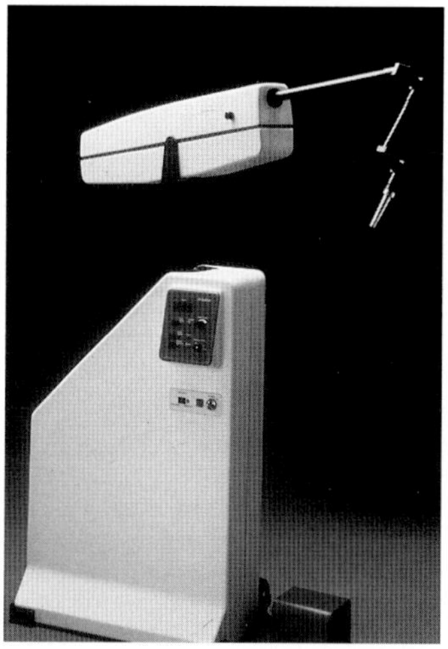

8.3

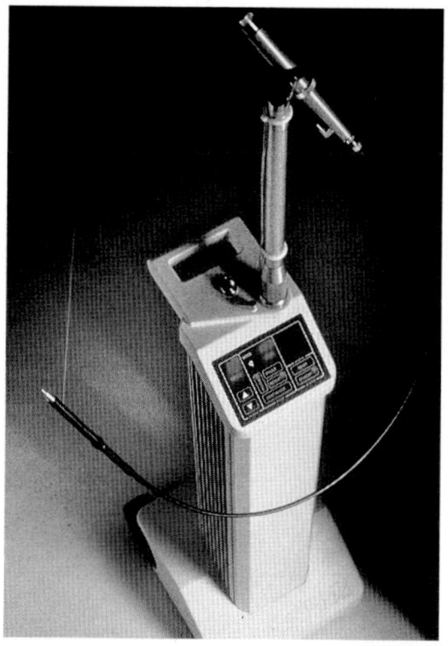

8.4

Fig 8.3 An articulated arm CO_2 laser (Coherent, Palo Alto, CA).

Fig 8.4 Flexible waveguide delivery system (Luxar Laser Corp, Bothell, WA) showing a hollow waveguide.

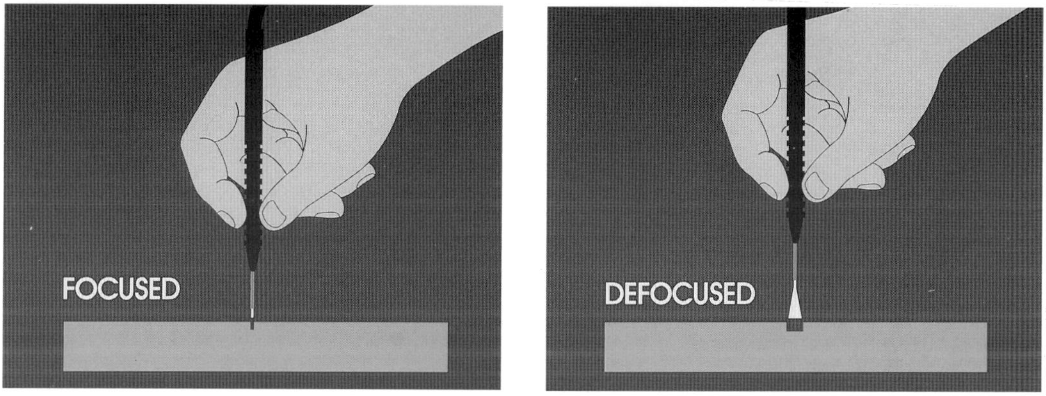

Fig 8.5 The CO_2 laser with hollow waveguide technology used in both focused **(a)** and defocused **(b)** modes of delivery. Note the short focal distance to tissue.

times cumbersome nature, CO_2 laser systems that use articulated arms are often difficult to use within the oral cavity. With articulated arm systems and those that use hand-held technology, the focal distance to tissue can vary from 1 to 3 cm.

Because the CO_2 laser beam is invisible, a red helium:neon (He:Ne) laser beam is built in coaxially for use as an aiming light. Aiming an invisible light at tissue from a distance is not only difficult, but adjacent tissues are at risk of being inadvertently hit by the laser beam. As of 1990, certain CO_2 laser systems use a hollow waveguide technology for delivery of the CO_2 laser beam. This type of delivery system can completely eliminate the need for articulating arms, since the beam is delivered through a flexible tube about 1. 2 mm in diameter (Fig 8.4). In addition, different tips can be attached to the waveguide to suit the specific surgical requirements. Furthermore, due to this technology, the beam is delivered closer to the tissue, which allows the operator to see exactly where the beam is being delivered (Fig

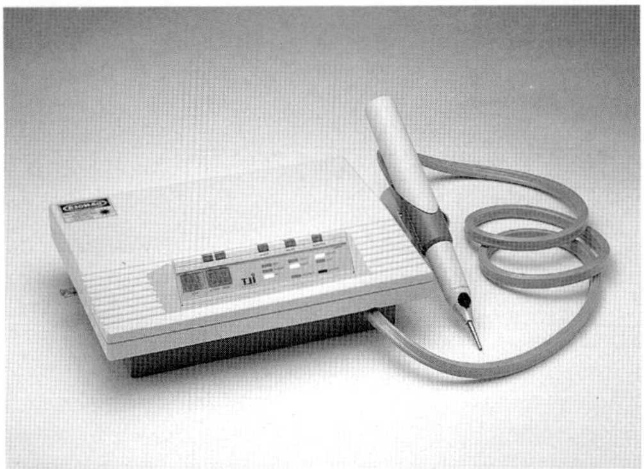

Fig 8.6 A portable hand-held CO_2 laser system (ILT Laser Corp, Salt Lake City, UT).

8.5). This state-of-the-art technology for oral delivery antiquates most articulated arm systems and, most importantly, provides ease of access to all areas of the oral cavity.

In hand-held carbon dioxide laser systems, the actual laser tube or cavity is within the handpiece. The handpiece is connected to a central control panel and power unit via a cord (Fig 8.6). These units are usually the smallest CO_2 lasers available for dentistry and the most portable. However, their ease of access lies somewhere between the articulated arm units and the hollow waveguide units.

Carbon dioxide lasers have a great affinity for any tissue with a high water content, regardless of tissue color. They are therefore very efficient for surgical procedures and perform well in cutting wet tissues such as those in and around the oral cavity. Their penetration depths are minimal (0.2 to 0.3 mm in oral tissues).

In incisional or excisional biopsies, the CO_2 laser is used as a precise cutting tool. In an excisional biopsy, the surgical outline is carefully mapped out, including normal margins at all borders of the lesion. Initially the laser is placed in a cutting or focused mode, held perpendicular to the tissue, and follows the predefined surgical outline. By means of a tissue pickup, a border of the outline is raised and the lesion is then undermined with traction-countertraction, as would be done with a scalpel. Power settings may vary depending on the laser used and the skill of the operator. On the average, power settings most commonly used range from 4 to 6 W.

Once the lesion has been removed, the area is left to heal by granulation. Incisional biopsies are performed in exactly the same manner as excisional biopsies. As with conventional procedures, normal margins are included. Depending on the size of the biopsy specimen, the wound is either left to granulate or closed with an appropriate suturing technique. The laser is an excellent alternative for the removal of lesions such as irritation fibromas present on the buccal mucosa or tongue, or for the removal of epuli.

Carbon dioxide lasers can be used impressively in the noncontact mode for the so called "laser peel" or whitening procedure. The peeling technique is usually used to remove certain vesiculobullous lesions or other surface lesions that involve a relatively large surface area. This is accomplished by using the laser in a highly defocused mode, and at lower power settings, usually 2 to 3 W maximum. One starts with the beam highly defocused and distanced from the tissue, initially with no effect being seen on the tissue plane. Then the beam is gradually brought closer into focus, but still in the defocused mode, until the tissue takes on a whitened appearance and begins to blister. This blistering appears to occur at the basement membrane of the tissue. This whitening technique is then extended over the rest of the lesion to be peeled. The whitened area can be easily grabbed with a tissue pickup or a hemostat, and the area peeled back to expose the underlying tissue for visualization. If more of the lesion still remains, the area can be further peeled or ablated as necessary. This is done with complete visualization because of the hemorrhage-free nature of the laser wound.

Ablation is a term used to describe the method of "painting away" a lesion or tissue removal by the laser. This is another noncontact surgical application of lasers. In the ablation mode, the tissue is simply vaporized. When performing an ablation of an inflammatory papillary hyperplasia of either the palate or the maxillary ridge, for example, the laser affords much greater control than either a blade or electrosurgery. The scalpel is very limited in this situation since it is extremely difficult to negotiate the curves of the palate and the ridges in somewhat straight lines and sharp angles. Because of the extent of the area of tissue removed, such as when the entire palate is involved, there can be a fair amount of hemorrhage when the procedure is performed with conventional methods. By comparison the laser allows one to perform the procedure with a dry field, giving excellent visibility. Curves and mucobuccal folds are easily negotiated with the laser. Power settings generally range from 2 to 12 W depending on the thickness of the tissue and operator technique. Depending on the delicacy of the procedure, various timed and chopped modes can also be used. Chopping or pulsing can reduce thermal damage to surrounding tissues as explained in Chapters 2 and 3.

When ablating surface lesions that extend more deeply into tissue, it becomes necessary to remove the lesion layer by layer. During surface ablation with the laser, a carbonized layer or char forms on the surface that must be removed before deeper layers can be ablated.

Once an area with these type of lesions is lased, the resulting char layer can be wiped away with a wet sponge, revealing the surgical area of either exposed epithelium or underlying muscle or connective tissue. With this exposure and dry field, the lesion can be visualized, and, if necessary, this process of lasing and wipe down can be continued until normal-appearing tissue is exposed. At this point, a final char layer is applied. Also, by moving in and out of focus, one can remove more or less of the lesion as necessary.

Specific parameters such as power settings, timed modes, gated modes, and when to use continuous modes are covered in greater detail in Chapter 10, which addresses the clinical application of CO_2 lasers specifically.

Fiberoptic Delivery Systems and Techniques

Lasers with wavelengths shorter than 2,500 nm can be delivered through an optical fiber. Of the lasers currently available for dentistry, included in this category are the argon, Nd:YAG, and Ho:YAG lasers. These lasers can be either true pulsed lasers, as in the case of a free-running pulsed Nd:YAG and Ho:YAG, or can be continuous wave lasers with the option of a gated pulse, eg, argon and Nd:YAG. Fiberoptic lasers then can be pulsed, gated, or continuous wave. After a beam has passed through a hollow wave guide or fiber, it is no longer coherent. The fiber acts to direct the photons along the long axis of the fiber, and as photons hit the outer surface of the fiber they are reflected back into the fiber by a reflective coating, thus some photons have a different travel distance as they "bounce" along the inside of the fiber. The greater the diameter of the fiber, the greater the variation of distances traveled by the photons. These differences in direction and interference patterns within the fiber result in variations in power density and spatial orientation at the point of delivery of the beam vs that observed at the source where the beam exits the laser tube. Consequently, beams delivered through optical fibers are described in terms of beam profile or character. The beam of light emitted from the fiber or waveguide remains highly directional with a relatively high energy density, but it is not truly coherent. The interaction of the fiber with the beam as previously described is said to cause depolarization of the beam. This will not generally have any clinical significance for the operator, but is presented here to clarify some of the technical terms that a practitioner may encounter in the scientific literature.

Lasers that are currently used in dentistry all produce tissue effects that are photothermal in nature. The laser is used to create a thermal wound that results from cutting, vaporizing, and coagulating tissue. The biologic tissue effect is influenced by many factors, but is primarily a result of the power density, wavelength, optical characteristics of the tissue, and duration of application. The power density is determined by the power used, diameter of the fiber, spot size, and distance from the tissue. The wavelength used determines the absorption model, which is the material that best absorbs the particular wavelength. The characteristics of the tissue and the pigments that are present influence the energy absorption. The time of application also influences the resultant tissue effect.

As the laser radiant energy is applied to the tissue, some of the energy is reflected, some is absorbed, some is scattered into the tissue, and some is transmitted through the tissue to the extinction depth. The absorbed energy heats the tissue, and there is a volume of tissue affected with a temperature gradient within that volume of tissue. The temperature is greatest closest to the fiber tip and diminishes deeper into the tissue. There is a unique pattern of this irradiation volume for each wavelength and tissue, depending on whether the application is made in contact or noncontact. In addition, the irradiation volume changes for each type of contact fiber used, depending on whether the application is pulsed, gated, or continuous wave. Learning how these variations affect the irradiation volumes will lead the practitioner to understand and anticipate the resultant biologic effects.

Most bare fibers consist of a glass rod core made of silica-quartz, with an outer surface cladding that has a different refractive index from the silica-quartz fiber, and an outer protective vinyl jacket. The standard fibers measure 6 to 12 feet in length and come in a variety of diameters, ranging from 50 to 600 μm. As the fiber diameter decreases, the potential energy densities increase, fiber flexibility increases, and the potential for lateral fracture of the fiber decreases. Most practitioners find the smaller fibers ideal for noncontact surgery because of the higher energy densities, eg, 50,000 J/cm^2 emitted at the tip, but smaller diameter fibers are considered undesirable for contact surgery because they are too flexible. The larger fibers are acceptable for low-energy density applications, eg, photopolymerization, but energy densities are too low for contact surgery. Compared to smaller fibers, they are very stiff and create difficulties for access in the mouth. The midsize fibers offer the most desirable overall characteristics, with fibers in the 300-μm range being most favored by experienced practitioners.

In addition to bare fibers, there are also a wide variety of other fiber styles. Neodymium:YAG contact fibers are available with sculptured tips that concentrate

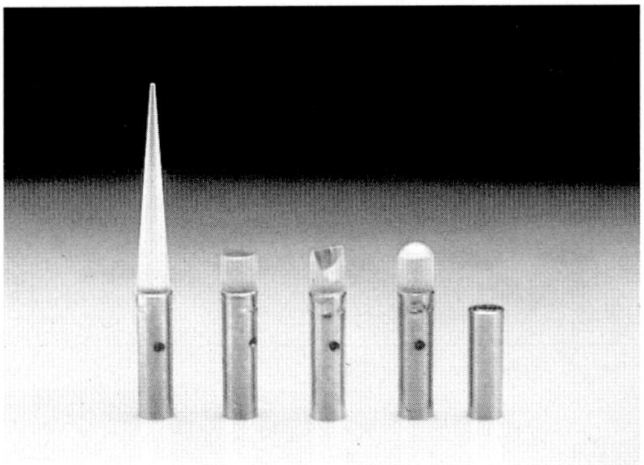

Fig 8.7 A series of sculptured laser tips (Premier Laser Systems, Irvine, CA).

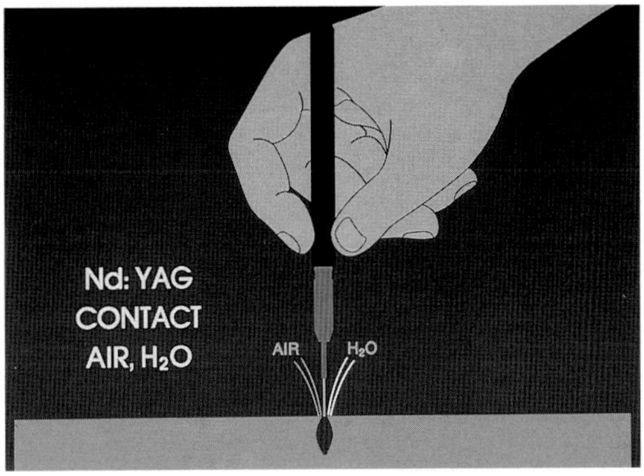

Fig 8.8 Diagram of a Nd:YAG laser with an air-and-water spray.

or disperse the energy in the tissue (Fig 8.7). Special sapphire-coated tips are also available that act to absorb the laser energy within the tip and create a "hot-tip" effect that acts like electrocautery on the tissue. There are several differently styled tips to cut, vaporize, and coagulate the tissue. Near-contact tips are available for the argon laser. These special fibers deliver the beam through a glass tube–like scalpel that brings the beam almost into contact with the tissue.

Handpieces for holding and aiming the fibers come in a variety of styles and sizes. A good handpiece should be lightweight with a positive gripping surface, withstand frequent autoclaving, and accommodate a variety of disposable cannulas. For contact applications, some practitioners prefer a fiber locking mechanism in the handpiece, while many prefer simpler designs with fewer parts. The handpiece should be comfortable to hold and allow easy physical and visual access to the mouth. The tip of the fiber is held in the handpiece with a disposable needle or cannula; many practitioners prefer Ultradent mini-tips (Ultradent, Salt Lake City, UT). It is best to use disposable cannulas.

Some handpieces are available with an optional air-and-water spray (Fig 8.8). The water spray is intended to cool the target tissue and reduce lateral thermal damage. It also flushes the coagulated tissue debris from the surgical site and prevents the coagulum from building up on the fiber tip. Water spray is contraindicated for the Ho:YAG laser because the holmium wavelength is well absorbed by water, and the water would interfere with the tissue effect. The Nd:YAG wavelength is not well absorbed by water, thus water may be used. Cooling, however, will interfere with a "hot-tip" effect, which is very efficient with this wavelength. If water is used, it will require greater amounts of energy to provide the desired tissue effects. In the case of argon, this wavelength is least affected by water, and a water spray is highly beneficial in cooling the tissue to reduce lateral thermal damage and to keep the fiber tip clean. The use of the water spray will vary depending on the wavelength and the surgical technique.

A "hot tip" improves cutting efficiency for low-power Nd:YAG instruments but requires cleaning or cleaving the fiber when the operator wishes to create a different tissue effect. As the carbonized tissue remnants build up on the fiber tip, it becomes necessary to wipe the fiber tip periodically during the procedure. This can easily be accomplished with a damp cotton sponge, taking care to treat the fiber tip as a contaminated surgical sharp. Some procedures may require the operator to cut, vaporize, coagulate, and provide hemostasis at different points of the procedure; or the operator may want to change from contact to a noncontact application mode. The carbonized tissue remnants on the fiber tip will diminish the energy output at the fiber tip for other applications and should be removed.

Laser energy diverges from the tip of a bare fiber at about 15 degrees, creating larger spot sizes with increasing distances from the fiber tip to the target tissue. Consequently, most fiber-delivered lasers use a coaxial aiming beam. This is particularly helpful for noncontact applications since it allows the operator to visualize the target site on the tissue. It is also important for lasers in the infrared invisible range for the same reason. Neodymium:YAG and Ho:YAG lasers use a red visible helium:neon or He:Ne beam at 632 nm and up to 5-mW power. Argon lasers use either an attenuated argon blue-green visible aiming beam, or He:Ne, depending on the model. The aiming beam is helpful in noncontact applications, but experienced clinicians may sometimes prefer to work without it. Most dental lasers have a switch that allows the operator to work with or without the He:Ne aiming beam.

During a bare fiber procedure when there is a degradation of power, or when switching from a "hot-tip" technique to another, or at the completion of a procedure, the fiber tip should be cleaved. If the tip is a sculptured or sapphire-coated tip, it should be cleaned and sterilized. To cleave a bare fiber first, strip some of the vinyl jacket if necessary, then scribe the silica-quartz fiber with the cleaving instrument. The best technique is to lay the fiber on a flat hard surface, scribe the fiber with light pressure on the top surface, and rotate the fiber and scribe the opposite surface at the same distance from the fiber tip. Gently separate the tip with a slightly lateral tugging motion. A good cleave will direct the energy in a perfect circle. A poor cleave will demonstrate multiple areas of scattered light around the target spot. Focusing the aiming beam on a hard surface at a distance of about 2 cm will demonstrate the quality of the cleave. A poor cleave will require greater energy for a desired tissue effect and result in more lateral thermal damage to the tissue. Achieving a satisfactory cleave requires patience and practice. Never cleave a fiber tip holding it in your hand—the fiber tip is a contaminated sharp object that can easily puncture latex and skin. Handle and dispose of the severed fiber tip with other contaminated surgical sharps.

Contact surgery relies on two different principles. The first technique is the creation of a "hot-tip" effect, either with sapphire-coated sculpted tips or by allowing carbonized tissue remnants to build up on the bare fiber tip. With the other principle, a clean tip is placed in contact with the tissue and relies on the pigment or the water present in the target tissue to absorb the laser energy. With either technique, the presence of charred tissue on the fiber tip or char created on the tissue surface increases the absorption of the laser energy and the resultant tissue effects. Char can be eliminated with a water spray, and then slightly more energy will be required to provide time-efficient results. When a fiber is placed in contact with the tissue, there is tactile control feedback for the operator. Keeping the fiber in one spot will gradually heat a growing mass of tissue in that spot, ie, the irradiated tissue volume will increase in size. This may be helpful for removing a relatively large tissue mass. However, most contact applications involve the sculpting or incising of tissue. In this application, the fiber is kept in steady motion and removes tissue in its path. The addition of movement extends the irradiation volume into a trough or elongated crater. By controlling the amount of exposure to the tissue, an incision can be created by directing the fiber along the same path either with one slow stroke or with multiple faster strokes. Covering larger tissue surface areas with the fiber tip will result in broader tissue removal and sculpting. This technique would be applicable for gingivoplasty.

Reducing the exposure energy allows the operator to create hemostasis in most surgical sites in the mouth. Moving the fiber along the tissue surface tends to create drag on the fiber tip unless sufficient energy densities are used to provide rapid cutting. The extent of fiber drag varies with each wavelength and fiber style and generally increases if carbonized tissue remnants are allowed to build up on the tip. Some operators prefer contact laser surgery for the tactile control, while others prefer noncontact surgery to eliminate the fiber drag interference. Faster sweeping motions can help eliminate some of this drag. It should also be kept in mind that working with Nd:YAG lasers in a noncontact or defocused mode can cause deeper tissue damage.

Contact vs Noncontact Modes

Noncontact surgery relies completely on the pigments and water present in the tissue that are responsible for the absorption model of each wavelength. Directing sufficient energy densities to the target tissue will then create the desired tissue effect. The creation and appearance of char on the tissue surface will also increase the energy absorption at the surface and will improve the efficiency. Directing the energy at one spot will gradually heat an increasing mass of tissue, and moving the energy along a path with single or multiple strokes will create an incision. Painting a large area with the energy will contour and sculpt tissue. Decreasing the energy will allow the operator to coagulate and create hemostasis in most surgical sites in the mouth. Noncontact surgery requires significantly greater power settings than contact surgery for the fiberoptic delivered lasers to achieve the equivalent tissue effect. The fiber tip must be well cleaved and kept free of debris. With proper technique, the results are the same as those for contact surgery; the techniques and principles are similar, only the feel is different. During noncontact surgery, the clinician operates with visual control with the aid of an aiming beam or by observing the tissue effect being created.

Surgical Characteristics of Argon Lasers

Argon is a visible wavelength laser with primary wavelengths of 488 and 514.5 nm. Argon can be delivered in a gated pulse or continuous wave mode, with bare fibers or near-contact scalpels, with or without a water spray, and in contact or noncontact applications (Figs 8.2a and 8.9). The tissue absorption model for argon is hemoglobin and hemosiderin, two pigments that are found in abundance in most oral soft tissues. Specific surgical techniques will vary considerably from one operator to another because of the versatile characteristics of the argon wavelengths. A typical cutting, vaporizing, coagulating procedure can be accomplished with the 300-μm bare fiber. With water spray and a power of 1.30 W in

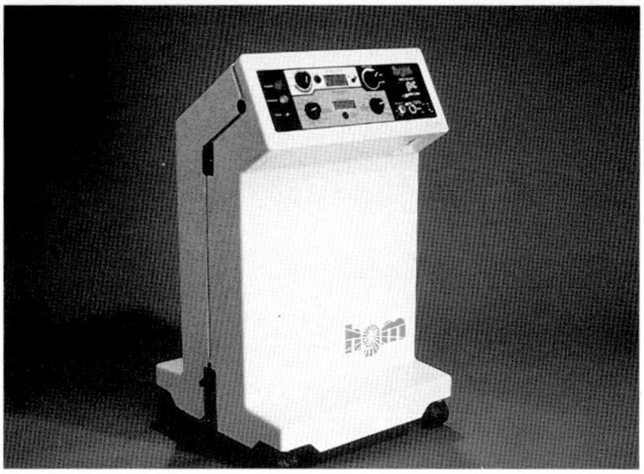

Fig 8.9 An argon dental laser (HGM Laser Corp, Salt Lake City, UT).

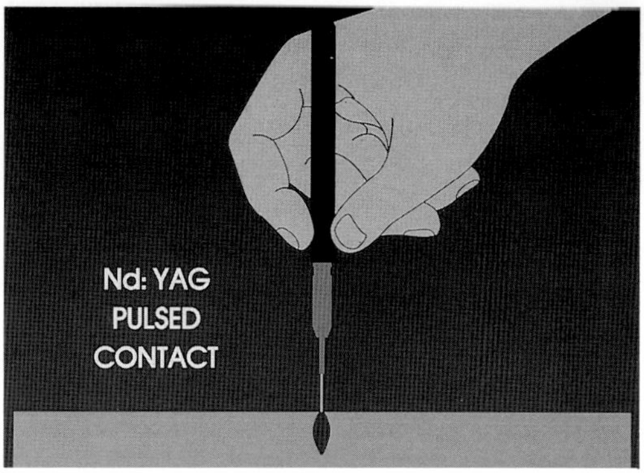

Fig 8.10 Diagram of a pulsed Nd:YAG laser.

continuous wave mode, the fiber will cut tissue with moderate speed when placed in contact with oral soft tissues. To vaporize and sculpt tissue, the fiber is kept about 5 mm out of contact. To coagulate and provide hemostasis, bring the fiber out of contact at a distance of about 1 cm. With distance as the only variable, all of these tissue effects can be accomplished with the same fiber and power setting. A water spray is always recommended during oral soft tissue procedures with the argon laser. However, these same effects can all be accomplished without water spray. Further variations make it possible to accomplish these same procedures either in contact or noncontact by varying the power setting, in gated pulse or continuous wave, or with different fiber sizes. The combination of variables to produce the same tissue result is endless and is determined primarily by the operator's individual preferences.

Surgical Characteristics of Nd:YAG Lasers

The Nd:YAG is a near infrared laser with a primary wavelength of 1,064 nm. The tissue absorption model is based on the pigments melanin and hemoglobin. Neodymium:YAG lasers are available in a free-running pulsed mode (Fig 8.10) or continuous wave with gated pulse options. Neodymium:YAG can be used either with a bare fiber, sculptured and/or sapphire-coated tip, with or without water spray, and in contact or noncontact applications (see Fig 8.2c). Some Nd:YAG lasers can be used with or without an air-and-water spray, or with various combinations of air-and-water cooling (Fig 8.11). A typical cutting, vaporizing, and coagulating procedure can be performed with a low-power, free-running pulsed Nd:YAG laser and a 320-μm bare fiber.

With an energy of 2.50 W and 20 Hz, up to 3.00 W and 100 Hz, the fiber is brought into contact with the tissue. The fiber will cut the tissue with slow-to-moderate speed. By allowing the carbonized coagulum to build up on the fiber tip without a water spray, the cutting and coagulating efficiency will be improved. By varying the energy and application time, coagulation and hemostasis can also be accomplished with this technique. Higher powered free-running pulsed Nd:YAG lasers can also accomplish these same tissue effects with

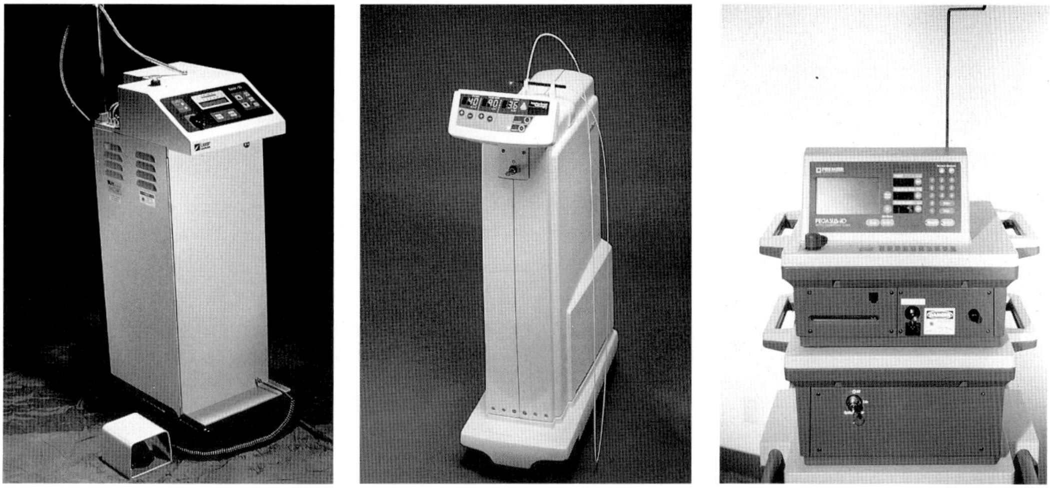

Fig 8.11 Various Nd:YAG dental lasers. **(a)**, Laser 35 with air-and-water spray (Medical Laser Technologies); **(b)**, Pulsemaster, free-running pulsed laser (American Dental Technology, Troy, MI); **(c)**, Pegasus laser with sculptured and coated tips (Premier Laser Corp, Irvine, CA).

higher power levels and a water spray without the "hot-tip" effect. By varying the power level, all of these effects can be accomplished in a contact application. Continuous wave Nd:YAG instruments can also be used to accomplish these same results with moderate power levels and sculpted and/or sapphire-coated tips. Sculpted tips direct the energy either by focusing or diffusing it into the tissue, depending on the shape of the tip. Sapphire-coated tips on the other hand absorb the laser energy and create a "hot-tip" effect. The fiber must be in contact with the tissue at all times the laser is activated, otherwise the tip will overheat and disintegrate. By varying the power levels and the shape of the tip, all of the desired tissue effects can be accomplished.

It is not recommended that continuous wave Nd:YAG laser energy for noncontact applications, and particularly bare fiber noncontact applications, be applied in the mouth. In these applications, the depth of tissue penetration and the irradiation volume is greatly increased and may result in undesirable tissue effects (see Fig 8.2b). While this provides excellent surgical applications in other areas of the body, eg, during gastrointestinal procedures where coagulation necrosis is intentional, it is not recommended for oral soft tissue applications at this time. There are a wide variety of Nd:YAG laser instruments available for dentistry and a wide variety of surgical techniques that can be applied based on operator preferences.

Surgical Characteristics of Ho:YAG Lasers

Ho:YAG is an infrared laser with a wavelength of 2,100 nm. The tissue absorption model is primarily water. Holmium:YAG is available in a free running pulsed mode, and typically delivered with a 300-μm bare fiber (Figs 8.2b and 8.12). A typical cutting, vaporizing, and coagulating procedure can be accomplished with the pulsed mode and the 300-μm fiber. With an en-

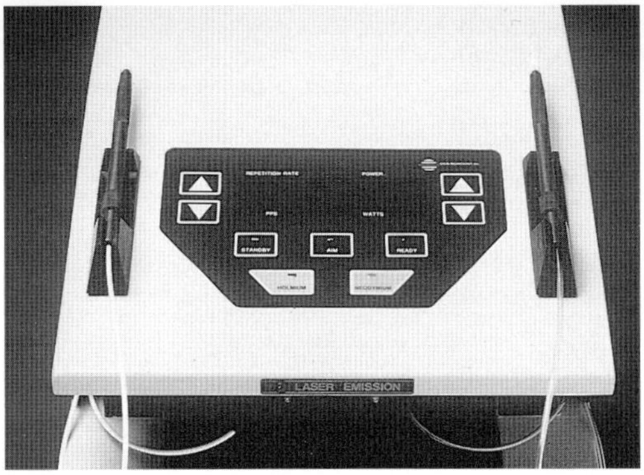

Fig 8.12 A combination Nd:YAG and Ho:YAG laser. Both lasers are housed in the same unit (Excel Quantronics, Hauppauge, NY).

ergy setting of 1.75 W and 10 Hz, the fiber will cut tissue with moderate-to-fast speed when brought into contact with the tissue. By reducing the energy density, the fiber will readily coagulate most tissues. By further reducing the exposure energy, hemostasis can be accomplished in most surgical sites in the mouth. The water absorption model for Ho:YAG and the abundance of water in most oral soft tissues make the Ho:YAG laser an efficient instrument without creating a "hot-tip" effect. This wavelength cuts and coagulates well with a clean fiber tip, which translates to less drag on the fiber for the operator. Most clinicians prefer the contact techniques for this wavelength.

While fiberoptically delivered lasers have improved accessibility in the mouth, it is important to realize that not every procedure can be accomplished with a laser alone. Contact and noncontact laser applications improve traditional surgical techniques. Excellent results can be achieved by combining the advantages of laser technology with traditional instruments and materials.

Acknowledgments

Special thanks to Bill Brown, Wendy Ochs, Alan Anderson, and David Sparks.

Part III

Current Applications of Lasers in Dentistry

Current Applications of Lasers in Dentistry

In the preceding chapters, the fundamental concepts of lasers provided an understanding of lasers as electro-optic devices. The practical aspects of laser operation, such as how laser light is generated, what may occur when laser light interacts with tissue, and some current concerns about laser education, safety standards, and regulations, provide the background needed by practitioners to more fully understand the basic principles of the clinical applications of lasers.

The chapters in Part III introduce the laser as a surgical tool or instrument. Although they are not surgical instruments in the classical sense, lasers may be used to replace traditional dental instruments for a variety of purposes. Traditionally, the procedures commonly performed in dentistry involve the mechanical action of rigid metal instruments to either cut, drill, or abrade hard and soft tissues. Dental treatment can be simplified to be understood as the process of removing infected or pathologic tissue either by drilling or cutting away the diseased component. Lasers may be effectively used in dentistry due to their ability to cut, incise, and ablate hard and soft tissues.

Other inherent properties of laser light, such as selective absorption, coagulation, sterilization, and stimulatory effects on vital structures offer some advantages over traditional techniques, making lasers the treatment of choice in certain situations. The potential benefits derived from laser treatment depend largely on the unique properties of laser energy at a particular wavelength and its interaction with dental tissues.

It is important to recognize that to apply this new technology to dentistry, the results must be not only similar or equivalent to results of established technology, but superior. Still the question remains—will experimental methods of treatment be tolerated in vivo? Caution is required in interpreting the results of experimental or clinical reports. It is important not to prematurely assume the applicability of a particular treatment before sufficient evidence substantiates both its safety and efficacy. It is also important to recognize the limitations of our current understanding of the long-term effects of laser energy on oral tissues and the mechanisms by which lasers affect biologic systems.

The chapters in this section are organized by laser type but not according to relative applicability or importance. Although many of the contributors to this section possess knowledge and experience in several laser types, most have distinguished themselves by their work with a particular wavelength. While some practitioners may suggest their preference for a particular wavelength or system for an application, the reader should be aware that most dental surgical procedures are not exclusive to specific laser systems or manufacturer brands. The reader will also observe that there is overlap between the various procedures presented in this section. This is simply because all lasers currently used in dentistry have been approved by the Food and Drug Administration for soft tissue surgery. The argon laser has also been approved for the polymerization of composite resin restorative materials.

Most of procedures described can be performed effectively by any type of laser regardless of wavelength (Table I). Listed in the table are some of the most common procedures and laser types currently being used or approved for use in dentistry. Ap-

Table I. Clinical Applications of Lasers in Dentistry

Clinical Application	Argon	CO_2	Ho:YAG	Nd:YAG
Maxillary midline frenectomy	X	X	X	X
Lingual frenectomy	X	X	X	X
Crown lengthening	X	X	X	X
Biopsy	X	X	X	X
White lesions	?	X	?	?
Malignant lesions	X	X	X	X
Aphthous ulcers	X	X	X	X
Coagulation	X	X	X	X
Hemorrhage disorders	X	X	X	X
Caries removal	?	X	?	—
Caries detection	X	—	—	X
Degranulation	X	X	X	X
Guided tissue regeneration	X	X	X	X
Analgesia	—	—	—	X*
Distal wedge	X	X	X	X
Tuberosity reduction	X	X	X	X
Scaling	X	—	X	X
Hypersensitivity	X	X	X	X
Gingivectomy	X	X	X	X
Gingivoplasty	X	X	X	X
Inflammatory papillary hyperplasia	—	X	—	—
Epuli	X	X	X	X
Vestibuloplasty	X	X	X	X
Implant exposure	X	X	?†	?†
Troughing	X	X	X	X
Composite curing	X	—	—	—

*Must be a pulsed Nd:YAG laser; †More research needed; ? Either no available information or additional research needed.

proval of lasers for treatment of hard tissues, including enamel, dentin, cementum, and bone, is still pending, and some procedures may be considered experimental in some countries. Unless otherwise stated, most dental procedures in this section are presented for illustrative purposes and are not exclusive to a particular laser system.

Lasers in Dentistry is intended to be used by an international audience, therefore some of the information and clinical applications may be viewed as experimental in some jurisdictions. Acceptable standards of practice vary based on regional norms. Ultimately, it is the responsibility of the dental practitioner to provide appropriate forms of treatment based on the specific needs of their patients. Before using lasers for any clinical procedures, including those presented here, practitioners should acquire the necessary skills by completing a formal dental laser training course. Practitioners should also contact their local governing boards about the suitability of laser use for the particular procedures they intend to perform.

As we approach the twenty-first century, we in dentistry are faced with the challenge of mastering a rapidly changing technology. Exploring and understanding the possibilities will enable us to discover better ways to serve our patients and to grow professionally. Entry into the second millennium means adapting to this ever-changing technology, an evolution from simple mechanics to the boundless era of electro-optics.

Chapter Nine

Surgical Applications of the Argon Laser

V. Kim Kutsch and Richard J. Blankenau

The argon laser, the active medium of which is argon gas, was first used in medicine in the 1960s. Energy passing through the laser's ion gas laser head and reflective mirrors generates coherent visible light with primary wavelengths of 488 and 514.5 nm. This laser light is then directed through flexible silica-quartz fibers and easily delivered to any accessible site of the body. Medicine recognized the special properties of this blue-green visible light, and the argon laser has become a valuable instrument in many specialties, including ophthalmology, otolaryngology, gynecology, and dermatology.

Specific Argon Laser-Tissue Interactions

The visible blue-green argon laser light wavelengths of 488 and 514.5 nm have specific interactions with tissues. In physical terms, the peak absorption of blue-green light is in red pigment such as hemoglobin; thus, the laser energy is well absorbed in pigmented tissues in general, and specifically in tissue with an abundance of hemoglobin, hemosiderin, and melanin. Argon laser energy is not well absorbed by enamel and dentin or other nonpigmented tissues eg, fibrotic tissues, and it is very poorly absorbed by water. These characteristics make argon laser energy very useful for cutting, vaporizing, coagulating, and providing hemostasis on gingiva and oral mucosa within the oral cavity (Dixon et al, 1986; Hohenleutner et al, 1991; Neumann et al, 1991). This can be accomplished with relative ease without the laser energy being absorbed by the teeth adjacent to the target tissue.

The argon laser can be applied with a contact or noncontact technique. An advantage of the argon laser is the versatility achieved by moving the fiber closer to or further from the tissue. As the laser fiber is moved from contact to further away from the target tissue, the power density decreases, lowering the resultant tissue temperature, which diminishes the ultimate tissue effect. The tissue effects from the argon laser are thermal in nature. As the tissue is progressively heated from body temperature, the following effects occur, respectively: reversible warming or hyperthermia, coagulation, welding, vaporization, cutting, charring, and rapid cutting. The practitioner can alter the tissue effect from cutting to vaporizing to coagulating by changing the power density at the tissue surface by moving the fiber in and out of focus with the target tissue. This characteristic of the argon laser results in appreciable versatility in its use.

Characteristics of Argon Laser Instruments

When activated, the argon laser cavity generates considerable heat, which is either air-cooled with a baffle and fan or liquid-cooled with an external fluid source (generally water) or internally contained with a radiator and fan. Newer argon lasers also control heat by operating by power on demand, where the laser head is activated only for the duration of a given pulse.

Most argon lasers are powered with a 220-V electrical source; however, some lower-powered 110-V units are available. Microprocessors in the argon lasers offer either continuous wave operation or a gaited pulse mode, with the shortest pulse available being 0.01 sec. For general dental purposes, a clinician will need an instrument with a maximum continuous energy output of about 2.0 W (Table). Fiberoptic delivery systems are available with a diameter range from 50 to 600 μm as well as with contact laser scalpel handpieces. Other options, eg, external meters, pulse counters, He:Ne aiming beams, etc, are also readily available.

Argon lasers are class IV medical devices and are subject to FDA, ANSI, and OSHA safety standards. Eye or skin exposure to direct or scattered visible radiation should be avoided. Argon laser protective lenses are orange and must be worn by the patient and all persons in the treatment room.

Argon Laser–Assisted Root Planing and Curettage

In gingival curettage, the inner wall of the periodontal pocket is debrided to convert a pathologic gingival attachment to a state of health (Boucher, 1988). Curettage removes the pathologic sulcular epithelium, leaving a new wound site to allow for healing and a return to physiologic health.

Table. Settings for Commonly Used Procedures in Treatment

Mode	Power (W)	Fiber	Purpose
Continuous	0.080	300 μm	Caries illumination
10 s	0.500	300 μm	Photopolymerization
Continuous	0.50–1.00	300 μm	Hemostasis
Continuous	1.00–1.25	300 μm	Gingival retraction
Pulsed	0.500–0.850	300 μm	De-epithelialization
Continuous	1.00–1.80	300 μm	Gingivectomy/gingivoplasty
Continuous	1.00–2.25	Laser scalpel	Frenectomy
Continuous	1.00–2.25	Laser scalpel	Incision/excision
Continuous	1.00	300 μm	Oral lesion therapy
Continuous	0.50–1.00	300 μm	Tissue welding

Closed gingival curettage is instrumentation by way of the lumen of the pocket to remove the soft tissue wall of a pocket and the connective (fibrous) tissue, subjacent to the level of the alveolar crest (Grant et al, 1988). Application of laser energy for curettage is the photocoagulation or vaporization of soft or fibrous tissue within the periodontal pocket subjacent to the alveolar crest. Curettage is normally performed in conjunction with root scaling and planing to remove calcified deposits and plaque. This nonsurgical debridement also disrupts and removes the pathologic bacteria that have invaded the sulcular epithelium and underlying gingival connective tissue (Henry et al, 1992a, b).

The argon laser may be used as an alternate instrument to remove the sulcular epithelium and disrupt the invading bacteria. The fiber is inserted into the periodontal pocket, directed toward the epithelial lining, and photocoagulation and vaporization (laser de-epithelialization) are performed in a thorough manner. Applied with pulsed energies, this procedure can normally be performed without the use of local anesthesia. After de-epithelialization and hand instrumentation, the laser fiber is returned to the sulcus to provide disruption of bacterial recolonization and to provide hemostasis.

Initial laser instrumentation is performed with the 300-μm fiber. It is inserted into the sulcus, with a pulse duration of 0.05 sec (interval between pulses, 0.20 sec), resulting in a pulse rate of 4 Hz. Begin with an energy of 500 to 750 mW, adjusted in increments of 50 mW, based on the patient's comfort level. Thoroughly expose the sulcular epithelium with the laser radiation. Direct the tip of the fiber toward the epithelium, and avoid prolonged contact with the root surface and alveolar bone. The power densities at the fiber tip will range from 700 to 1,200 W/cm^2, producing tissue temperatures of 50°C to 90°C. At these power densities, the argon laser will not efficiently cut fibrous tissue, but care should be taken not to destroy the existing periodontal attachment. During this procedure, always provide high-speed evacuation within 2 cm of the operative site. Topical anesthetic may be applied to increase patient comfort, but most patients tolerate this procedure very well without any anesthesia.

After the initial exposure, about 30 to 45 sec per tooth, the power level can be increased to 0.75 to 0.85 W. The most efficient de-epithelialization occurs at this energy level with the 300-μm fiber. Some practitioners prefer the 600-μm fiber for this procedure, but the 300-μm fiber approximates the size of most periodontal probes and can be inserted into any sulcus with less difficulty. Spend about 45 to 60 sec in each pocket, or until the sulcus has been thoroughly exposed. The preferred technique is to sweep the fiber along the epithelium, being careful not to exert too much lateral force on the fiber, which may result in fiber breakage. Some patients may tolerate continuous wave delivery instead of the pulsed mode, which will be more time efficient.

During this procedure, the coagulated epithelium will be clearly evident and may need to be wiped from the fiber tip with a sterile 2 × 2 cotton gauze. The charred epithelial remnants may also be left on the fiber tip, which will create a "hot-tip" effect, where the laser energy is being absorbed by the charred material heating the tip of the fiber. This can also be an efficient technique for de-epithelialization. Additional variations of this procedure would be to add a water spray to the operative site. This will cool the tissue, reduce the risk of lateral tissue damage, and flush the coagulated epithelium from the site, keeping the fiber tip clean. It will also, however, slow the thermal efficiency to the tissue debridement and may require an increase in power setting. The energy will need to be adjusted according to patient comfort, amount of tissue pigmentation present, and the fibrous quality of the gingival tissues.

The advantages in using a laser to assist in root planing and curettage include: increased patient comfort during the procedure with reduced need for local anesthesia; reduced postoperative complications, discomfort, inflammation, and edema, with reduced need for postoperative analgesics; conservative yet thorough depithelialization; hemorrhage control in the operative field; bacterial reduction in the sulcus; and improved patient acceptance of treatment and follow-up. Laser wounds also delay epithelial response, allowing more access time for the periodontal ligament cells to attach to the root surface during the healing and reattachment phase.

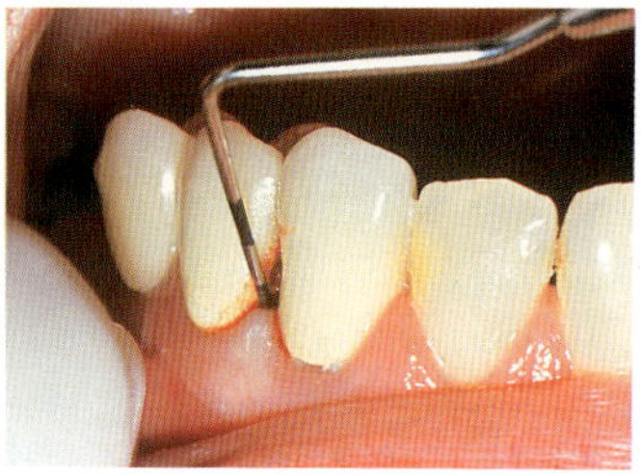

Fig 9.1a Preoperative probing maxillary right canine.

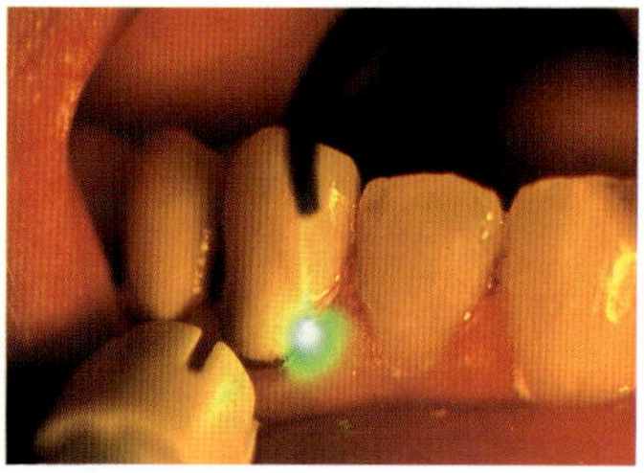

Fig 9.1b Argon laser fiber performing de-epithelialization.

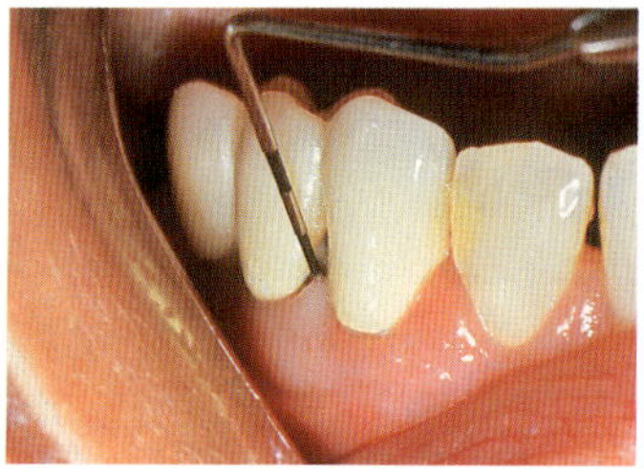

Fig 9.1c Appearance 28 days after surgery.

Case 1

A 37-year-old white woman had class II periodontal disease. She was a cigarette smoker, but otherwise her medical history was unremarkable. The patient presented with generalized 3- to 5-mm pockets with some bleeding on probing, isolated minor alveolar bone loss, and minimal mobility. The first step in treatment was a preliminary debridement with root planing and curettage. The periodontal pocketing was evident on the distofacial region of the maxillary right canine (Fig 9.1a). The 300-µm fiber was placed into the sulcus to perform the de-epithelialization (Fig 9.1b), and the irradiation volume of the visible green 514.5-nm wavelength laser energy was evident. This was followed with conventional instrumentation, in this case a Gracey curette, to accomplish the root planing. At 28 days after surgery, the tissue appearance had improved (Fig 9.1c).

Laser-assisted root planing and curettage have been greatly debated within the periodontal specialty. The purpose of this material is not to argue the indications and contraindications based on the published scientific literature, but to provide the practitioner with an adequate description of the technique for this application.

Argon Laser–Assisted Gingival Retraction

Argon laser energy has peak absorption in hemoglobin, thus lending itself to providing excellent hemostasis and efficient coagulation and vaporization of oral tissues. These characterisitics are beneficial for retraction and hemostasis of the gingival tissue in preparation for an impression during a crown and bridge procedure (Kutsch, 1993).

Following traditional preparation of the teeth, the argon laser is used to provide hemostasis and retract the gingival tissue. With a 300-μm fiber, and a power setting of 1.0 W, continuous wave delivery, the fiber is inserted into the sulcus in contact with the tissue. In a sweeping motion, the fiber is moved around the tooth. It is important to contact the fiber tip with the bleeding vessels. Provide suction in the field; most clinicians prefer a water spray. This technique, which will provide a power density of 1,400 W/cm^2 at the fiber tip and create tissue temperatures of 90°C to 100°C, will coagulate the small bleeding vessels and remove the sulcular lining epithelium, allowing for a clean impression.

Variations of this technique include different-sized fibers and energy settings, with or without the water spray. The water rinses the field of blood and allows for good exposure of the open vessels; otherwise all of the energy would be absorbed in the surface of the blood and the underlying vessel would be unaffected. The water also rinses the coagulated epithelium from the site and helps keep the tip of the fiber clean, as well as cooling the tissue and reducing lateral thermal damage. Like the laser-assisted curettage procedure, by not using water spray and allowing the charred epithelial remnants to remain on the fiber tip, a "hot-tip" effect can be created, increasing thermal efficiency. Some clinicans also prefer to provide the hemostasis out of contact, with a water spray to flush the blood from the sulcus. Depending on the amount of pigment and vascularity present in the tissue, the power may be adjusted up or down slightly. Some clinicians use the argon laser for hemostasis only and provide retraction with a retraction cord. This technique works very well, and the impression cord needs to remain packed for only 3 to 4 min before taking the final impression. The argon laser may be used at this point for crown lengthening by gingivectomy or gingivoplasty to further expose the crown margins. The power may be increased to 1.25 W for faster tissue removal.

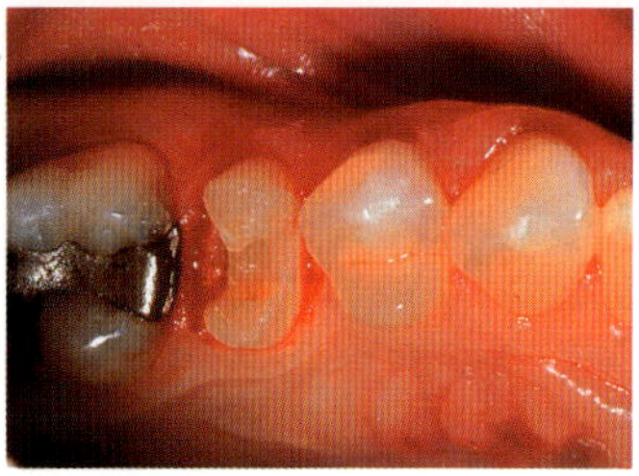

Fig 9.2a After traditional preparation for a three-quarters precious-metal crown.

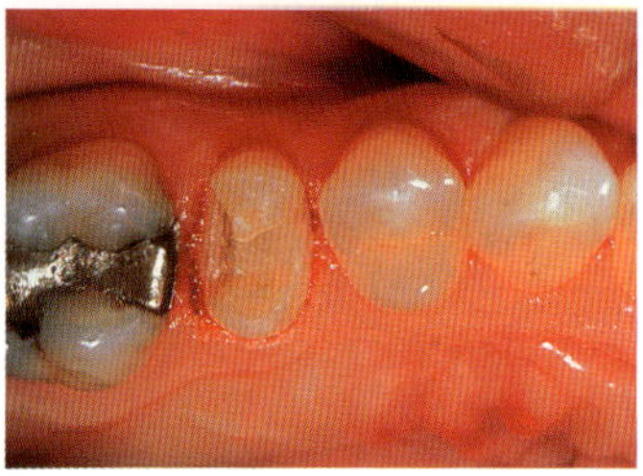

Fig 9.2b Retraction complete and ready for the final impression.

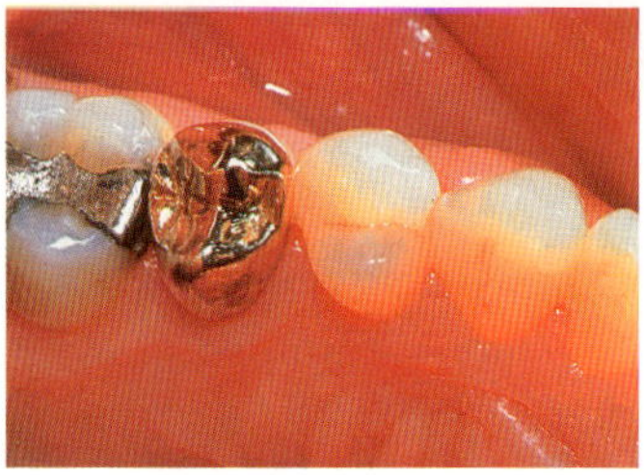

Fig 9.2c Restoration and gingival tissues 28 days after surgery.

Case 2

A 47-year-old white man with an unremarkable medical history presented with a failing restoration on the maxillary second premolar. The existing restoration and decay were removed, and the tooth was prepared for a three-quarters precious-metal crown. The sulcular epithelium had been traumatized, and there was bleeding in the sulcus (Fig 9.2a). The 300-μm fiber was used in contact, at 1.0 W, continuous wave, to provide hemostasis. The hemostasis was immediate with the argon laser, and the total operating time in the sulcus was less than 30 sec. For gingival tissue retraction, the operating time increased to about 60 sec. Without a water spray, the epithelial remnants build up on the fiber tip. On completion of the hemostasis and retraction procedure, the sulcus was clean and the tissue was slightly retracted without excessive thermal damage or charring (Figs 9.2b and c). The tissue appeared very healthy around the final restoration 28 days after surgery (Fig 9.2d). Using a laser to provide hemostasis and gingival retraction results in excellent conservative care and significant time savings for the clinician.

Gingivectomy/Gingivoplasty

The removal and recontouring of gingival tissues can be easily accomplished with the argon laser. The laser can be used as a primary surgical instrument to remove excessive gingival tissue, whether diseased, secondary to drug therapy or orthodontic treatment, or congenital. The laser will remove the tissue and provide hemostasis and tissue weld the wound.

When rapidly removing tissue or creating incisions with a laser, as a general rule, local anesthesia will be required. Some clinicians will use a form of topical anesthetic and then cool the tissue with a water spray. For time efficiency, however, it is better to begin with the aid of local anesthesia. Like the de-epithelialization and retraction procedures, there is a variety of techniques to accomplish the desired tissue removal. While all of the variations are effective, the clinician must develop a technique he or she is comfortable with. A recommended technique is to use the 300-μm fiber in contact, at 1.0 to 1.8 W, continuous wave, with a water spray. This will create power densities of 1,400 to 2,600 W/cm^2 at the fiber tip and tissue temperatures of 100°C to 150°C. The power will need to be adjusted in this range based on the pigmentation and fibrous characteristics of the patient's tissue. The goal is to accomplish efficient tissue removal with minimal thermal damage to the surrounding tissues. The fiber is placed against the tissue, and in a sweeping motion the tissue is either coagulated or it is incised. Because the argon wavelengths are not well absorbed by hard tissues, no special precaution is necessary to protect the teeth and alveolar bone. However, these tissues should not be carelessly exposed.

General variations of this technique include different fiber sizes, power levels, with or without water spray, and/or a "hot-tip" effect, and in or out of contact. For the gingivectomy procedures, combinations of all of the variations can be effective depending on the clinician's developing preferences. Most clinicians prefer a contact technique with a 300-μm fiber.

Case 3

A 17-year-old white girl had redundant gingival tissue on the maxillary anterior teeth (Fig 9.3a). With local anesthesia, the argon laser was used to perform the gingivectomy procedure and expose these teeth. A 300-μm fiber was used with 1.3 W, continuous wave, in contact to remove the tissue. No water spray was used, which resulted in a "hot-tip" effect but also a slight charring of the tissue. The bloodless tissue removal and visible irradiation volume of the argon laser was clearly evident (Fig 9.3b). (A water spray would have reduced the amount of charring to the lateral tissues, which would have resulted in slightly less inflammation during the healing phase.) After tissue removal, the gingiva had the typical appearance of a laser thermal wound (Fig 9.3c). The tissue exhibited excellent health 28 days after surgery with healing completed (Fig 9.3d).

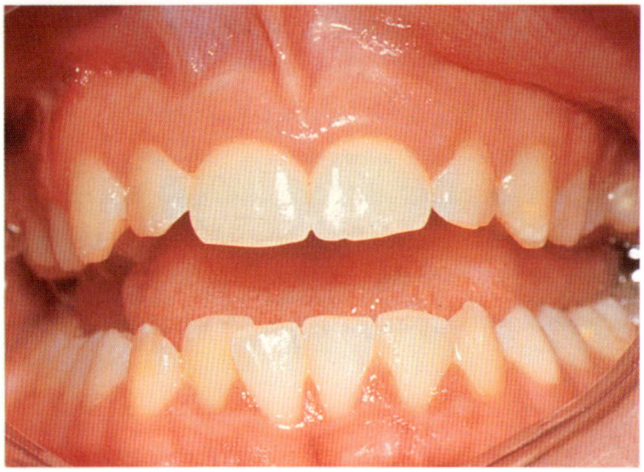

Fig 9.3a Preoperative appearance of the maxillary anterior teeth.

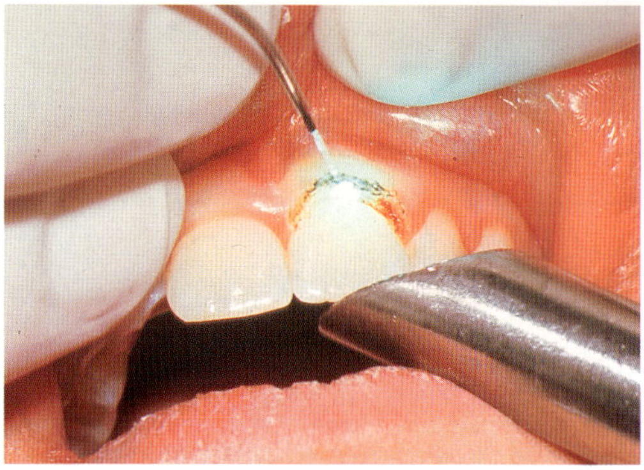

Fig 9.3b Argon laser ablating the excessive gingival tissues.

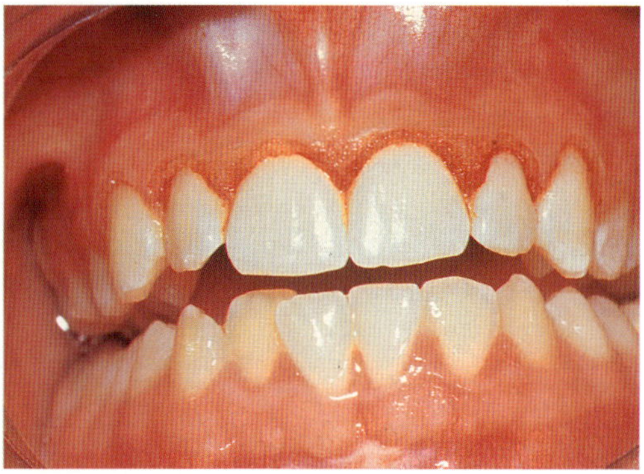

Fig 9.3c Immediately after surgery.

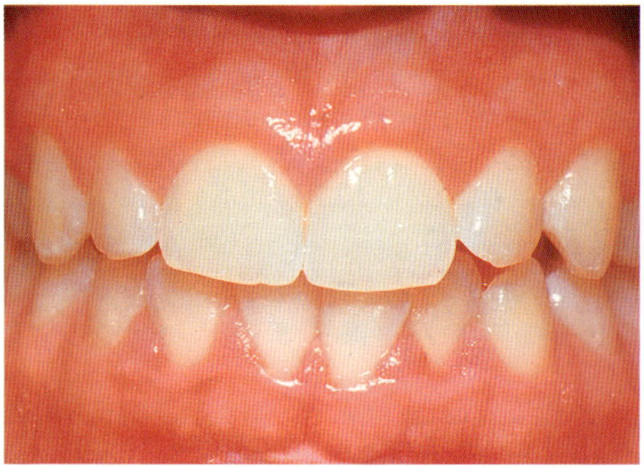

Fig 9.3d Final healing at 28 days after surgery.

The advantages in using a laser for these types of surgical procedures include a bloodless field, fewer postoperative complications, reduced postoperative discomfort, and a patient perception that these wounds heal faster. While this perception is not necessarily true, because of the significantly reduced postoperative discomfort the patient experiences an easier recovery. There is generally no need to place a periodontal dressing on these wounds, sutures are rarely required, and postoperative analgesics are rarely prescribed. Again, the laser provides excellent and conservative care.

Laser-Assisted Frenectomy

The argon laser is a valuable tool in performing frenectomy procedures. While the argon laser is very effective in cutting fibrous tissue at higher energies, it is also particularly beneficial for lingual frenectomies because of the hemostatic properties of argon laser light. The use of the argon laser during these procedures results in efficient tissue removal with a bloodless field.

As with all surgical techniques for the argon laser, there are numerous effective combinations of treatment parameters. However, as with all procedures, one technique generally enjoys the most popularity. Frenectomy is a procedure that is very well suited to surgical contact laser scalpel handpieces. Rather than use a bare fiber, a contact laser scalpel is the instrument of choice. With the laser set at 1.0 to 2.25 W, continuous wave delivery, the laser scalpel is placed on the frenular tissue, which is excised. Water spray may be used, but evacuation is always provided in the surgical site to remove the plume. This will result in power densities of 1,400 to 3,200 W/cm^2 and result in tissue temperatures of 100°C to 175°C. The tissue is removed with conventional standards for incision design. Care is taken not to damage vital structures in the surgical envelope, eg, Wharton's ducts. The frenum can literally be cut away. Excellent hemostasis occurs, sutures are not required, and the patient experiences minimal discomfort during the healing period.

The goal of the surgery is to release the attachment with minimal damage to the surrounding tissues. The laser power will need to be adjusted within the suggested range, based on the pigmentation and fibrous characteristics of the tissue and the desired speed of cutting.

Variations of this technique involve the use of bare fibers, in or out of contact, and with or without water spray. Some clinicians prefer to perform noncontact surgery with the argon laser. However, this requires application of higher powers, larger spot sizes, less precision and control, and generally results in more damage to the surrounding tissues. The goal of all laser surgeries is to perform the task efficiently with the least amount of energy, and result in as little tissue damage as possible.

Oral Lesion Therapy

The ability of laser energy to vaporize and coagulate surface tissue makes the argon laser an adjunctive instrument in treating a variety of oral lesions. The laser can be used to remove the surface epithelium and necrotic tissue cells from aphthous ulcers and herpetic lesions, and it can be used to coagulate and excise vascular lesions of the lip and oral mucosa (Sexton et al, 1993). The goal of the laser therapy is to remove the necrotic tissue from the surface, reduce the size of the lesion, disinfect the remaining wound, and create a conservative thermal laser wound that will heal with less postoperative discomfort and fewer complications. Oral lesion therapy tends to be one of the more uncomfortable procedures performed with a laser; therefore, a topical anesthetic is generally applied.

The recommended technique involves using the laser out of contact, creating a spot size large enough to cover the entire lesion. Any size fiber may be selected, although for simplicity we prefer to use the 300-μm bare fiber. Set the laser at 1.0-W, continuous wave, and begin exposing the lesion. Adjust the energy setting up or down slightly for patient comfort. Time of application becomes the variable factor between patients. A 5-mm spot size with 1.0 W of power will create power density of 5 W/cm^2, resulting in tissue temperatures of 60°C after 30 sec of application, and continued application will result in higher tissue temperatures adequate to begin a slow ablation of the surface cell layer. It generally takes from 2 to 3 minutes to coagulate a 5- to 8-mm diameter aphthous ulcer. The laser is applied until the lesion has a dessicated appearance and the necrotic cells have a glazed appearance. With this level of thermal change in the tissue, an aphthous ulcer will generally heal in 4 to 5 days, regardless of the age of the lesion. While an untreated aphthous ulcer will heal in 10 to 14 days without any treatment, after laser therapy the patient will be much more comfortable than if the lesion was not treated.

Always provide evacuation in the operative field. Variations of the technique involve different size fiber and energy settings. Some clinicians prefer to operate in contact and coagulate and even char the surface of the lesion. This results in greater tissue damage, however, and requires a longer healing phase. Because laser wounds tend to heal with little discomfort and few complications, the patient will experience significant and immediate relief from the oral lesions, many of which are quite painful. Little else can be offered as true treatment for these lesions.

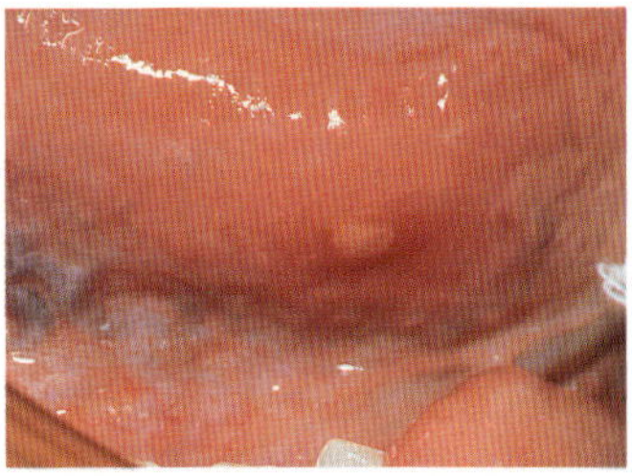

Fig 9.4a An aphthous ulceration of the tongue of 4 days duration.

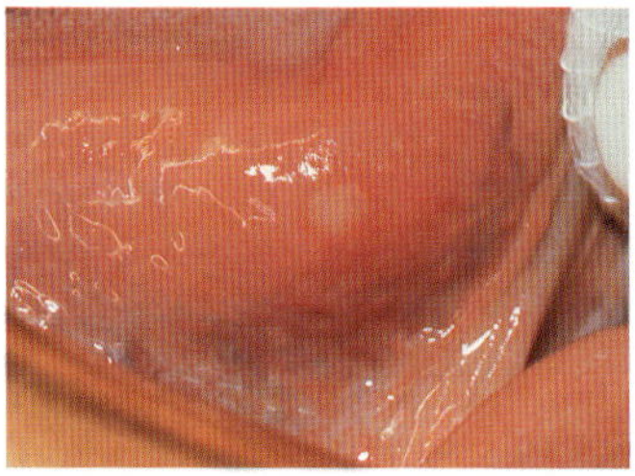

Fig 9.4b Immediate postoperative view of the lesion.

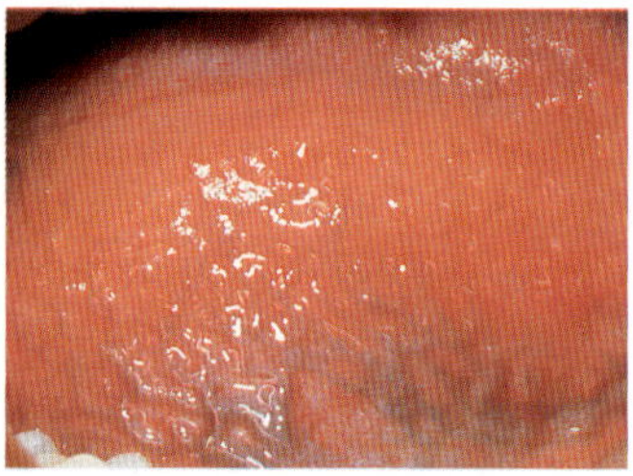

Fig 9.4c Complete healing appearance of the lesion at 5 days after surgery.

Case 4

A 47-year-old hispanic woman had an aphthous ulcer on the lateral inferior border of the tongue. The lesion was about 4 mm in diameter and of 4 days duration (Fig 9.4a). The argon laser energy was applied at 1.0-W energy, continuous wave, with the 300-μm fiber out of contact, at a distance far enough to create a spot size to cover the entire lesion. Immediately following the laser therapy, in this instance applied for 2 minutes, the lesion was reduced in size and had a glazed appearance. There was a dramatic reduction in the amount of visible inflammation surrounding the lesion (Fig 9.4b). At 5 days after surgery, there was complete healing and the patient reported no discomfort during the remaining 5 days (Fig 9.4c).

The argon laser provides potential therapy for lesions of the mouth, whether of viral, bacterial, or traumatic origin. This procedure is efficient and the results are predictable.

Argon Laser Tissue Welding

Argon lasers have been used in medicine for vascular tissue welding, the fusing of vascular tissues by laser thermal welding. Argon laser welding has been proven superior to sutures in thin- and thick-walled vessels (White et al, 1986). It has been reported to be effective in sealing both large vessels as well as arteriovenous anastomoses (White et al, 1987a, b, c). Argon laser welding has been used in arterial incisions (Kopchok et al, 1988; Crew et al, 1989). It appears that the mechanism for tissue welding is based on cross-linking or degrading extracellular matrix proteins (Murray et al, 1989). Argon laser vascular welding requires the approximation of tissue in a bloodless interface with low power, about 0.5 to 1.0 W. The use of laser energy has the advantage of fewer foreign body reactions due to the absence of suture material; preservation of the mechanical properties of the tissues; decreased intimal hyperplasia, and unrestricted enlargement of growing vessels. The argon laser can also be expected to provide hemostasis and seal bleeding vessels that are up to 1.5 mm in diameter. These characteristics make the argon laser an important surgical tool for hemostatic control and tissue welding in dentistry.

The argon laser can be used as an adjunctive instrument to coagulate bleeding vessels and provide a bloodless surgical field; approximate and weld scalpel incisions and flaps; weld the tissue surface during excisional procedures; as well as create primary incisions. By moving the fiber in and out of focus to change the power densities, the argon laser can easily be used to cut, vaporize, or coagulate tissue during a surgery.

To provide hemostasis and coagulate bleeding vessels, the blood must be removed from the field by rinsing with water, or the fiber tip must contact the vessel end. When welding the tissue surface of an excisional procedure, the fiber can be held out of contact and directed over the wound site with a water spray to remove the blood, or the fiber tip can be brushed lightly and rapidly in contact with the tissue surface. The fiber of choice is the 300-μm bare fiber, with the power set at 1.0 W, continuous wave delivery. This will create a power density of 1,400 W/cm^2, and moving the fiber tip quickly over the tissue surface will create the 50°C to 70°C temperature needed to weld the surface. The tissue should be free of bleeding and have a glazed appearance. Creating a wound that has a significant amount of blanched coagulated tissue is a result of using too much energy or too long of an application. The power setting and time of application should be adjusted appropriately for each patient.

With experience, the clinician will get a feel for how the power density and application time relate to the tissue temperature and resultant effects. Because the typical surgical instruments clinicians have used are mechanical and the laser is noncontact, most clinicians are initially uncomfortable with lasers. The laser is a precise beam of light that creates nonspecific thermal effects in the tissue, and the operator must learn to manipulate and control these thermal effects.

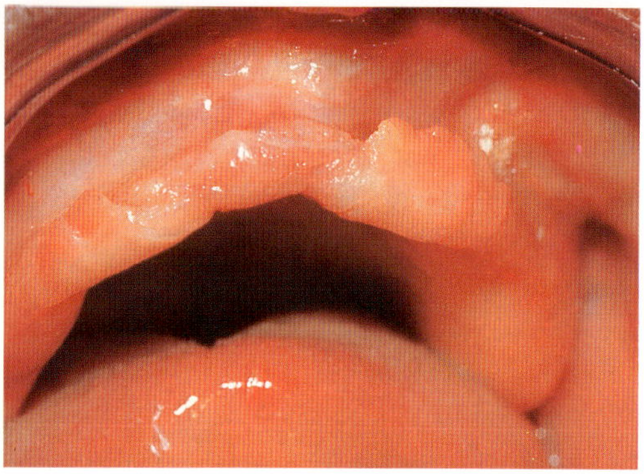

Fig 9.5a Preoperative appearance of the maxillary epulis lesion.

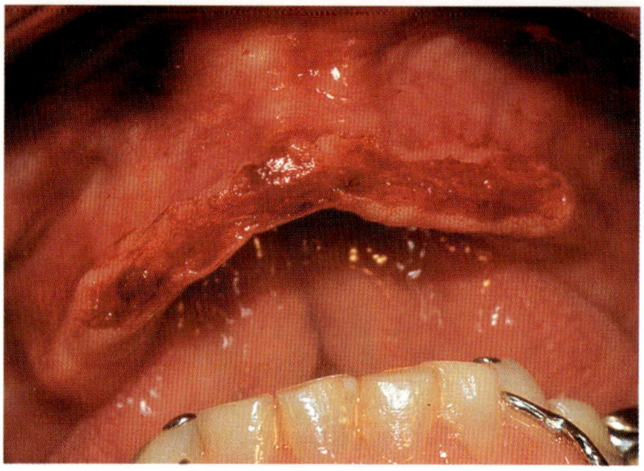

Fig 9.5b Immediately following laser welding.

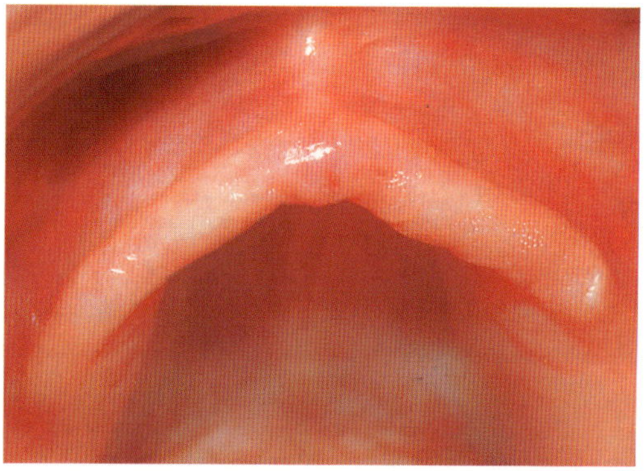

Fig 9.5c Appearance at 28 days after surgery.

Case 5

A 49-year-old white man with an unremarkable medical history and an edentulous maxilla presented with a large epulis lesion on the anterior alveolar ridge (Fig 9.5a). With local anesthesia, the lesion was removed with a scalpel. The wound site was then welded with the argon laser, in contact, 300-µm fiber, 1.0 W, with evacuation, for a total operating time of 2 minutes. The wound appeared glazed after the laser welding and there was excellent hemostasis (Fig 9.5b). The wound then healed without complication or discomfort and at 28 days after surgery was completely healed (Fig 9.5c).

The argon laser can be used to weld all incisions and excisions of oral soft tissues. This results in excellent treatment and healing for all surgical sites, including biopsy and tissue donor sites.

Excision of Traumatic Hemangioma

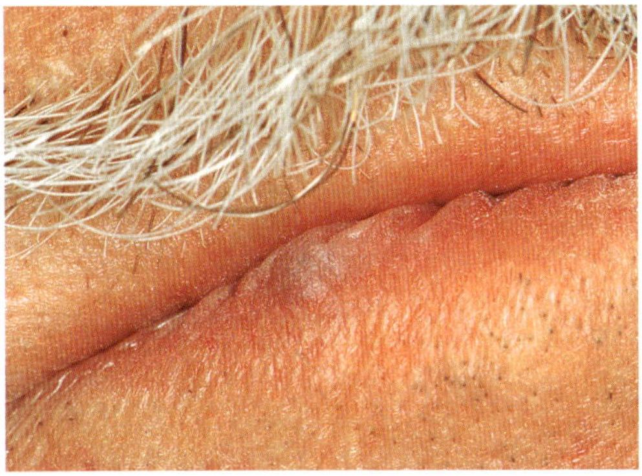

Fig 9.6a Labial hemangioma before treatment.

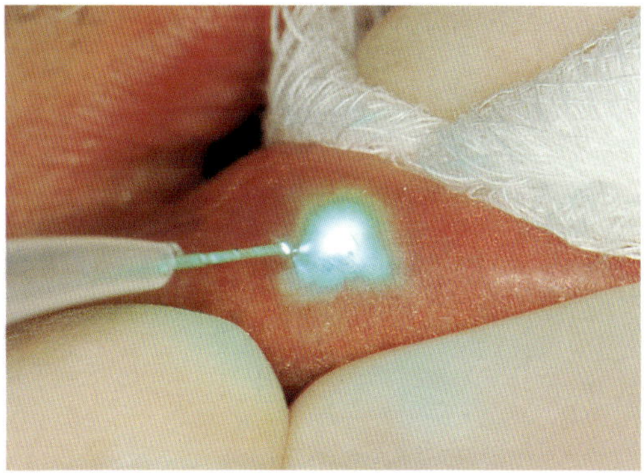

Fig 9.6b Excision of lesion (contact mode).

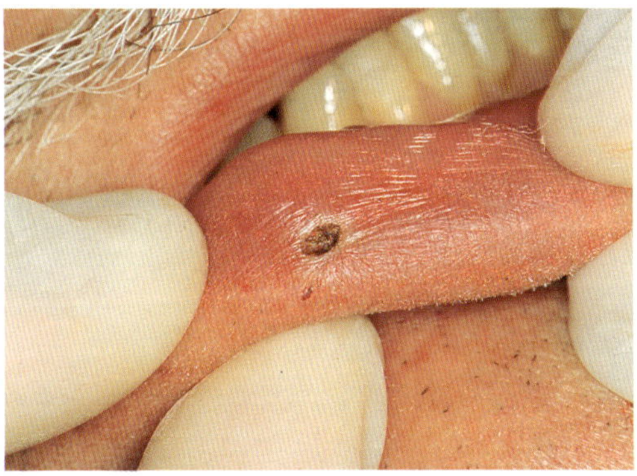

Fig 9.6c Immediate postoperative appearance. Note complete hemostasis.

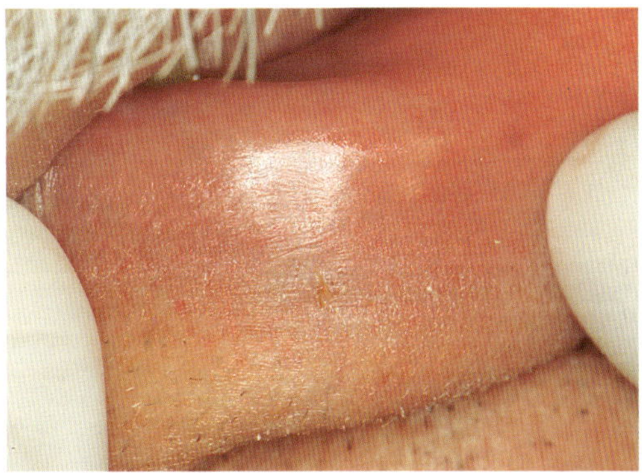

Fig 9.6d Normal appearance 2 weeks postoperatively.

Case 6

A 65-year-old man sustained an injury to his lower lip 9 months previously that resulted in the formation of a hemangioma (Fig 9.6a). The argon laser, operating at 2 W with a 200-µm fiber, was used to remove the hemangioma (Figs 9.6b and c). Two weeks postoperatively, healing was complete (Fig 9.6d). This procedure was performed with local anesthesia. The patient tolerated the procedure very well and required no postoperative analgesia.

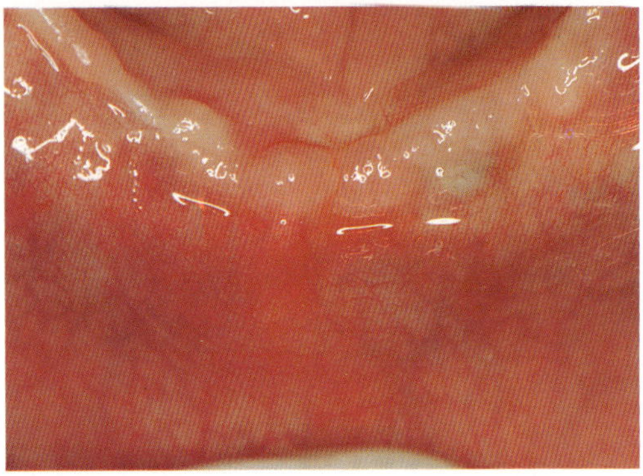

Fig 9.7a Mandibular ridge following stage 1 healing phase.

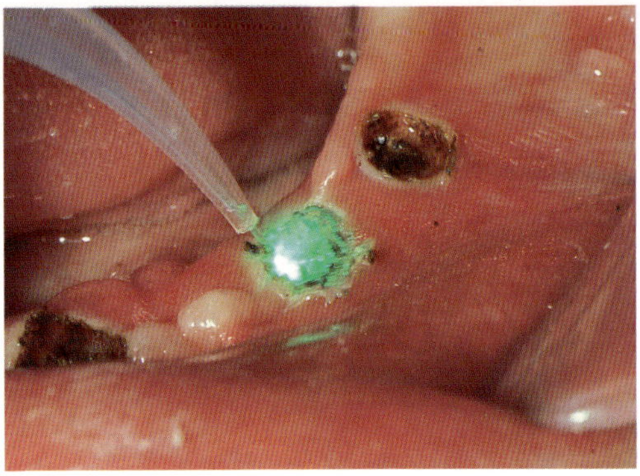

Fig 9.7b Exposure of integrated implants by argon laser recovery.

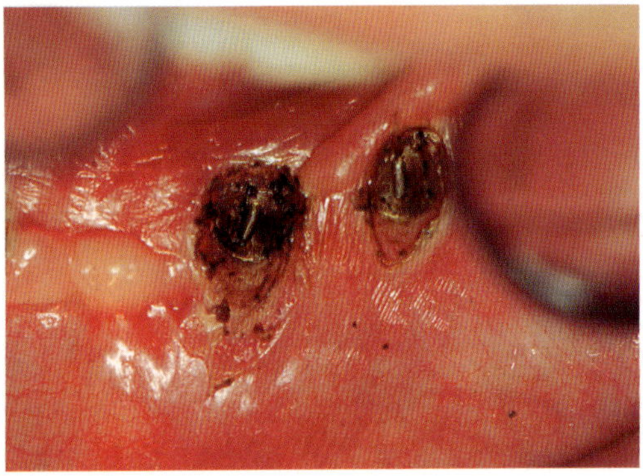

Fig 9.7c Surgical site with implants exposed and gingival recontour.

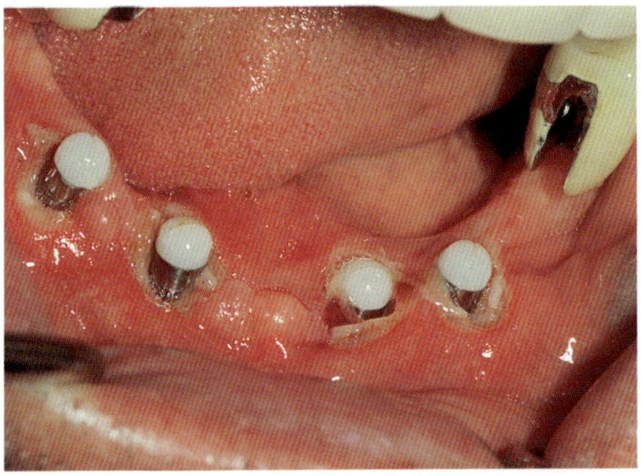

Fig 9.7d Two-week postoperative appearance.

Implant Recovery

Following the placement of an implant and its integration into the osseous substrate, the current method of treatment is to surgically uncover the implant, wait for the tissues to heal, and then proceed with impressions and the fabrication of the restoration. The reason for the delay is to facilitate the impression-taking process. The use of an argon laser can greatly expedite this procedure because the implant can be uncovered and the impressions can be obtained at the same appointment. This is possible because the laser allows for a bloodless field, the laser does not harm the implant, and argon laser-treated tissue margins do not recede during or after healing. Soft tissue overgrowth occurs following implant placement (Fig 9.7a). The argon laser is used to remove the soft tissue overlying the implants (Figs 9.7b and 9.7c). Two weeks postoperatively, healing was complete in this patient (Fig 9.7d). This surgery was performed with local anesthesia, and no postoperative recovery problems were noted.

Conclusion

The argon laser has been an invaluable surgical tool for medicine. The advantages of having a single instrument that will cut, vaporize, and coagulate are well-recognized by many medical specialties. The argon laser offers the same versatility to dentistry. When examining the total potential clinical applications of these argon wavelengths, the future role of this laser in dentistry is self-evident. It has applications in most dental specialties and is a valuable instrument for the general practitioner.

As the clinical cases indicate, the argon laser provides a broad range of surgical applications for dentistry. Additionally, because of the unique properties of the 488-nm and 514.5-nm wavelengths, a number of nonsurgical procedures are possible, which are further described in Chapter 16.

Acknowledgments

Special thanks to Bill Brown, Wendy Ochs, Alan Anderson, and David Sparks.

References

Boucher CO. Current Clinical Dental Terminology. A glossary of accepted terms in all disciplines of dentistry. St. Louis: Mosby;1988.

Crew JR, Stertzer SH, Myler RK, et al. Blood vessel welding by laser: preliminary clinical application. J Invasive Cardiol 1989;1:77–83.

Dixon JA, Davis RK, Gilbertson JJ. Laser photocoagulation of vascular malformations of the tongue. Laryngoscope 1986;96:537–541.

Grant DA, Stern IB, Listgarten MA (eds). Periodontics in the tradition of Gottlieb and Orban. Gingival and subgingival curettage: curettage of the pocket wall. St. Louis: Mosby;1988:749–760.

Henry C, Dyer B, Judy M. Selectivity of argon laser on phototoxicity of microbes. ISLD 3rd Int Congress 1992a:4.

Henry C, Dyer B, Judy M. Phototoxicity of argon laser on prevottella and porphyromonas. ISLD 3rd Int Congress 1992b:28.

Hohenleutner U, Landthaler M. Traditional tattooing of the gingiva: successful treatment with the argon laser. Arch Dermatol 1990;126(4):547.

Kopchok G, White RA, White G, et al. CO_2 and argon laser vascular welding: acute histologic and thermodynamic comparison. Lasers Surg Med 1988;8:584–588.

Kutsch VK. Lasers in dentistry: comparing wavelengths. J Am Dent Assoc 1993;124:49–53.

Murray L, Su L, Kopchok G, White RA. Crosslinking of extracellular matrix proteins: a preliminary report on a possible mechanism of argon laser welding. Lasers Surg Med 1989;9:490–496.

Neumann KA, Knobler RM. Treatment of oral mucous cysts with an argon laser. Arch Dermatol 1990;126(6):829–830.

Sexton J, O'Hare D. Simplified treatment of vascular lesions using the argon laser. J Oral Maxillofac Surg 1993;51:12–18.

White RA, Abergel RP, Lyons R, et al. Biological effects of laser welding on vascular healing. Lasers Surg Med 1986;6:134–141.

White RA, Kopchok G, White GH, Klein SR, Uitto J. Laser vascular anastomotic welding. In White, Grundfest (eds): Lasers in Cardiovascular Disease. Chicago: Year Book Med Publishing Co, Inc;1987a:103–115.

White RA, Kopchok G, Donayre C, et al. Large vessel sealing with the argon laser. Lasers Surg Med 1987b;7:229–235.

White RA, Kopchok G, Donayre C, et al. Argon laser welded arteriovenous anastomoses. J Vasc Surg 1987c;6:447–453.

Chapter Ten

Clinical Applications of the CO_2 Laser

Robert M Pick, M. Anthony Pogrel, and Hong Sai Loh

Like most lasers, the CO_2 laser offers the clinician a variety of advantages: little or no bleeding, a dry operating field, excellent visibility, possible reduction in operative time, reduced swelling, improved coagulation, reduced pain, decreased scarring, little or no need for sutures, little chance for mechanical trauma, little chance for bacteremia, and high patient acceptance. Because the CO_2 laser operates in a noncontact mode, one of its greatest advantages is its outstanding ability to easily negotiate curves and folds in the oral cavity. An ideal example of this advantage would be the ablation of inflammatory papillary hyperplasia of the palate.

Biopsies

Carbon dioxide lasers are used effectively for both incisional and excisional biopsies (Pecaro et al, 1983; Frame, 1984; Pick et al, 1985; Pick and Pecaro, 1987; Pick, 1993; Pick and Powell, 1993). An important principle to remember is that even though the clinician is using a laser, all the surgical principles of the respective procedure must be strictly followed. As with biopsies performed conventionally, both normal and pathologic tissues should be removed.

With a focused mode, an incision is made in the biopsy area. For most CO_2 lasers, the power settings will be in the range of 4 to 6 W. An edge is grasped with a tissue pickup, and with traction/countertraction, the lesion is undermined with the beam in the focused mode. The specimen is then removed and placed in the appropriate fixative solution, sent for pathologic evaluation, and read for histopathologic examination and diagnosis (Pick et al, 1985; Pick and Pecaro, 1987; Pick and Miserendino, 1989; Pick, 1993; Abt et al, 1987; Flynn et al, 1988; Gaspar and Szabo, 1989a). In most instances, sutures are not needed and the laser wound is left to heal by secondary intention (Fig 10.1). A char layer of varying degrees will be present over the wound site. It is recommended that only a light char layer be applied, since heavy char layers lead to more patient discomfort. The laser also works extremely well for the excison of vascular lesions such as oral hemangiomas (Apfelberg et al, 1985).

The amount of tissue destroyed lateral

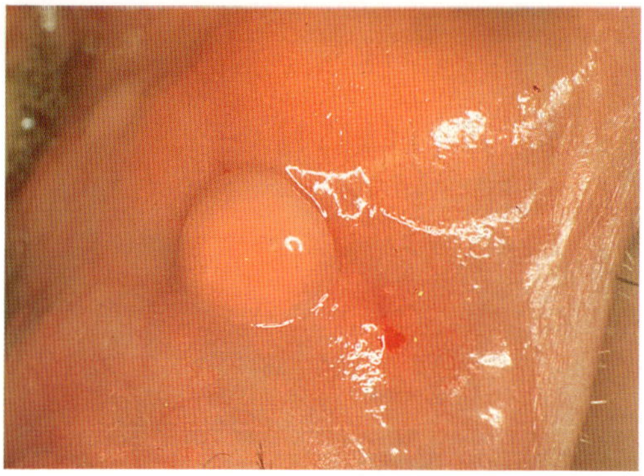

Fig 10.1a An irritation fibroma on the buccal mucosa.

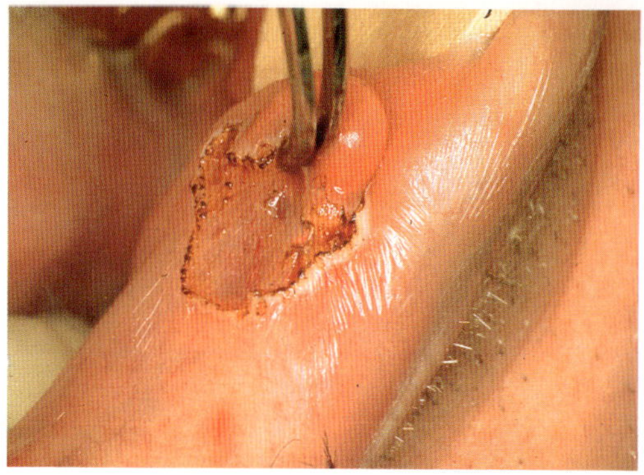

Fig 10.1b An excisional biopsy is performed with a CO_2 laser at 5 W of power, continuous wave mode. Note the hemorrhage-free nature of an area that normally bleeds copiously.

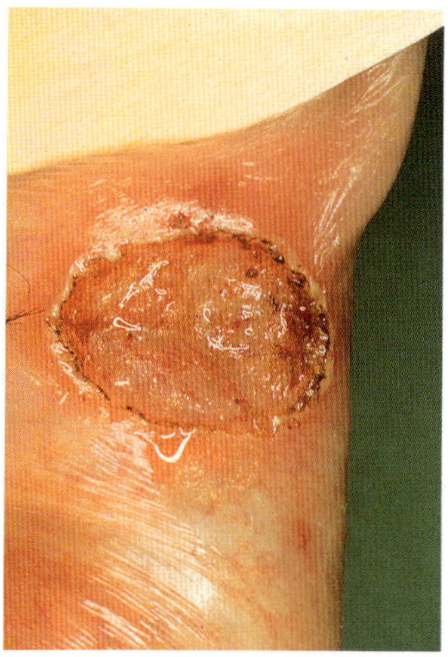

Fig 10.1c The specimen is removed, the underlying surface is dry, and there are no sutures placed to close the wound.

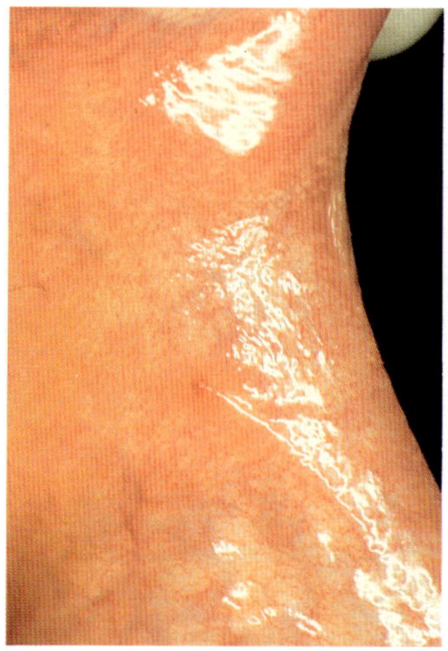

Fig 10.1d Six weeks after surgery.

to a CO_2 laser excision is of considerable importance in assessing the rate and quality of wound healing. This factor is of paramount importance since all excised lesions must be submitted for histologic examination. If there is a wide area of lateral tissue damage, it may affect the accuracy of the histologic examination results. Studies have shown that the width of laser-damaged tissue varies with the type of tissue being treated and is probably a function of the water content of the tissue; ie, the higher the water content, the smaller the zone of tissue damage (Pogrel et al, 1990a). Tissue damage appears to vary from approximately 45 μm for salivary gland tissue and fat and 90 μm for epithelium. Thus, one must allow for up to 0.10 mm of tissue to be valueless for histologic examination, and the pathologist must be made aware that the specimen has been laser-excised. In general, however, histologic examination of laser-excised tissue is not a problem. (Fisher and Frame, 1984; Fig 10.2).

Tongue Lesions

Lesions present on the tongue can be removed quite impressively with the CO_2 laser. In an area where conventional biopsies would cause immediate and copious blood flow, the laser removes most of these lesions bloodlessly and without the need for sutures. Although one of the advantages of using the laser is that sutures are not usually necessary, in certain tongue lesions sutures are still recommended. For example, when lesions are deep rather than superficial, or when large portions of the tongue are being removed such as in a hemiglossectomy, undermining of the borders and suturing are performed routinely (Pecaro and Garchume, 1983; Basu et al, 1988; Barak et al, 1990).

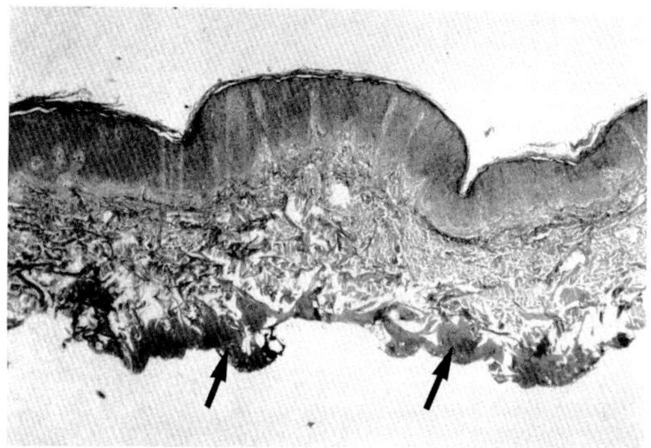

Fig 10.2 Deep surface of a laser-excised biopsy specimen. Note the thin margin of laser-damaged tissue (arrows), which measures between 60 μm and 80 μm. The tissue is mainly a loose connective tissue. (Hematoxylin and eosin, x 100.)

Average indicated power settings for excision of lesions of the tongue will range from 3 to 12 W of power depending on the size and bulk of the lesion to be removed.

White Lesions, Vesiculobullous Lesions, and Premalignant Lesions

Most of these lesions can be removed with the CO_2 laser once the biopsy has been taken or the diagnosis established. Examples include lichen planus, erosive lichen planus, benign mucous membrane pemphigoid, sublingual keratosis, and various hyperkeratotic growths. White lesions on the buccal mucosa, palate, and especially the floor of the mouth can be easily ablated with lasers.

For the various white lesion ablations, it has been our experience that the CO_2 laser is the most applicable laser because of its ability to ablate tissue rapidly in the defocused mode with minimal underlying tissue damage. Also, at lower powers (3 to 4 W) and in the highly defocused mode, the CO_2 laser allows the tissue to blister and causes certain lesions to separate at the basement membrane, allowing the clinician to "laser peel" the lesion away (see Chapter 8). If more of the lesion is found remaining, it can be further ablated or peeled away.

This technique works exceptionally well with the various forms of lichen planus. Traditional methods of treating lichen planus include application of various medications and steroid therapy, which have limited success. Itching and burning and a lack of tolerance for hot and spicy foods are often the chief complaints accompanying these lesions (Loh, 1992). After laser treatment, most of these patients are immediately symptom-free, without recurrence for months to years. The clinical appearance of lesions such as lichen planus often improves quite dramatically (Fig 10.3). If symptoms do recur, the process is so benign that patients often do not object to retreatment (Pecaro and Garchume, 1983; Pick and Pecaro, 1987; Chu et al, 1988; Gaspar and Szabo, 1989b; Chiesa et al, 1990).

An alternative to the peel technique is surface vaporization or ablation of the lesion down to the required depth once the biopsy has been obtained. This technique is particularly applicable to large areas of leukoplakia or keratosis of all varieties where surgical excision would result in major problems with morbidity and reconstruction. Surface vaporization to a depth of approximately 0.5 mm will normally result in good secondary reepithelization with normal mucosa. Sublingual keratosis, with its relatively high malignant transformation rate (Pogrel, 1979), lends itself very well to laser vaporization (Frame, 1984). The duct of the submandibular gland (and parotid gland, if applicable) can be transected with relatively few problems. This is because the duct is normally wider than the laser beam, so it will not be sealed by it. Because of the relative lack of swelling after laser surgery, the duct will not be obstructed postoperatively and will continue to secrete from a more proximal opening.

Aphthous Ulcers

One of the more remarkable laser benefits is the relief of the painful symptoms associated with aphthous ulcers. This is accomplished with resounding success. The exact mechanism by which this occurs is not known. It appears that an aphthous wound, which is painful, is converted to a laser wound, which is nonpainful. Immediately after laser treatment, patients experience relief. This may be accomplished with topical anesthetic or without anesthetics. The laser is set to its lowest indicated setting, usually 1 to 2 W. The laser is brought into a highly defocused mode where minimal energy is being delivered to the site and then the beam is brought closer to the aphthous ulcer until the patient just begins to feel a slight sensation of discomfort or heat. At this point, using a circular motion, the aphthous ulcer is lased from its center to just beyond the erythematous halo. Slight surface alteration of the aphthous ulcer will be noted (Colvard and Kuo, 1991).

Herpetic Lesions

Carbon dioxide lasers have been used effectively for symptomatic relief of herpetic lesions. The results are immediate and the lesions tend to heal more quickly. The technique is exactly the same as that for the removal of aphthous ulcers. However, extreme caution should be exercised in these cases since the herpes virus may be transmitted via the laser plume. Although there have been no reports in the dental

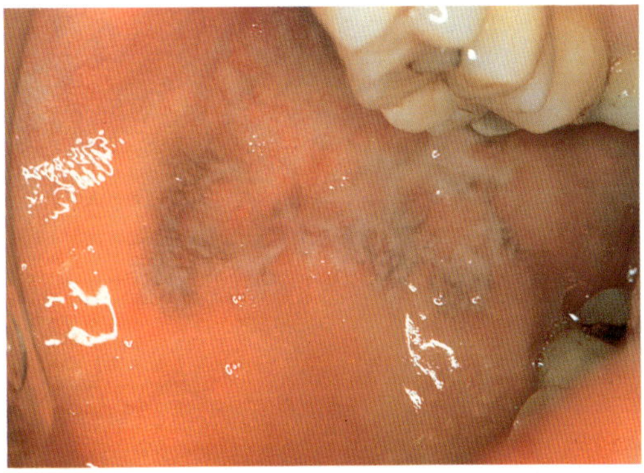

Fig 10.3a Lichen planus on the buccal mucosa.

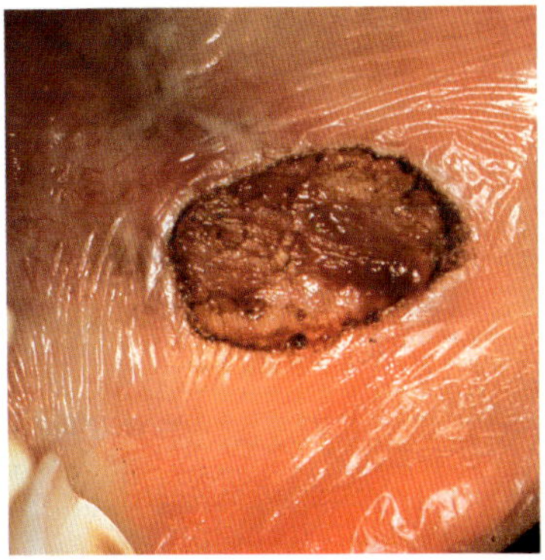

Fig 10.3b Immediately after incisional biopsy. Note the lack of bleeding in an area that would normally bleed easily.

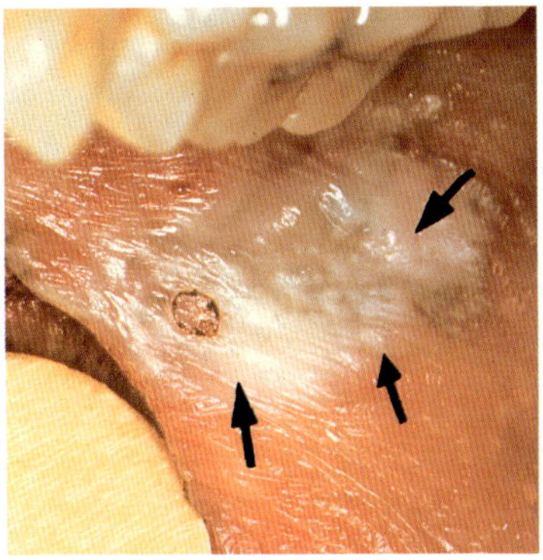

Fig 10.3c Because the patient had a chief complaint of a burning and itching sensation, the rest of the lesion is removed. Note the blistering of the tissue caused by the laser (arrows).

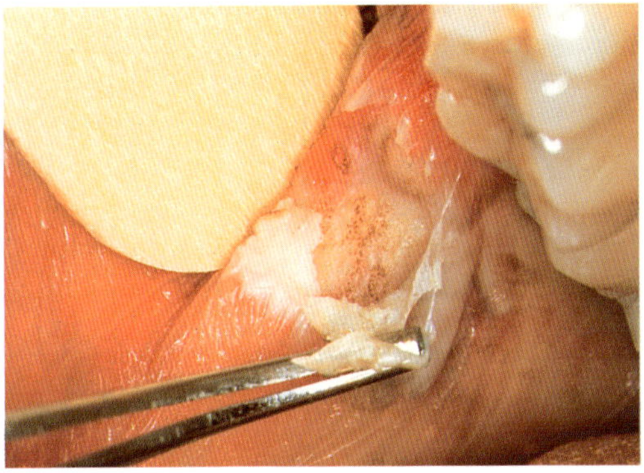

Fig 10.3d After blistering or whitening of the tissue, the lesion can be easily peeled away.

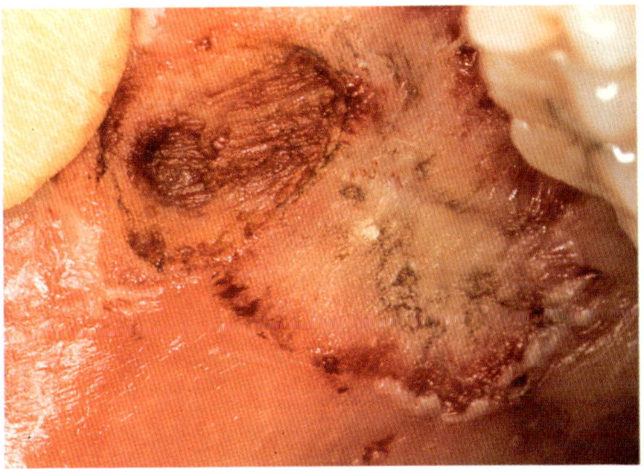

Fig 10.3e Immediately after peeling. A light char layer will be placed and the wound is left to heal by secondary intention.

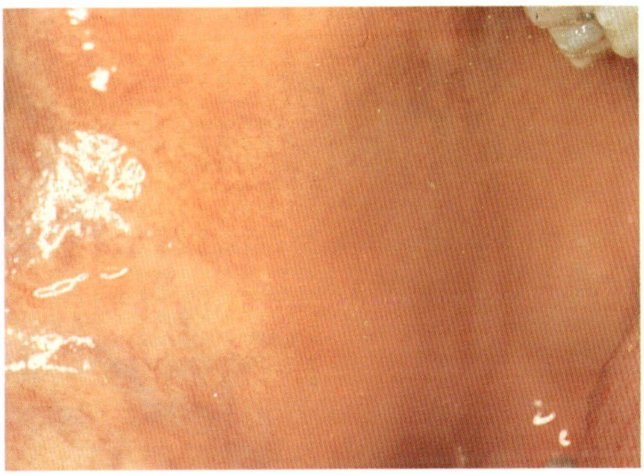

Fig 10.3f Twelve weeks after lasing. As with all cases of lichen planus, the patient is informed of the possibility of recurrence.

literature of this occurence, the spread of the virus is possible. Because verruca viruses can be spread via the plume, lasers should be used with caution for the removal of herpetic lesions.

Coagulation

For coagulation of bleeding areas, coagulation of soft tissue graft donor sites, or other small, oral bleeding areas, CO_2 lasers can be effective. One of the greatest concerns to the dentist is postoperative bleeding from the donor site after soft tissue grafting. Once laser coagulation is achieved, the chances for postoperative bleeding are minimal to nonexistent. For active bleeding sites, argon, Nd:YAG, and Ho:YAG are the lasers of choice, in that order. In nonbleeding areas, to prevent subsequent bleeding, all lasers are applicable. To coagulate an active bleeding site with a CO_2 laser, the bleeding must first be momentarily stopped. This is usually easily accomplished via pressure or the administration of additional anesthetic. Once the hemmorhage has stopped, with low power settings of 3 to 4 W and a defocused mode, the area is lased until a light char layer is noted (Pick and Pecaro, 1987; Pick and Miserendino, 1989; Pick, 1990).

Exposure of Implants (stage II)

Carbon dioxide lasers work exceptionally well for uncovering implants whether they be single or multiple fixtures. For this indication, the CO_2 laser simply vaporizes the overlying tissue until the surgical healing cap is reached. This is accomplished with a defocused mode, a circular motion, and an indicated power setting of 3 to 6 W. This can also be referred to as a "cookie-cutter" approach. The opening can then be easily contoured and enlarged as needed. When applicable, the laser eliminates the need for a flap and suturing, and reduces the level of postoperative discomfort that would normally be associated with this procedure (Fig 10.4). However, conventional flap procedures may be performed in cases in which there is a need for apically positioning a flap or for uncovering implants within osseous structures. When regeneration material, such as Gore-Tex augmentation filters, need to be recovered, the laser is not recommended.

Removal of Granulation Tissue

The CO_2 wavelength can also be used to remove granulation tissue either for periodontal "clean-out," or for degranulating any wound site present. In certain furcation areas, circumferential defects, intrabony defects, and three-wall defects, where stubborn tissue tags can persist, the laser can help either entirely to degranulate or partially degranulate these areas. Caution must be taken not to damage root surfaces or osseous structures. Carbon dioxide lasers with hollow waveguides are recommended for this purpose since the tip can be easily directed to the site to be degranulated. The laser should be used in the focused or near-focused mode, and power settings should be adjusted from 1 to 2 W of indicated power with possible gating of the beam. When working in areas of larger openings or better accessibility, higher power settings can be used but, again, with caution. Other wavelengths such as argon or Nd:YAG may prove to be more practical for this application.

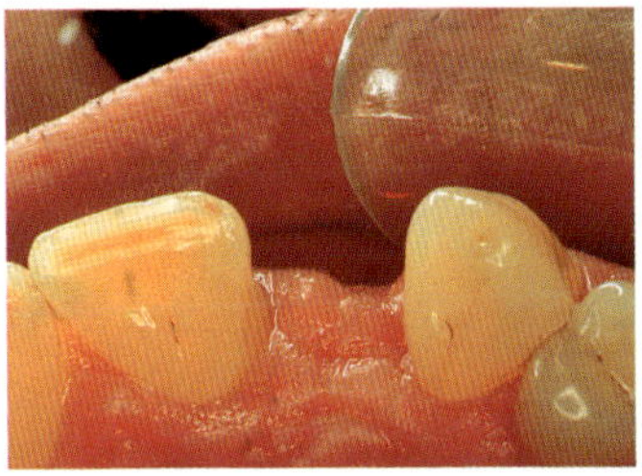

Fig 10.4a Implant exposure (stage II) of a screw-type fixture placed 4 months earlier.

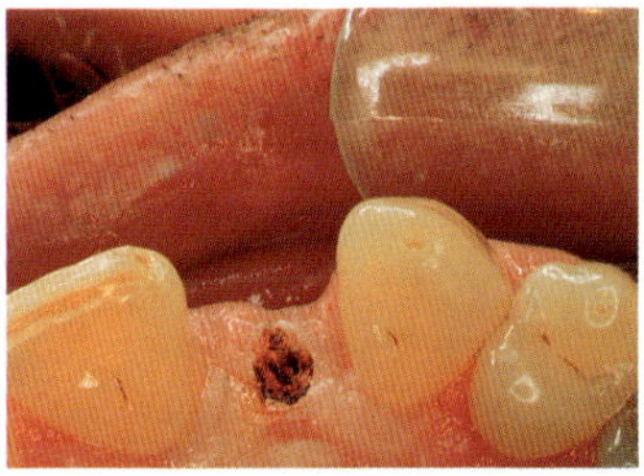

Fig 10.4b With 6 W of indicated power, a slightly defocused mode, and the "cookie-cutter" approach, the laser is used to expose the implant.

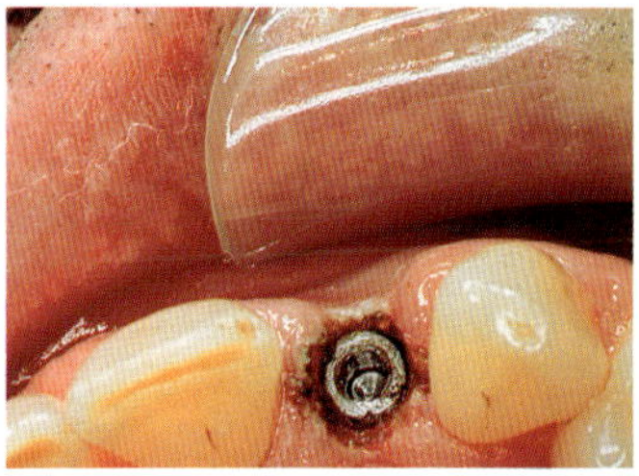

Fig 10.4c The collar is removed in the usual fashion and the implant is checked for osseointegration.

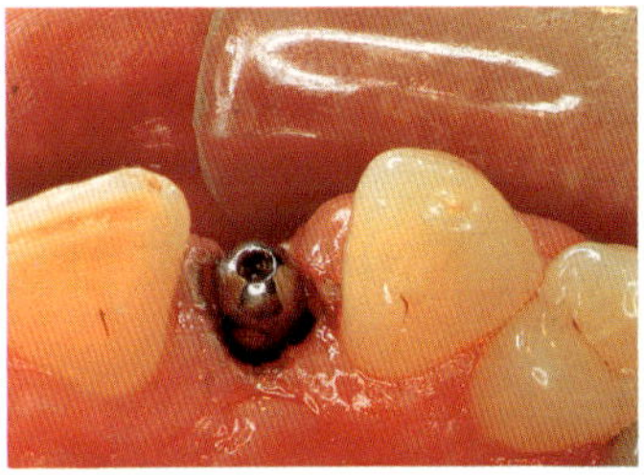

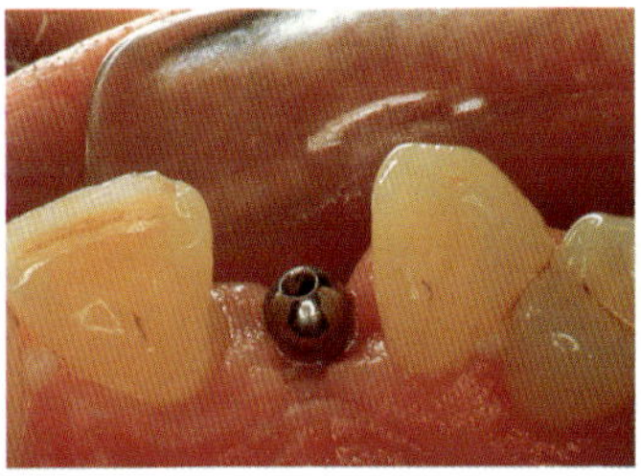

Figs 10.4d and e The final healing cap is placed **(d)**, and 3 weeks later **(e)** the patient is ready to proceed with restorative therapy.

Frenectomy

There is no better use for the CO_2 laser than for maxillary midline or lingual frenectomies. In maxillary midline frenectomy, the frenum is simply vaporized with the CO_2 laser. In lingual frenectomy, the tip of the tongue is grasped, tension is placed, and from the greatest concavity of the frenum moving posteriorly, the frenum is simply vaporized until the desired effect is achieved. Indicated power settings for both frenectomies are usually 4 to 5 W and in the slightly defocused mode (Figs 10.5 and 10.6). When the CO_2 laser is used for these procedures, operative time is reduced, requiring 35 seconds to 2 or 3 minutes. With these procedures, patients can almost be guaranteed a pain-free postoperative course. For both maxillary and lingual frenectomies, there is a tremendous advantage with this method since sutures do not have to be removed from the nonkeratinized movable oral mucosa at 1 week, which can be difficult and irritating to the patient (Pick and Miserendino, 1989; Pick, 1993; Pick and Powell, 1993).

Crown Lengthening

Lasers can be used very efficaciously for crown lengthening (removal of excessive gingival display) due to excessive soft tissue or a passive eruption problem. When patients have clinical crowns that appear too short or when they have an uneven gingival line producing an uneven smile, excessive tissue can be easily and quickly removed without the need for blade inci-

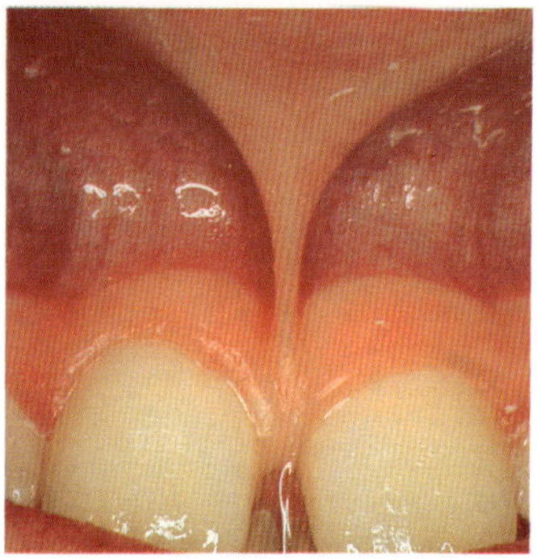

Fig 10.5a Maxillary midline frenum causing pull on the marginal and interdental papilla.

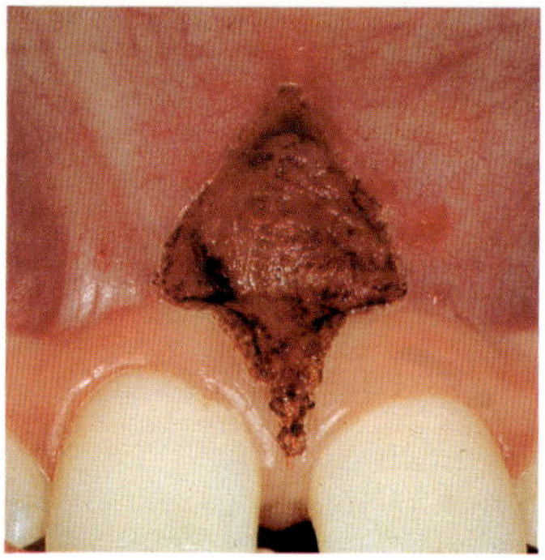

Fig 10.5b Immediately after CO_2 lasing of the frenum. Note the char layer and the lack of sutures.

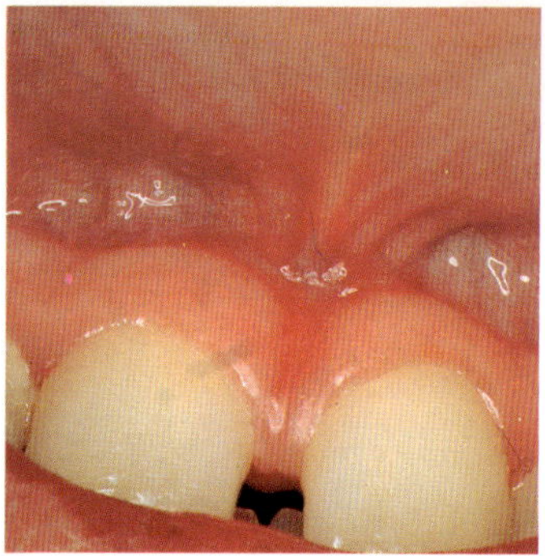

Fig 10.5c Two months after surgery. Note the new position of the frenum.

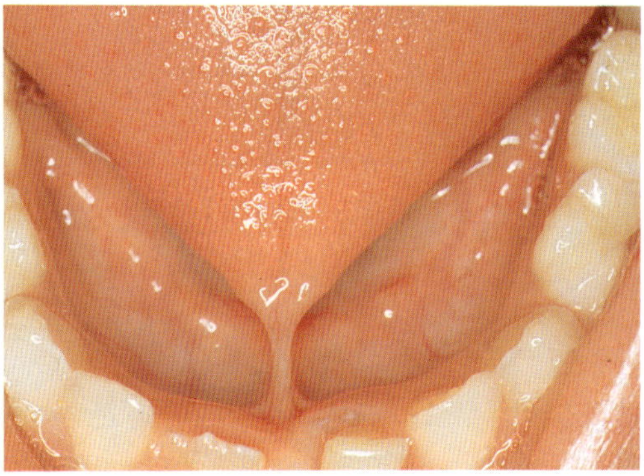

Fig 10.6a A 7-year-old boy with a tongue-tie.

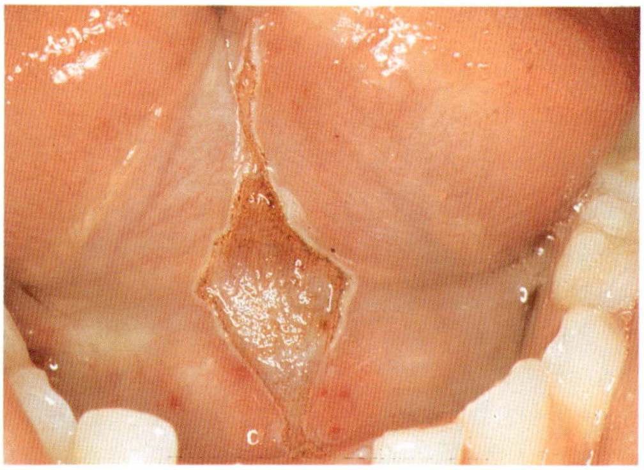

Fig 10.6b After the administration of local anesthesia, the tip of the tongue is grasped with a tissue forceps and, using 4 W of defocused power, the CO_2 laser is used to vaporize the frenum. Note the lack of bleeding.

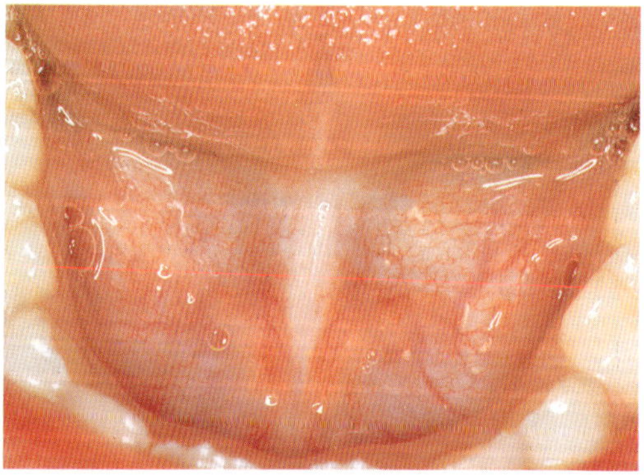

Fig 10.6c Eight weeks after lasing.

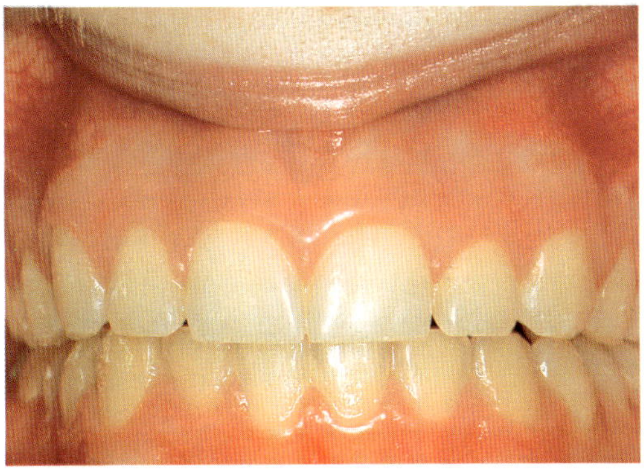

Fig 10.7a A 16-year-old girl presenting with a chief complaint of her teeth being too short in appearance.

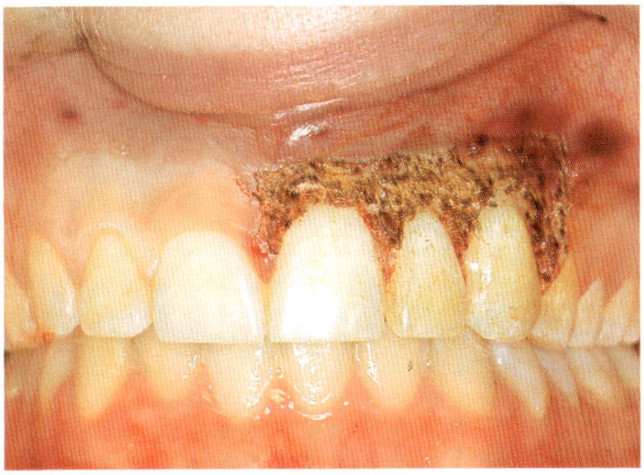

Fig 10.7b After CO_2 lasing of the left half to the cementoenamel junction.

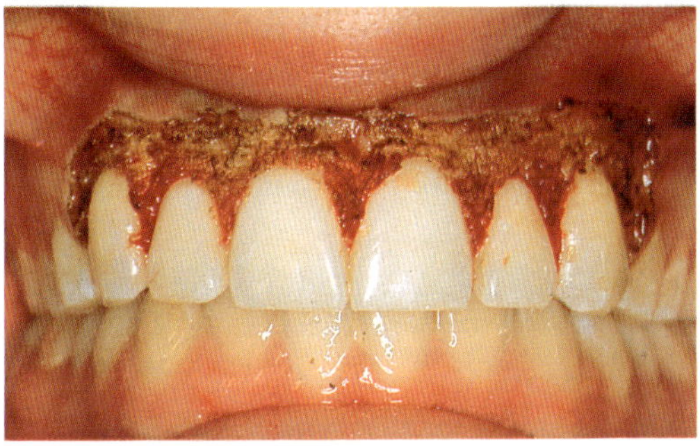

Fig 10.7c After complete lasing of the excessive tissue.

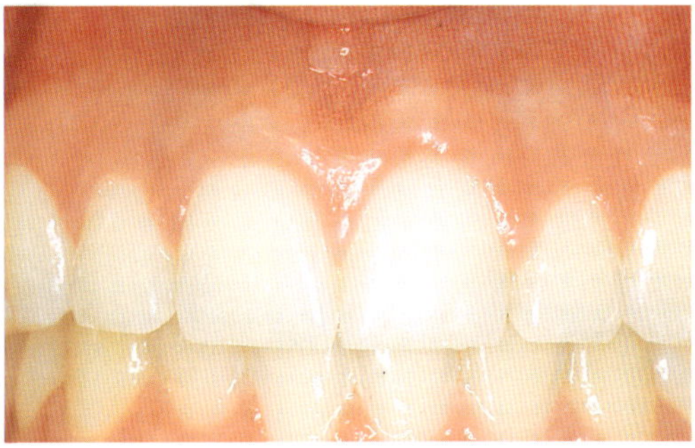

Fig 10.7d Six weeks after laser surgery.

sion, flap reflection, or suturing (Fig 10.7). Power settings are usually from 3 to 6 W of indicated power, with the beam moving from a focused to a defocused mode as necessary. To protect underlying tooth structure, a no. 7 wax spatula is used in the sulcus. As lasing continues, the spatula is moved in conjunction with the laser. One must first sound the area to determine the position of the cementoenamel junction relative to the crest of the tissue. If this distance is short, there is a good chance that the clinical crown and the anatomic crown are approximately the same. Therefore, when this situation arises, conventional crown lengthening must be performed to assure that the biologic width is not violated (Pick and Miserendino, 1989; Pick, 1993; Pick and Powell, 1993).

Distal Wedge and Tuberosity Reduction

For soft tissue distal wedge and tuberosity reduction procedures, lasers offer many advantages. Common problems often associated with these procedures are the limited access for proper protocol, and the absence of keratinized tissue, especially true in the areas distal and lingual to the lower second and third molars. Furthermore, every clinician who has performed maxillary distal tuberosity reductions has faced the following scenario: once the wedge is prepared and the tissue is thinned, the flaps overlap. These in turn must be further trimmed, often more than once, and often after further trimming the flaps are too short to approximate. Furthermore, these can prove to be difficult areas for access to suturing. The laser allows the operator to simply vaporize or cut away the tissue as needed until the desired end result is achieved. Indicated power settings range from 4 to 7 W, with the beam moving from a focused to a defocused mode as needed for vaporization and fine tissue removal.

Hypersensitivity

Lasers have proven to be very effective in reducing or completely eliminating temperature sensitivity, especially that due to cold. The exact mechanism for the various wavelengths is not yet known. It would appear that in some way they effectively seal the dentinal tubules. For the CO_2 laser, the beam is used in the highly defocused mode and at low indicated power settings, 1 to 2 W, sometimes gated. Some operators place a fluoride gel over the root surface first before lasing. Although purely anecdotal, the reported results, which come from numerous operators and institutions, are impressive.

Gingivectomy

When patients present with oral problems of tissue overgrowth, pseudopockets, or hyperplasias from various causes, lasers can be effectively used to perform laser gingivectomies (Fig 10-8). Tissue overgrowths can occur secondary to medication side effects, such as those from phenytoin, cyclosporine, nifedipine, and others, from idiopathic causes, poor oral hygiene, or from orthodontic hardware with or without poor oral hygiene. With CO_2 lasers, the excessive tissue may be easily vaporized. For larger hyperplasias, the CO_2 wavelength is the definite choice due to its speed.

Depending on the delivery system, tooth protection is sometimes needed. This can be accomplished with a periosteal elevator or no. 7 wax spatula placed in the pocket or sulcus so that when lasing is complete the beam hits the instrument rather than the tooth. Indicated power settings range from 4 to 10 W, depending on the thickness of the tissue, and the beam is used in both the focused and defocused mode. Near tooth margins, the beam is used in the focused mode to precisely contour the gingival margin. Away from the gingival margin, the beam is used in the defocused mode to simply ablate or vaporize the excess tissue. For mentally handicapped adults and children, this is an outstanding modality since it allows for a relatively benign postoperative course for a patient who otherwise does not understand why there may be bleeding and pain (Pick et al, 1985; Pick and Pecaro, 1987; Pick and Miserendino, 1989; Pick, 1993; Pick and Powell, 1993; Abt et al, 1987).

Gingivoplasty

For either small tissue aberrances seen after periodontal surgery or small areas of reverse tissue architecture with an otherwise healthy periodontium, CO_2 lasers are very effective in performing gingivoplasty. These are extremely fast procedures, often requiring no local anesthetic or only a topical anesthetic, and they almost always cause patients no postoperative

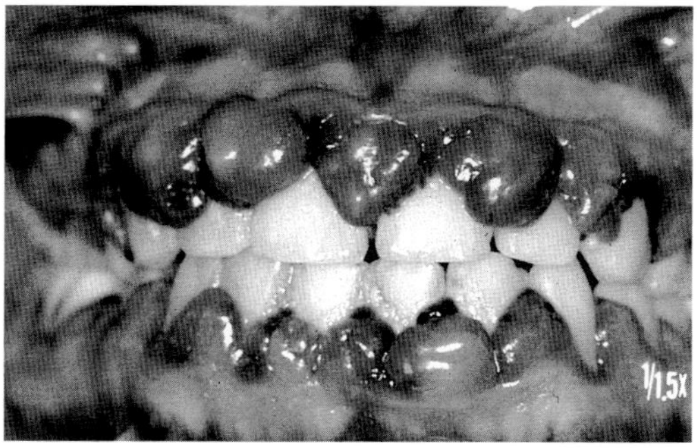

Fig 10.8a A 22-year-old mentally handicapped woman presenting with phenytoin hyperplasia. Note the degree of inflammation in the tissues and the heavy plaque build-up.

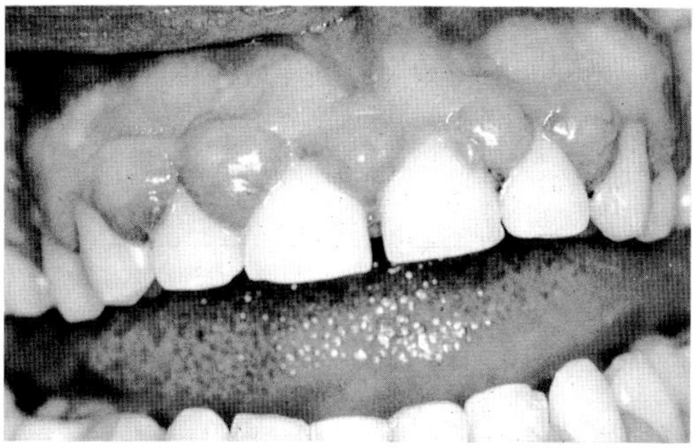

Fig 10.8b After full mouth scaling and root planing and oral hygiene instruction and reinforcement. There is a reduction in inflammation and swelling, but the hyperplasia remains.

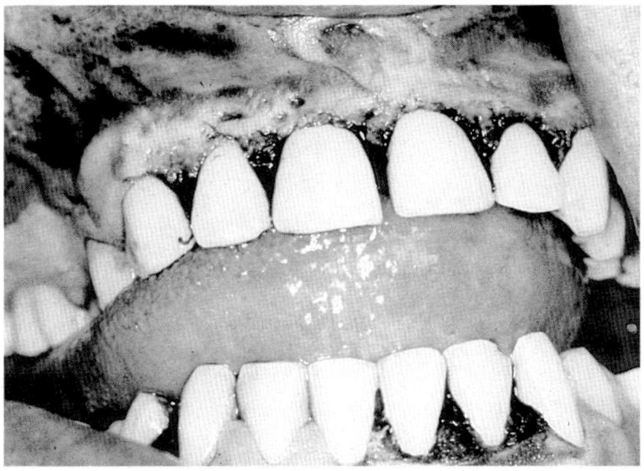

Fig 10.8c Immediately after lasing.

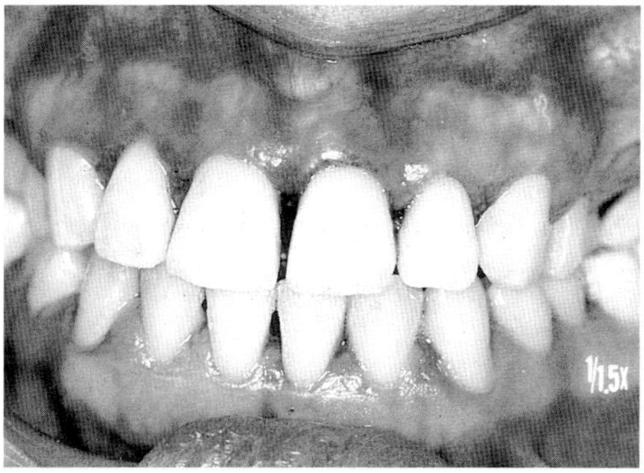

Fig 10.8d Just under 4 weeks after CO_2 lasing. Due to the patient's handicap, home care is lacking. Peridex was eventually prescribed.

complications of any kind. The laser is usually used in both the focused and defocused mode, with indicated power settings ranging from 2 to 5 W, depending on the size of the lesion.

Preprosthetic Surgery

For removal of epuli, inflammatory papillary hyperplasia, vestibuloplasty, or other preprosthetic surgical needs, once again CO_2 lasers are a superb alternative to the conventional modalities (Pecaro and Garchume, 1983; Pick and Pecaro, 1987; Pick and Miserendino, 1989; Pick and Powell, 1993, Stanley, 1988; Pogrel, 1989). Patients with ill-fitting dentures often develop hyperplastic folds over time. Other prosthodontic problems that frequently occur are high frenum attachments, scarred and keratotic tissue formations, and a shallow vestibule. These are detrimental to the proper functioning of a denture prosthesis. Preprosthetic surgery is advisable in these situations to provide a better soft tissue–bearing base. Conventional surgical techniques commonly produce extensive bleeding, which limits visualization and often requires su-

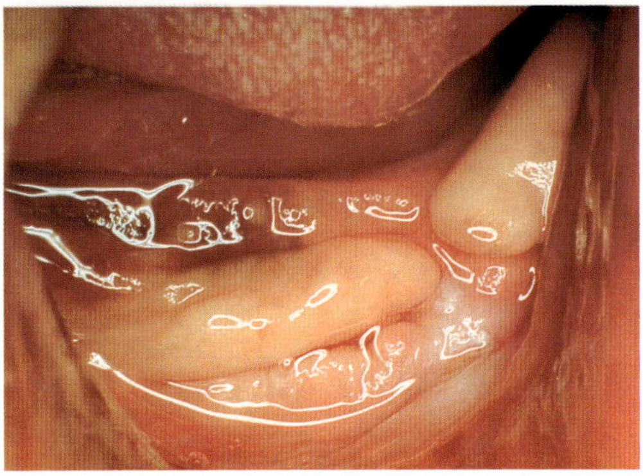

Fig 10.9a Two large epuli are seen in the mandibular anterior region secondary to an ill-fitting denture.

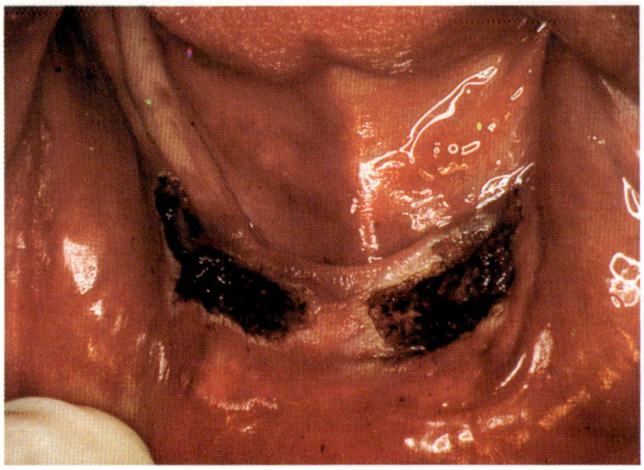

Fig 10.9b Immediately after lasing. The epuli were removed via excisional biopsies.

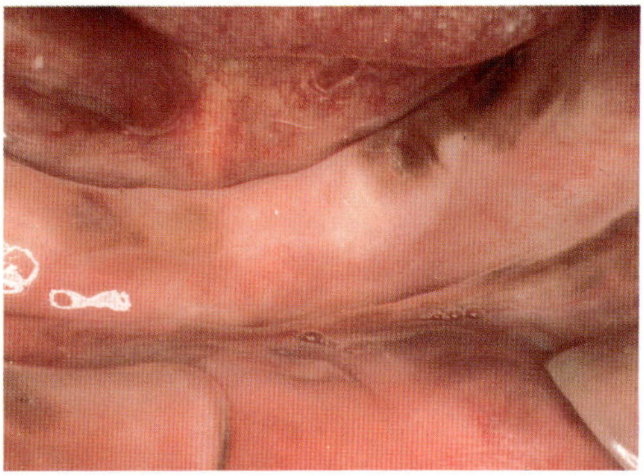

Fig 10.9c Six weeks after surgery.

turing. When the area involved is large, there is often significant postoperative pain, and grafting is sometimes necessary to cover the wound. In some situations, contracture of the wound on healing compromises the result. For example, inflammatory papillary hyperplasia can be removed either with a blade or electrosurgery effectively, but the laser offers the advantage of negotiating curves and folds easily, no bleeding during or after the procedure, a dry field, speed, minimal scarring, contracture, and reduced-to-absent postoperative pain and swelling for the patient. Furthermore, there is near-normal color and texture of the wound compared to the surrounding tissues. Suturing is rarely needed and, consequently, the normal anatomic contour is preserved (Keng and Loh, 1992). Submucous dissections can also be undertaken to eliminate frenal attachments or to deepen the vestibular sulcus. It is a simple bloodless and effective procedure. A dampened gauze pad is used to apply tension as the laser beam is swept across the sulcus area. There is no need to cover or protect the wound with a stent since healing is usually uneventful.

In removing an inflammatory papillary hyperplasia, first an area is lased with 4 to 6 W of indicated power in the defocused mode. The resulting char layer that forms can be wiped away and the underlying tissue inspected. If more tissue must be removed, this process of lasing and wipe down is repeated until the desired amount of tissue is removed. Epuli are removed in an excisional biopsy manner as previously described (Fig 10.9). For the larger preprosthetic lesions, such as inflammatory papillary hyperplasias, the CO_2 laser is recommended due to its speed and effectiveness in vaporization (Pick, 1993).

Malignant Lesions

Malignancies found in the oral cavity can be removed with CO_2 lasers. They offer the advantages of minimal bleeding, swelling, and less postoperative pain, especially considering that large areas of tissue are often removed. Surgical margins are similar whether a malignant lesion is excised with a laser or a scalpel and should be at least 1 cm clear of the lesion and 2 cm if possible. With a bloodless field, more precise cancer surgery can often be performed. A focused mode is usually used and indicated power settings range from 4 to 10 W. A potential advantage that can be hypothesized is that the chance for seeding the lesion and subsequent metastasis may be minimized or eliminated because lasers have the ability to seal blood vessels and lymphatics, depending on the lesion. Animal studies have confirmed this hypothesis (Lanzafame et al, 1986a, b), as have a small number of clinical studies (Adams and Price, 1979; Nagorsky and Sessions, 1987). Still other studies have failed to confirm this finding (Rhys-Williams and Carruth, 1988). As with surgical treatment of all malignancies, surgical protocol must be followed.

Gingival Troughing

One of the more recent areas of application for the CO_2 laser is gingival troughing. Lasers can be used to create a trough around a tooth before impression-taking. This can entirely replace the need for retraction cord, electrocautery, and the use of hemostatic agents. The results are predictable, efficient, minimize impingement on the epithelial attachment, cause less bleeding during the subsequent impression, minimize postoperative problems, and reduce chair time. Ganz (1992) recommends the following protocol:

1. Preparing the tooth with a shoulder to or just below the gingival margin.
2. Indicated power settings from 2 to 5 W, continuous wave mode, and primarily a focused mode. The tip should be kept parallel to the long axis of the tooth to avoid charring the tooth structure.
3. With a small diamond-tipped bur, the shoulder is beveled within the trough. Because of the high degree of visibility achieved, this is easily accomplished.
4. A transitional restoration is fabricated prior to obtaining the impression.
5. The impression is obtained with an elastomeric material of choice. As always, the tissue should be healthy, the biologic width not violated, and good physiologic contours on the provisional restoration achieved (Ganz, 1992).

Hemorrhagic Disorders

Carbon dioxide lasers have been used effectively to treat patients who have various intraoral lesions compounded by hemorrhagic disorders (Pecaro and Garchume, 1983). These disorders include hemophilia, idiopathic thrombocytopenia purpura, and Sturge-Weber syndrome (Fig 10.10) (Pick and Pecaro, 1987; Pick and Miserendino, 1989; Pick, 1990, 1993). Although these patients are still cross-matched for blood, they lose minimal amounts of blood because of the coagulative effects of lasers.

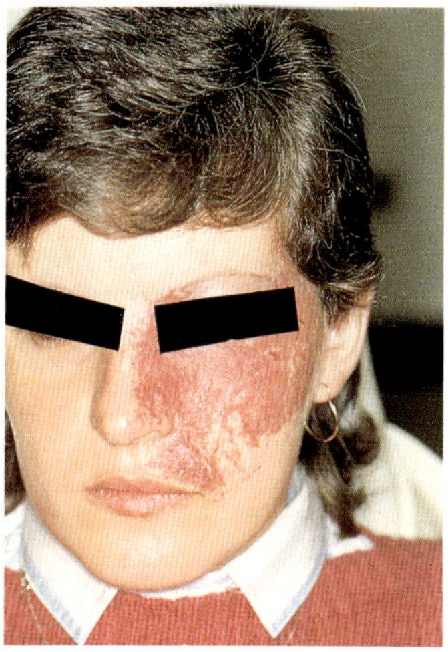

Fig 10.10a A patient with Sturge-Weber syndrome. Her port wine stain follows V–II.

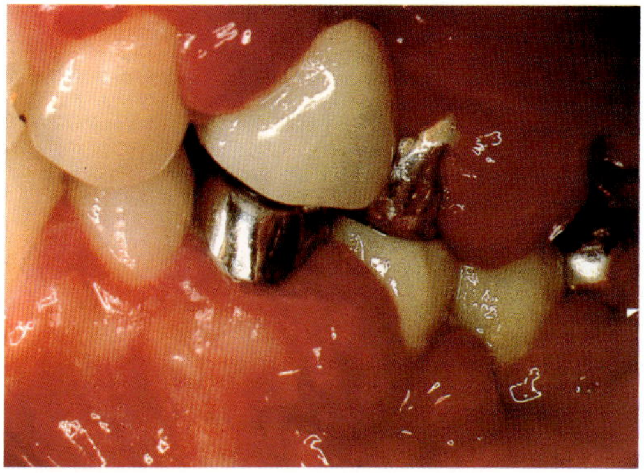

10.10b

Figs 10.10b–d The patient presents with numerous intraoral pyogenic granulomas on the affected side only. Immediately after lasing **(c)** and 6 weeks after surgery **(d)**. A total blood loss of 2 mL was measured.

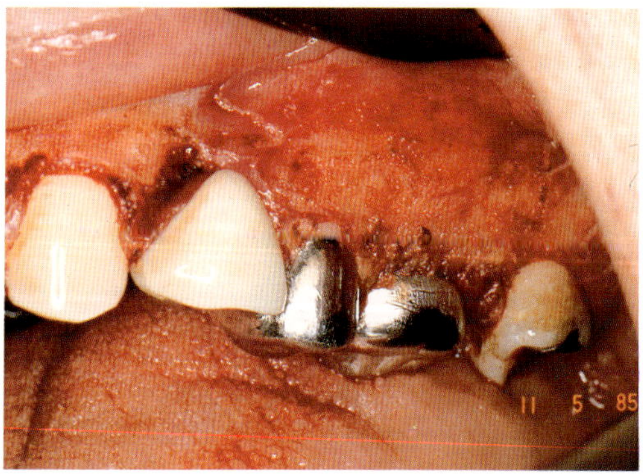

10.10c

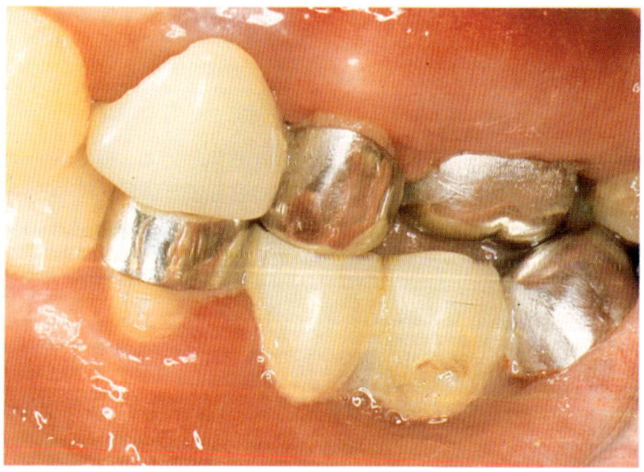

10.10d

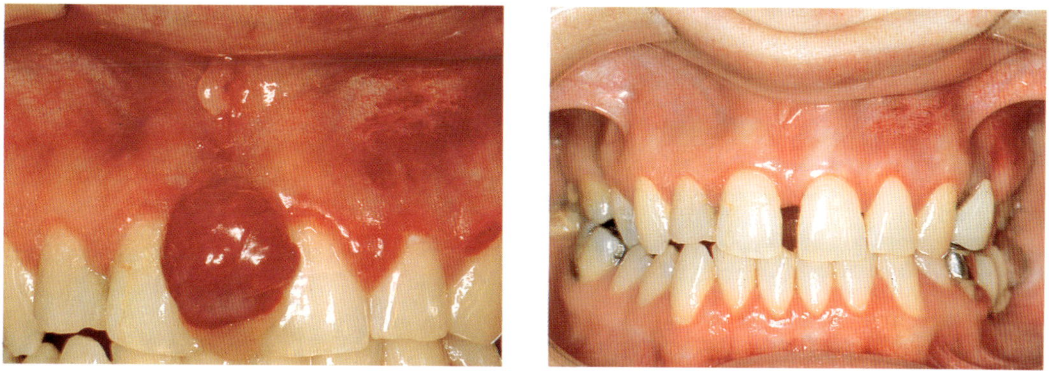

Figs 10.10e and f Before and after lasing in the maxillary midline.

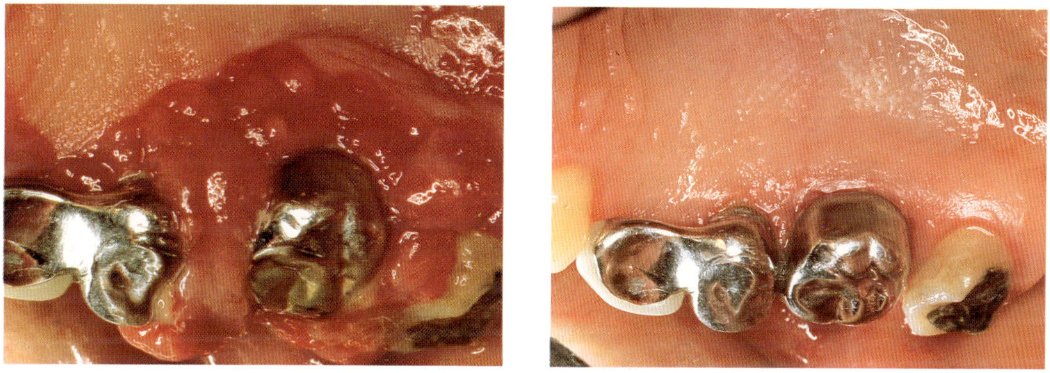

Figs 10.10g and h Before and after lasing on the palate.

References

Abt E, Wigdor H, Lobraido R, Carlson B, Harrison D, Pyrcz R. Removal of benign intraoral masses using the CO_2 laser. J Am Dent Assoc 1987;7:33.

Adams EL, Price NM. Treatment of basal-cell carcinomas with a carbon dioxide laser. J Dermatol Surg Oncol 1979;5:803–806.

Apfelberg DB, Maser MR, Lash H, White DN. Benefits of the CO_2 laser in oral hemangioma excision. Plast Reconstr Surg 1985;75:46–50.

Barak S, Kaplan I, Rosenblum I. The use of the CO_2 laser in oral and maxillofacial surgery. J Clin Laser Med Surg 1990;8:69.

Basu MK, Frame JW, Rhys-Evans PH. Wound healing following partial glossectomy using the CO_2 laser, diathermy and scalpel: a histological study in rats. J Laryngol Otol 1988;102:322–327.

Chiesa F, Tradati N, Sala L, et al. Follow up study of oral leukoplakia after carbon dioxide laser surgery. Arch Otolaryngol Head Neck Surg 1990;116:177–180.

Chu FWK, Silverman S, Dedo HH. Carbon dioxide laser treatment of oral leukoplakia. Laryngoscope 1988;98:125–130.

Colvard MD, Kuo P. Managing aphthous ulcers: laser treatment applied. J Am Dent Assoc 1991;122:51.

Fisher SE, Frame JW. The effects of the carbon dioxide laser on tissues. J Br Oral Maxillofac Surg 1984;22:414–425.

Flynn MB, White M, Tabah RJ. Use of carbon dioxide laser for the treatment of premalignant lesions of the oral cavity. J Surg Oncol 1988;37:232–234.

Frame JW. Treatment of sublingual keratoses with the CO_2 laser. Br Dent J 1984;156:243–246.

Ganz CH. Laser dentistry: A prosthodontic perspective. Dentistry Today 1992;11:62–79.

Gaspar L, Szabo G. Removal of benign oral tumors; and tumor-like lesions by CO_2 laser application. J Clin Laser Med Surg 1989a;7:33.

Gaspar L, Szabo G. The use of the CO_2 laser in the therapy of leukoplakia. J Clin Laser Med Surg 1989b;7:27.

Hall RP, Hill DW, Beach WD. Carbon dioxide surgical laser. Ann R Coll Surg Engl 1971;48:181–188.

Keng SB, Loh HS. The treatment of epulis fissuratum of the oral cavity by CO_2 laser. J Clin Laser Med Surg 1992;10:303–306.

Lanzafame RJ, Rogers DW, Naim JO, Herrera HR, De Franco C, Hinshaw JR. The effect of CO_2 laser excision on local tumor recurrence. Lasers Surg Med 1986a;6:103–105.

Lanzafame RJ, Rogers DW, Naim JO, DeFranco CA, Ochej H, Hinshaw JR. Reduction of local tumor recurrence by excision with the CO_2 laser. Lasers Surg Med 1986b;6:431–441.

Loh HS. A clinical investigation of the management of oral lichen planus with CO_2 laser surgery. J Clin Laser Med Surg 1992;10:445–449.

Nagorsky MJ, Sessions DG. Laser resection for early oral cavity cancer. Ann Otol Rhinol Laryngol 1987;96:556–560.

Patel CKN, McFarlane RA, Faust WL. Selective excitation through vibrational energy transfer and optical maser action in N_2-CO_2. Physiol Rev 1964;13:617–619.

Pecaro BC, Garchume WJ. The CO_2 laser in oral and maxillofacial surgery. J Oral Maxillofac Surg 1983;41:725–728.

Pick RM, Pecaro BC, Silberman CJ. The laser gingivectomy. The use of the CO_2 laser for the removal of phenytoin hyperplasia. J Periodontol 1985;56:492–496.

Pick RM, Pecaro BC. Use of the CO_2 laser in soft tissue dental surgery. Laser Surg Med 1987;7:207–213.

Pick RM, Miserendino LJ. Lasers in dentistry. J Clin Laser Med Surg 1989;7:33.

Pick RM. Lasers in soft tissue dental surgery, laser surgery: advanced characterization, therapeutics, and systems II, progress in biomedical optics. SPIE 1990:1200:416.

Pick RM. Using lasers in clinical dental practice. J Am Dent Assoc 1993;24:37–47.

Pick RM, Powell GL. Lasers in dentistry. Dent Clin North Am 1993;37:281–296.

Pogrel MA. Sublingual keratosis and malignant transformation. J Oral Pathol 1979;8:176–178.

Pogrel MA. The carbon dioxide laser in soft tissue preprosthetic surgery. J Prosthet Dent 1989;61:203–208.

Pogrel MA, McCracken KT, Daniels TE. Histologic evaluation of the width of soft tissue necrosis adjacent to carbon dioxide laser incisions. Oral Surg Oral Med Oral Pathol 1990a;70:564–568.

Pogrel MA, Yen CK, Hansen LS. A comparison of carbon dioxide laser, liquid nitrogen and scalpel wounds in healing. Oral Surg Oral Med Oral Pathol 1990b;69:269–273.

Rhys-Williams S, Carruth JAS. The role of the carbon dioxide laser in treatment of carcinoma of the tongue. J Laryngol Otol 1988;102:1122–1123.

Skelton H. Storage of water by various tissues of the body. Arch Intern Med 1927;40:140–152.

Stanley RJ. Actinic cheilitis: treatment with the carbon dioxide laser. Mayo Clin Proc 1988;63:230–235.

Chapter Eleven

Er:YAG Laser Effects on Oral Hard and Soft Tissues

Ulrich Keller and Raimund Hibst

The Erbium:YAG laser is a very promising laser system because the emission wavelength of 2.94 μm coincides with the main absorption peak of water, resulting in good absorption in all biologic tissues, including enamel and dentin. In 1988, the first description of Er:YAG laser effects on dental hard tissue indicated that effective ablation of healthy tissue, as well as carious lesions, is possible without thermal injury to the surrounding hard tissues (Hibst et al, 1988; Hibst and Keller, 1989). Since that time, a variety of investigations have been carried out on the removal of dental tissue (Willenborg, 1989), temperature effects, possible damage to the pulp, and on laser incision on oral mucosa and osteotomies of the jaws. An overview of in-vitro, animal study, and clinical investigations with the Er:YAG laser, the indications and possibilities, and the differences compared to other laser systems follow.

In-vitro Experiments

In all investigations, a flash-lamp-pumped Er:YAG laser in the free-running mode at 2.94-μm wavelength was used, with a total pulse duration of 250 μsec. The in-vitro experiments were performed on extracted human teeth that were 2-mm-thick sections and fixed in 4% formaldehyde.

Ablation Rates

To determine the efficiency of the laser ablation, both crater depth and mass loss were investigated for various conditions. First crater depth measurements revealed that ablation rates of more than 30 μm per pulse could be achieved for healthy hard tissue. For carious decay, the crater depth is somewhat greater. This is about two orders of magnitude higher than that for the ArF-excimer laser (Hibst et al, 1988; Keller and Hibst, 1989b; Paghdiwala, 1989; Neev et al, 1991). A comparison of various other lasers showed similar results only for the pulsed TEA CO_2 laser at 9.6 μm (Franetzki, 1991).

After exceeding the ablation threshold, the mass loss increases linearly with the radiant energy and is higher for dentin than for enamel (Fig 11.1). For pulses with 300 mJ each, the mass loss is about 40 μg for enamel and twice as much for dentin. Considering the tissue density of 2.9 g/cm^3

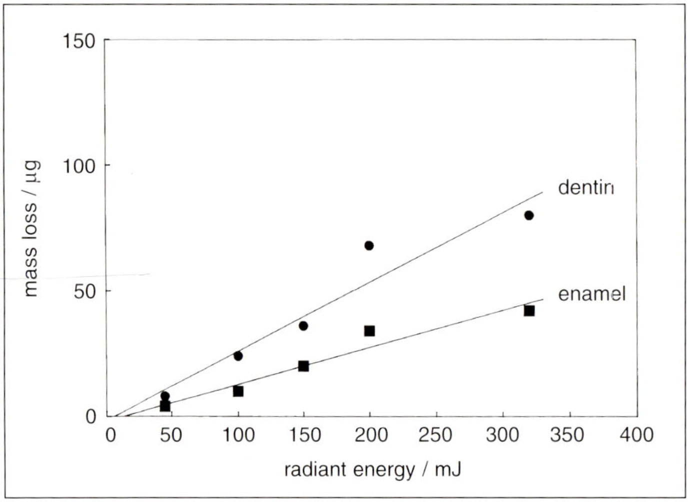

Fig 11.1 Mass loss of enamel and dentin after Er:YAG laser irradiation with various energies.

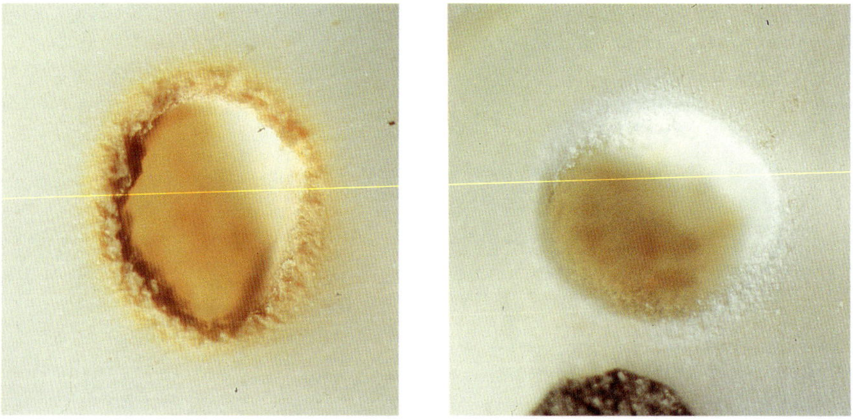

Fig 11.2 Microscopic view of Er:YAG laser–induced crater in dentin. **(a)**, Without water spray. Brownish rims as thermal side effects. **(b)**, With water spray, clean edges without discoloration.

and 1.9 g/cm^3, respectively, it can be calculated that 73 pulses of 300 mJ each are needed for ablation of 1 mm^3 of enamel and 25 pulses for ablation of 1 mm^3 of dentin. With a repetition rate of 4 Hz, less than 20 sec is necessary. Compared to the mechanical drill, the laser ablation of enamel takes about twice as much time, but it is short enough for clinical practice if cavity preparation is not too extensive.

Morphology

Previous studies with infrared laser systems like the continuous wave CO_2 or the Nd:YAG laser have reported the presence of zones of carbonization and necrosis. The width of these zones depends mainly on the absorption and the irradiation time. The cracks and melted and glazed surfaces after CO_2 and Nd:YAG laser treatment are signs of high temperatures

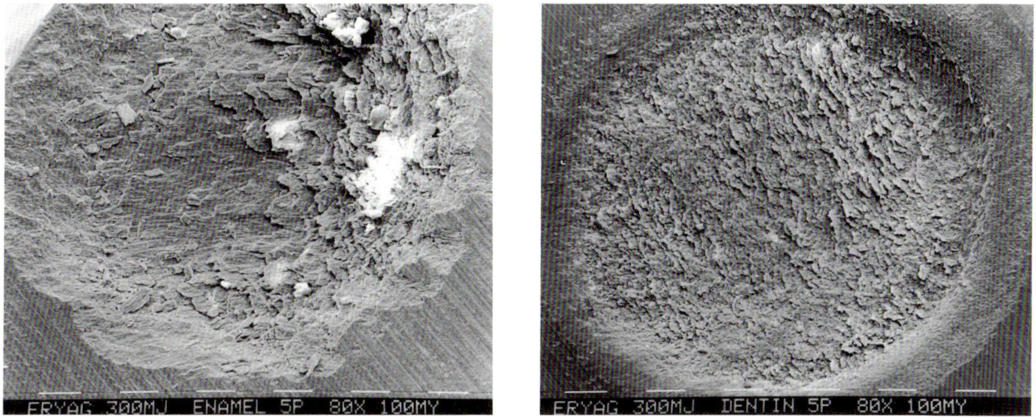

Fig 11.3 Er:YAG laser–induced crater in enamel and dentin (330 mJ, 5 pulses). Rough walls and crater bottom without thermal changes. **(a)**, Enamel, scanning electron microscopy (SEM) × 80. **(b)**, Dentin, SEM × 80.

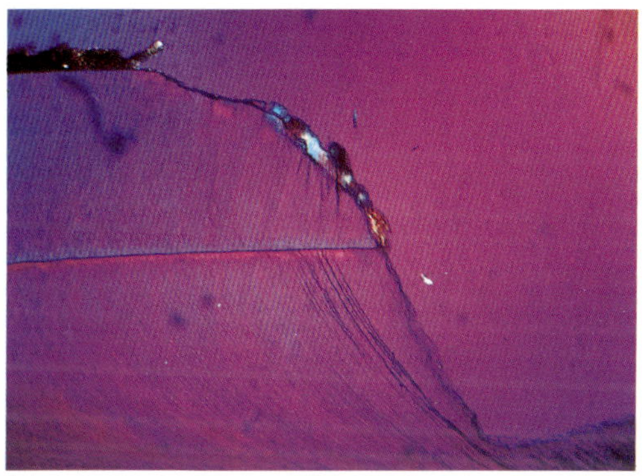

Fig 11.4 Undecalcified histologic tooth sample following Er:YAG laser irradiation (500 mJ, 4 Hz). Only a 20- to 40-µm layer of debris, changed in color, can be seen on enamel and dentin. Polarization microscopy, × 220.

caused by an evaporation process (Stern et al, 1972; Stern, 1974; Vahl, 1971).

In contrast after Er:YAG laser treatment no thermally induced changes can be seen, except a brownish rim if the dentin is desiccated by laser irradiation (Fig 11.2a). This discoloration can be avoided by moistening the tooth surface with a fine water spray. With this method, the Er:YAG laser irradiation leads to a clean hole with sharp edges to the surrounding hard tissues (Fig 11.2b) and with no signs of melting or cracking (Keller and Hibst, 1989a; Hoke et al, 1990; Kayano et al, 1991; Yamamoto et al, 1992). Only a zone of debris overlays the cavity surface, which can be identified as crystalline particles. The walls and the floor of the crater are rough, giving the impression that the mineralized tissues are ripped off (Figs 11.3 and 11.4). Investigations of the ablated material showed a corresponding morphology (Keller, 1989; Keller and Hibst, 1989a, b; Keller and Hibst, 1990).

The high ablation efficiency and the morphology can be explained by a thermally induced mechanical process. Water has a very high absorption for the Er:YAG laser light at 2.94 µm. Consequently, the incident Er:YAG laser radiation is absorbed in a thin surface layer, causing sudden heating and vaporization of the water. A high steam pressure then leads to microexplosions with erupting particles with a crater corresponding morphology. Because the tissue is not vaporized completely but only disintegrated into fragments, the radiant energy is converted efficiently into the ablation that alters the

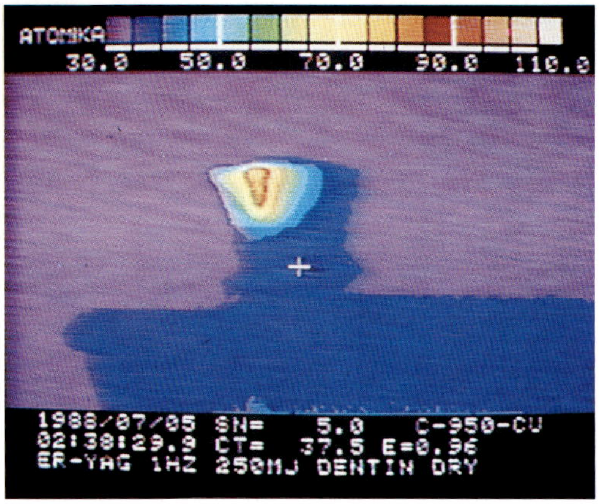

Fig 11.5 Thermal image of half-cut teeth with focused Er:YAG laser irradiation of dentin (250 mJ per pulse, 1 Hz) after 30 pulses.

morphological structure of the tissue. No melting process takes place that might lead to considerable heat damage to the surrounding tissues.

Temperature Measurements

Beside the efficiency and precise control of ablation, the temperature increase caused by laser treatment is of special interest (Paghdiwala, 1989). For a first experiment, longitudinal half-cut teeth were fixed in a cork plate and the roots were dipped in a water bath at a temperature of 37°C. The laser light was focused near the rim onto the top of the tooth, parallel to the sectional plane. The temperature across the surface was measured with a thermal camera with a close-up lens. Additionally, the temperature in the pulp was measured with a thermocouple.

The thermal images show that the temperature increase caused by a single pulse is limited to the tissues closest to the cavities (Fig 11.5). After about 2 sec, the temperature has nearly reached its starting point again. For multiple pulses, the heat effect is cumulative. The small, single pulse heat effect is safe, but the influence of pulse number and repetition rate requires a definition of maximum tolerable laser parameters (Keller, 1989; Hibst and Keller, 1990).

For a quantification of the heat effect and evaluation of possible pulp damage, a second series of temperature measurements was performed. In these experiments, a tooth cavity preparation with opening of the pulp chamber was simulated. Teeth were cut along the tooth axis into 2- or 4-mm-thick sections. With a mechanical bur, small holes were prepared at the back side and thermocouples were placed in the holes with a paste of very high thermal conductivity. Cavities were prepared with the Er:YAG laser beam aimed at the thermocouple. When the laser beam reached the thermocouple, irradiation was stopped.

The observed maximum temperatures rise with increasing radiant energy and repetition rates. The influence of the repetition rate is much more pronounced. With energies of 100 mJ to 300 mJ and repetition rates of 1 to 3 Hz, the maximum temperature increases in the range of 10 K to 25 K. These temperatures are recorded at the entry site, when the pulp is just opened by the laser beam (Hibst and Keller, 1990). Further investigations with the same experimental setup, but with a fine water spray during laser irradiation, revealed a significant reduction of temperature. The maximum temperature can be limited to 5 K, even for energies exceeding 400 mJ and a repetition rate of 2 Hz. The results of Hoke et al (1990) and of Burkes et al (1992) are comparable.

Under practical conditions, the heat effect, which is restricted to the cavity walls, is less in larger cavities than in smaller cavities. Therefore, the temperature increase will not exceed 5 K and pulpal damage can be avoided (Hibst and Keller, 1989, 1990; Keller and Hibst, 1992).

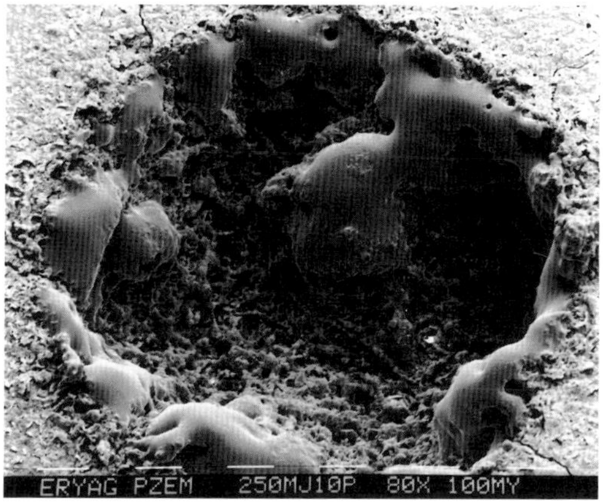

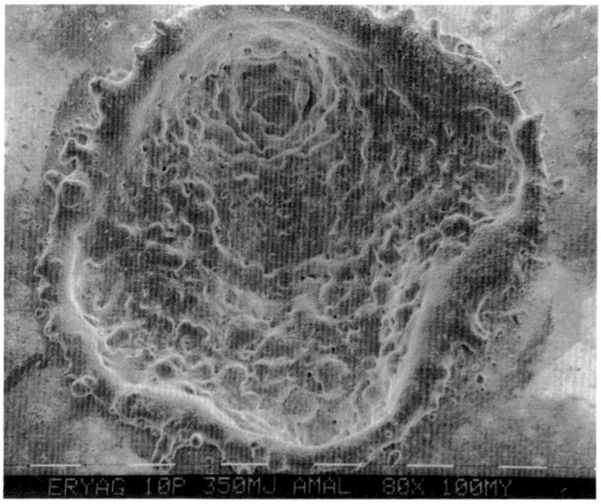

Fig 11.6 Filling materials after Er:YAG laser irradiation with 10 pulses. **(a)**, Phosphate cementum (250 mJ), SEM, × 80. **(b)**, Amalgam (350 mJ), SEM, × 80.

Removal of Dental Filling Materials

For practical use, it is not only important to remove primary decay with the laser, but also a variety of restorative materials. In many cases, patients have different kinds of filling materials with secondary carious lesions. Therefore, the effect of Er:YAG laser radiation on different restorative filling materials was also investigated (Hibst and Keller, 1991, 1992).

The ablation efficiency and precision of the Er:YAG laser was examined for the following restorative filling materials: phosphate cementum, carboxylate cementum, polymaleinate glass-ionomer cementum, polyketone (root canal filling material), composites (PMMA), and silver amalgam. Platelets from each material were prepared according to the manufacturer's instructions. The platelets were irradiated by the Er:YAG laser beam with energies ranging from 50 to 350 mJ. For each radiant energy, 10 pulses with a repetition rate of 1 Hz were applied. The ablation efficiency was determined by optical micrometry, and the morphology was examined with optical and electron microscopes.

All tested restorative filling materials can be effectively removed with the Er:YAG laser. Ablation efficiency is only slightly lower than that in enamel or dentin, except for silver amalgam. For this material, the ablation is possible only with energies exceeding 150 mJ.

The crater appearance strongly depends on the material. In composites, the crater walls are granular with a rough or even fissured surface. For glass-ionomer cementum, polyketone and phosphate cementum melting zones can be found. Temperature measurements confirm these results, but the temperature distribution is localized and can be decreased with a water spray. In contrast to these materials, the surfaces of amalgam craters look like waves as the result of a melting process (Fig 11.6). The melting zones indicate high temperatures during the ablation process.

It is possible to remove some types of dental fillings; however, amalgam should not be removed with the Er:YAG laser because of a high concentration of mercury in the escaping plume during ablation. It is not possible to remove gold fillings or ceramic restorations.

Animal Experiments

The intent of the first animal experiments on rats was to evaluate the physiologic reaction of pulp during Er:YAG laser application (Keller, 1989; Keller et al, 1991a). Following irradiation of tooth hard tissue with ruby, continuous wave CO_2, or Nd:YAG laser, high temperatures with consequent partial or total pulp necrosis can be observed (Stern et al, 1969; Lenz et al, 1977; Melcer et al, 1987; Serebro et al, 1987). There is no possibility for the pulp to conduct heat significantly to dentin and enamel because the mineralized structures act like heat isolators. Therefore, the pulp response to increasing temperatures results in a hyperemic reaction of the pulpal blood flow. This intensified blood circulation is reversible if the temperature ranges between 43°C and 49°C. If 49°C is exceeded, an irreversible pulp necrosis occurs. Furthermore, the temperature changes in the pulp are correlated with the perception of pain.

Changes in the microcirculation during laser irradiation can be measured with a laser Doppler flowmeter. A laser Doppler flow probe was adapted to the apical part of the lower incisors. The Er:YAG laser light was applied coronal or apical to the probe site, either by single pulses or by pulse trains from 2 to 10 pulses.

No reaction occurred during laser irradiation of the enamel or the superficial dentin. At the moment the zone of dentin and predentin near the pulp is reached, an immediate pulpal blood flow reduction is observed. This reduction is reversible within a few minutes. Even if the pulp chamber is exposed by the laser beam coronal to the probe, the same effect can be observed. No reactive hyperemia can be seen, which would be expected if temperatures exceed 43°C, and no systemic reaction results.

It must be concluded that no thermal damage to the pulp occurs during careful Er:YAG laser application. Laser amputation of the pulp can be performed without thermal side effects, such as coagulation of the pulp, when using single pulses or short pulse trains.

Long-Term Pulp Reaction

The aim of histologic investigations was to determine whether the pulp can be kept alive over a longer period after Er:YAG laser preparation (Keller, 1989; Keller and Hibst, 1991; Keller et al, 1992). In animal experiments on dog teeth, cavities were prepared with and without opening the pulp chamber. The Er:YAG laser energies ranged from 150 mJ to 500 mJ and repetition rates from 1 to 4 Hz. Preparations were done with and without a water spray. Two, four, six, and eight weeks postoperatively, a histologic evaluation was performed. The teeth were embedded in methacrylate and sectioned into 20- to 80-µm-thick undecalcified sections for light microscopic investigation.

No pulp reaction occurred for all laser parameters used in a cavity preparation in enamel or in dentin far from the pulp. Even after 6 weeks, no new dentin was visible.

If a tissue preparation near the pulp was used, an increased number of ectatic vessels was observed within 2 weeks postoperatively. When opening the pulp chamber, the coronal part of the pulp tissue near the lesion were found to be necrotic, but the odontoblasts on the edges of the laser defect were still alive.

Four weeks after laser treatment, the defects near the pulp showed a new zone of dentin in the adjacent pulp region. When the pulp chamber was opened 4 weeks postoperatively, a mineralized bridge of dentin had been produced by the vital pulp. Six and eight weeks postoperatively, the new dentin in the defects near the pulp and in the case of pulp opening was increased in thickness (Fig 11.7).

These experiments show that after Er:YAG laser irradiation to tissues not adjacent to pulp, no reaction occurs, and after laser irradiation to tissue adjacent to pulp or by opening the pulp chamber only local damage to the pulp occurs, which is comparable to the mechanical injury by the bur. The long-term histologic observations correspond to the results of the microcirculation studies of Er:YAG laser irradiation, as previously described. Compared to other laser systems, thermal injuries of the pulp, such as necrosis, can be avoided (Keller and Hibst, 1989a, b, 1992; Abt et al, 1992). The pulp is still viable in every case if suitable laser parameters and a water cooling system are used.

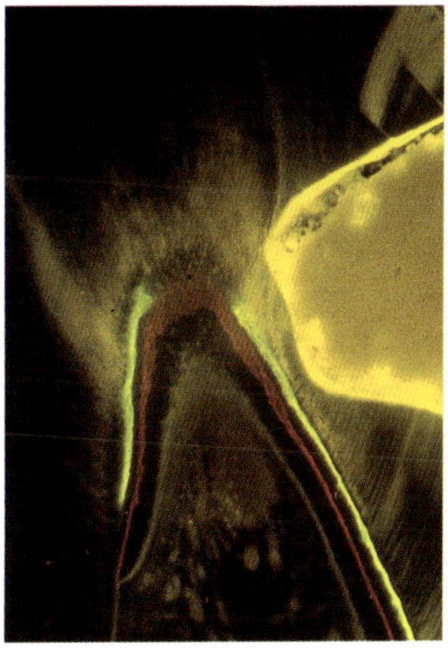

Fig 11.7 Undecalcified histologic section of a dog tooth 8 weeks after Er:YAG laser preparation. Dentin adjacent to pulp (300 mJ, 3 Hz). The newly produced dentin is marked by fluorescent colors. Fluorescence microscopy, × 85.

Bone Ablation

Like teeth, the mineralized matrix of bone consists mainly of hydroxyapatite. The water content and the hydroxyapatite are responsible for the high absorption of the Er:YAG laser light in bone. Some reports indicate that the Er:YAG laser has very promising potential for bone ablation (Nelson et al, 1988, 1989; Nuss et al, 1988; Walsh and Deutsch, 1989; Walsh et al, 1989; Hibst, 1992; Li et al, 1992). A precise and efficient tissue ablation with few thermal side effects offers this laser some advantages compared to other laser systems.

Er:YAG laser osteotomies with saline cooling were performed on beagle dogs. For comparison, bone cuts were undertaken with a continuous wave CO_2 laser and a mechanical bur. After 2, 4, 6, and 8 weeks, histologic evaluations of undecalcified sections of the treated bone samples showed only minimally damaged margins (Keller, 1989; Keller et al, 1991b). The wound healing corresponds to secondary fracture healing after mechanical bur osteotomy, without any delay (Fig 11.8). In contrast, the bone healing following continuous wave CO_2 laser osteotomy is delayed 3 to 4 weeks according to Small et al (1979) and Horch (1983). However, if

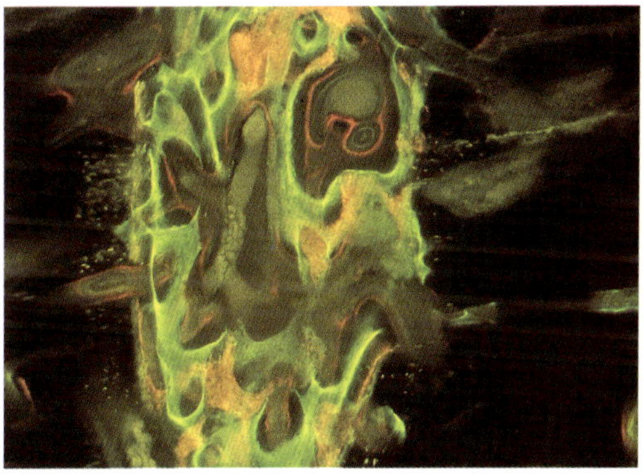

Fig 11.8 Undecalcified histologic section 6 weeks after Er:YAG laser osteotomy. Bone healing marked by fluorescent colors is comparable to that of bur osteotomy, but without delay. Fluorescence microscopy, × 85.

the CO_2 laser is used in the short pulsed mode at 9.6 μm, the healing period is nearly the same as that for the Er:YAG laser (Meyer et al, 1990).

These results can be explained by the different ablation processes. With the continuous wave CO_2 laser, only an evaporation process is responsible for bone ablation. A carbonization of the cut walls and consequently a delay in bone healing can be observed. For Er:YAG laser osteotomy, the process is comparable to thermomechanical ablation of dental hard tissue. Nelson (1989) reported a delay in wound healing following Er:YAG laser bone ablation similar to the observations after continuous wave CO_2 laser osteotomy. For our experimental conditions, however, bone healing after Er:YAG laser osteotomy followed the rules of normal fracture healing and was not delayed.

Possible clinical indications for the Er:YAG laser are apectomies (Paghdiwala, 1991), even during tooth replantation as reported for the CO_2 laser (Miserendino, 1988). Further applications are osteotomies of cysts and impacted teeth.

Oral Soft Tissue Ablation

Diagnosis and treatment of early stages of precancerous or malignant dysplasias of the mucosa are the best possibilities to improve the prognosis of oral carcinomas. These are indications for the continuous wave CO_2 or the Nd:YAG laser because they provide considerable thermal side effects, which help destroy tumors totally. Many extensive benign lesions, such as leukoplakia simplex and lichen planus simplex, should be removed without thermal injury. However, if a scalpel is used, plastic surgery is necessary to close up the wounds and is often followed by scar formation.

Previous reports by Pick et al (1985) and Pick and Pecaro (1987) have shown that in periodontal surgery, thermal-induced coagulation effects occur after CO_2 laser ablation and are undesirable because of the following retraction of the gingiva. These are further possible indications for the Er:YAG laser because of its special ablation effect.

In animal experiments on pig mucosa, lesions were produced by Er:YAG laser irradiation to study the ablation effect and subsequent wound healing (Keller, 1989; Keller et al, 1990). Additionally, incisions were performed with the CO_2 laser and the scalpel.

After focused Er:YAG laser irradiation, small and deep cuts with partial bleeding are seen. Shallow and large lesions are produced by defocused irradiation. In all cases, only a minimal damage zone of about 20 to 40 μm without carbonization occurs. Two days postoperatively, the wounds are closed in the epithelial parts. Eight days postoperatively, the epithelial wound healing is completed. The subepithelial fibrous tissue is not totally repaired at this time. This corresponds to the normal wound healing after surgical incision or excision by scalpels. In contrast, the CO_2 laser cuts show a delay in wound healing of 2 to 3 days because of the extended thermal damage zones.

The Er:YAG laser has indications in soft tissue surgery if no coagulation effect is desired, ie, removal of hyperplastic gingival tissue, periodontal surgery, and ablation of large benign lesions of the oral mucosa or the skin (Kaufmann and Hibst, 1989; Keller et al, 1990), without closing the wound by sutures. For removal of premalignant or malignant dysplasias of the oral mucosa, the delay in wound healing is of secondary importance. These are indications for continuous wave CO_2 or Nd:YAG laser vaporization.

Clinical Applications

For clinical treatment, the Er:YAG laser was used in a focused mode with energies ranging from 100 mJ to 500 mJ and repetition rates of 1 to 4 Hz. Additionally, the teeth were moistened with a water spray.

In an initial clinical study, 67 teeth of 33 patients were treated with a laser according to the guidelines of human rights of Helsinki. Buccal cavities were prepared, primarily because these locations are generally very painful for the patient. In all 67 treatments, there was no pain perception reported in 24 teeth and minimal pain in 38 teeth. In 29 of 41 teeth with deep cavities, only minimal pain was perceived. In a second study, the pain perception after laser preparation was compared with the pain after mechanical drilling. It was found that only 6% of the patients with laser cavities required local anesthesia in comparison to 11% of the patients with mechanically drilled cavities. In 83%, the bur was judged to be more uncomfortable and 88% of the patients would prefer the Er:YAG laser for further therapy. The pain perception during laser treatment was reduced; the pain was described as only like short needle sticks. No loss of vitality was observed. Initial clinical results of apectomy, osteotomy of cysts, impacted teeth, and the removal of oral mucosal lesions show similar good results.

Conclusion and Perspectives

In comparison to other laser systems, the Er:YAG laser is preferred for a variety of indications. The in-vitro experiments and the animal studies have shown that the Er:YAG laser can be used for the removal of healthy tooth hard tissue as well as carious decay with high efficiency and without thermal injury to the adjacent tissues. Restorative materials like composites and cements can be ablated without using the mechanical bur. Gold crowns and cast fillings cannot be removed because the laser beam is reflected. No ablation effect can be observed on ceramics; however, a great number of patients with primary or secondary caries can be treated with the Er:YAG laser (Figs 11.9 and 11.10). From the microcirculation studies, histologic investigations, and clinical applications it can be concluded that a laser cavity preparation is possible without or with only minimal toothache.

For caries therapy, a cavity preparation is possible without using the mechanical bur in primary carious lesions. With secondary carious lesions, filling materials should be removed first by the bur followed by laser preparation of the carious lesion. The advantage is a precise and less painful preparation.

Soft tissue ablation without delay of wound healing and removal of calculi without damaging the root are further potential indications for the Er:YAG laser in periodontics or in ablation of benign soft tissue dysplasias.

The Er:YAG laser is recommended for osteotomy, cyst removal, or apectomy because of excellent bone healing. The Er:YAG laser could be used in endodontics if a fiber is developed for root canal treatment.

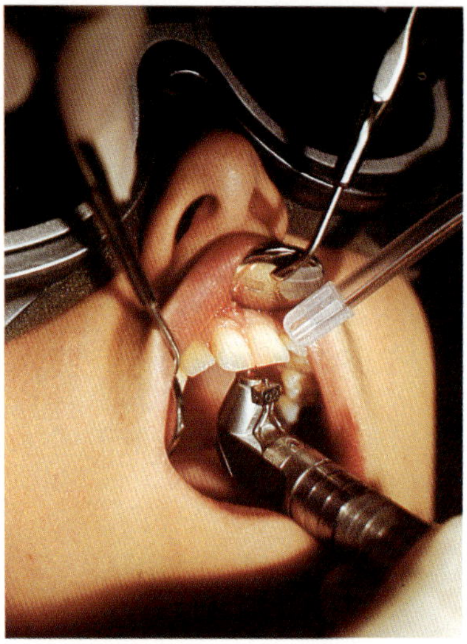

Fig 11.9 Er:YAG laser applicator in situ on the mesial wall of the left maxillary central incisor.

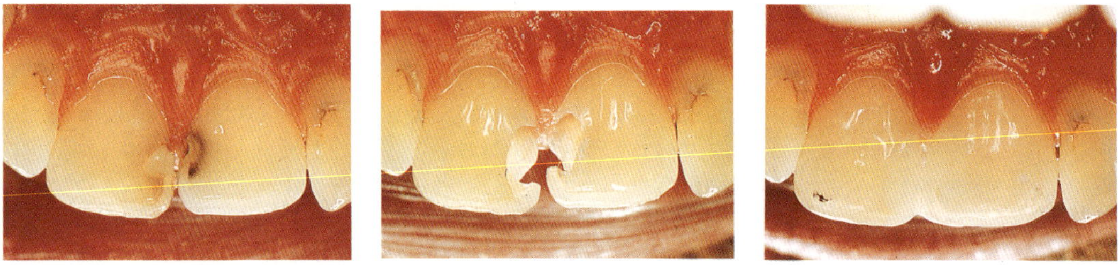

Fig 11.10 Er:YAG laser caries treatment of the maxillary central incisors. **(a)**, Primary caries decay in the right incisor. Secondary caries decay in the left incisor. **(b)**, After laser preparation, cavities with a laser-roughed zone in enamel. **(c)**, Teeth esthetically reconstructed with composites.

References

Abt E, Wigdor H, Walsh J, Brown J. The effect of the CO_2, Nd:YAG and Er:YAG lasers on dentin and pulp tissues in dogs. Laser surgery: advanced characterization, therapeutics, and systems III. Proc SPIE 1992;1643: 464–474.

Burkes EJ, Hoke J, Gomes E, Wolbarsht M. Wet versus dry enamel ablation by Er:YAG laser. J Prosthet Dent 1992;67:847–851.

Franetzki M. Laser in der Zahnmedizin. Magazin für ZMK 1991;3:9–14.

Hibst R, Keller U, Steiner R. Die Wirkung gepulster Er:YAG Laserstrahlung auf Zahngewebe. Laser Med Surg 1988;4:163–165.

Hibst R, Keller U. Experimental studies of the application of the Er:YAG laser on dental hard substances. I. Measurements of the ablation rate. Lasers Surg Med 1989;9:338–344.

Hibst R. Mechanical effects of erbium:YAG laser bone ablation. Lasers Surg Med 1992;12:125–130.

Hibst R, Keller U. Heat effect of pulsed Er:YAG laser radiation. Laser surgery: advanced characterization, therapeutics and systems. Proc SPIE 1990;1200:379–386.

Hibst R, Keller U. Removal of dental filling materials by Er:YAG laser radiation. Lasers in orthopedic, dental, and veterinary medicine. Proc SPIE 1991;1424:120–126.

Hibst R, Keller U. Laserbearbeitung von Zahnhartsubstanzen und zahnärztlichen Füllungsmaterialien. In

Waidelich W, Waidelich R, Hofstetter A (eds): Lasers in Medicine. Berlin-Heidelberg: Springer; 1992;288–291.

Hoke JA, Burkes EJ, Gomes ED, Wolbarsht ML. Erbium:YAG (2.94 μm) laser effects on dental tissues. J Laser Appl 1990;2:61–65.

Horch HH. Laser-Osteotomie und Anwendungsmöglichkeiten des Lasers in der oralen Weichteilchirurgie. Berlin: Quintessenz; 1983.

Kaufmann R, Hibst R. Pulsed Er:YAG- and 308 nm UV-excimer laser: an in vitro and in vivo study of skin-ablative effects. Lasers Surg Med 1989;9:132–140.

Kayano T, Ochiai S, Kiyono K, Yamamoto H, Nakajima S, Mochizuki T. Effect of Er:YAG laser irradiation on human extracted teeth. J Clin Laser Med Surg 1991;4:147–150.

Keller U. Die ablative Wirkung des Erbium:YAG Lasers an oralen Hart- u Weichgeweben. Habilitationsschrift Universität Ulm, 1989.

Keller U, Hibst R. Experimental studies of the application of the Er:YAG laser on dental hard substances. II. Light microscopic and SEM investigations. Lasers Surg Med 1989a;9:345–351.

Keller U, Hibst R. Zur ablativen Wirkung des Er:YAG Lasers auf Schmelz und Dentin. Dtsch Zahnaerztl Z 1989b;44:600–602.

Keller U, Hibst R. Ultrastructural changes of enamel and dentin following Er:YAG laser irradiation on teeth. Laser surgery: advanced characterization, therapeutics and systems. Proc SPIE 1990;1200:408–415.

Keller U, Hibst R, Mohr W. Tierexperimentelle Studien zur Laserablation von Mundschleimhauterkrankungen mit dem Er:YAG Laser. Oesterr Z Stomatol 1990;87: 475–480.

Keller U, Raab W, Hibst R. Die Pulpareaktion während der Bestrahlung von Zahnharztsubstanzen mit dem Er:YAG-Laser. Dtsch Zahnaerztl Z 1991a;46:158–160.

Keller U, Hibst R, Mohr W. Tierexperimentelle Untersuchungen zur Laserosteotomie mit dem Er:YAG-Laser. Dtsch Z Mund Kiefer Gesichtschir 1991b;15:197–199.

Keller U, Hibst R. Tooth pulp reaction following Er:YAG laser application. Lasers in orthopedic, dental, and veterinary medicine. Proc SPIE 1991;1424:127–133.

Keller U. Lasers in dentistry. Future trends in biomedical applications of lasers. Proc SPIE 1991;1525:282–288.

Keller U, Hibst R. Wirkungsweise und Indikationen des Erbium-YAG Lasers in der Zahn-Mund-Kieferheilkunde. Magazin für ZMK 1992;4:6–10.

Keller U, Hibst R, Mohr W. Histologische Untersuchungen der Pulpareaktion nach Er:YAG-Laserbestrahlung. Dtsch Zahnaerztl Z 1992;47:222–224.

Lenz P, Gilde H, Pyttel U. Morphologische Untersuchungen zur Wirkung der Laserstrahlung auf Pulpa und Mundschleimhäute. Dtsch Zahnaerztl Z 1977;32:508–511.

Li ZZ, Reinisch L, Van de Merwe WP. Bone ablation with Er:YAG and CO_2 laser: study of thermal and acoustic effects. Lasers Surg Med 1992;12:79–85.

Melcer J, Chaumette MT, Melcer F. Dental pulp exposed to the CO_2 laser beam. Lasers Surg Med 1987;7:347–352.

Meyer DR, Scholz C, Klanke J, Büchle A, Grothues-Spork M, Müller GJ, Siebert W, Dinkelaker F, Cierpinksi T. Der kurzgepulste CO_2 Laser mit 9,6 μm Wellenlänge im Vergleich zum Erbium:YAG Laser bei der Laserosteotomie. Laser Med Surg 1990;6:150–155.

Miserendino LJ. The laser apicoectomy: endodontic application of the CO_2 laser for periapical surgery. Oral Surg 1988;66:615.

Neev I, Liaw LL, Raney DV, Fujishige IT, Ho PT, Berns MW. Selectivity and efficiency in the ablation of hard dental tissues with ArF pulsed excimer lasers. Lasers Surg Med 1991;11:499–510.

Nelson JS, Yow L, Liaw LH, et al. Ablation of bone and methacrylate by a prototype mid-infrared erbium-YAG laser. Lasers Surg Med 1988;8:494–500.

Nelson JS, Orenstein A, Liaw LH, Berns MW. Mid-infrared erbium-YAG laser ablation of bone: the effect of laser osteotomy on bone healing. Lasers Surg Med 1989;9:362–374.

Nuss RC, Fabian RL, Sarkar R, Puliafito CA. Infrared laser bone ablation. Lasers Surg Med 1988;8:381–391.

Paghdiwala AF. Application of the erbium:YAG laser on hard dental tissue: measurements of the temperature changes and depth of cut. Proc ICALEO 88, Laser Institute of America, 1989;64:192–201.

Paghdiwala AF. Root resection of endodontically treated teeth by erbium:YAG laser radiation. Lasers in orthopedic, dental, and veterinary medicine. Proc SPIE 1991; 1424:150–159.

Pick RM, Pecaro BC. Use of the CO_2 laser in soft tissue dental surgery. Lasers Surg Med 1987;7:207–213.

Pick RM, Pecaro BC, Silverman CJ. The laser gingivectomy. The use of the CO_2 laser for removal of phenytoin hyperplasia. J Periodontol 1985;56:492–496.

Serebro L, Segal T, Nordenberg D, Gordil C, Bar-Lev M. Examination of tooth pulp following laser beam irradiation. Lasers Surg Med 1987;7:236–239.

Small IA, Osborn TP, Fuller T, Hussain M, Kobernick S. Observations of carbon dioxide laser and bone burr in the osteotomy of the rabbit tibia. J Oral Maxillofac Surg 1979;37:159–166.

Stern RH, Renger HL, Howell FV. Laser effects on vital dental pulps. Br Dent J 1969;127:26–28.

Stern RH, Vahl J, Sognnaes R. Lased enamel: ultrastructural observations of pulsed carbon dioxide laser effects. J Dent Res 1972;51:455–460.

Stern RH. The laser in dentistry: a review of the literature. J Dent Assoc S Afr 1974;29:173–179.

Vahl J. Der Laser und seine bisherige Anwendung in der Zahnmedizin. Hippokrates 1971;42:488–506.

Walsh JT, Flotte TJ, Deutsch TF. Er:YAG laser ablation of tissue: effect of pulse duration and tissue type on thermal damage. Lasers Surg Med 1989;9:314–326.

Walsh JT, Deutsch TF. Er:YAG laser ablation of tissue: measurement of ablation rates. Lasers Surg Med 1989; 9:327–337.

Willenborg GC. Dental laser applications: emerging to maturity. Lasers Surg Med 1989;9:309–313.

Yamamoto H, Kayano T, Ochiai S. Möglichkeiten der Er:YAG Laseranwendung in der Konservierenden Zahnheilkunde. In Vahl J, van Benthem H (eds): Laser in der Zahnmedizin. Berlin: Quintessenz; 1992.

Chapter Twelve

Clinical and Investigative Research on the Excimer Laser

Tim Liesenhoff

During the past 10 years, there have been attempts to remove dental hard tissues with Er:YAG lasers (Hibst and Keller, 1989; Keller and Hibst, 1989a, b; Walsh et al, 1989; Walsh and Deutsch, 1989). Preliminary studies seem to indicate that thermal side effects are greatly reduced with this type of laser. The Er:YAG laser beam is not easily transmitted through optical fibers and therefore is usually applied via mirror and arm delivery systems. A root canal preparation is not possible due to the lack of a suitable delivery system. In the early 1980s, the excimer laser gained clinical significance in refractive surgery on the eye and in angioplasty (Bende et al, 1988; Trokel et al, 1983).

Depending on the gas filling the excimer laser, it can be used at different wavelengths: most commonly, 193 nm, 248 nm, and 308 nm. The 308-nm excimer laser beam can be delivered through optical quartz glass fibers and has a sufficient transmission through water. The demand in dentistry is to find systems that make existing procedures easier and more effective, or even to make treatments possible that did not exist before. To evaluate side effects of the 308-nm excimer laser beam, it was necessary to find answers to the following questions: (1) is it possible to remove dental hard tissues with the 308-nm excimer laser; (2) what energy densities are necessary to ablate dental hard tissues; (3) what kind of ultrastructural changes in the dental hard tissues occur through the 308-nm excimer laser; and (4) what kind of temperature rises occur in the surrounding tissue due to the 308-nm excimer laser.

Many investigations have already been performed on the possible antimicrobial effects of carbon dioxide laser light (Adrian and Gross, 1979; Hardee et al, 1990; 1993; Hooks et al, 1980; McGuff and Bell, 1966; Melcer, 1982; Melcer, 1987; Miserendino, 1988; Miserendino et al, 1988; Staberg, 1983; Zakariasen et al, 1986; Zakariasen et al, 1989). The CO_2 laser produces the bactericidal effect by heat from vaporization. It has also been known for more than 30 years that ultraviolet (UV) light has a sterilizing effect. Unfortunately it is necessary to apply very long exposures of irradiation when using conventional UV light sources to influence bacterial growth. Since the excimer laser produces not only monochromatic but also coherent and collimated light, it was our intention to investigate the influence of the 308-nm excimer laser on bacterial growth.

If there is a bactericidal effect, it is of special interest to determine if it is dependent on the type of bacteria, the energy density, and/or the time of irradiation. Since the 308-nm excimer laser is guidable through optical quartz glass fibers and has a good transmission through water, it was also of interest to determine if root canal preparation is possible with the 308-nm excimer laser. We also wanted to know if it is possible to perform root canal treatment with the 308-nm excimer laser in humans. Since 308-nm excimer laser root canal treatment is a very expensive and time-consuming procedure, it was of special interest to determine if the unique cleaning and sterilizing effect of the 308-nm excimer laser could reduce the treatment to a single appointment without loss of success. Two techniques of preparation were performed. One group of patients was treated with an excimer laser root canal preparation only, and the other group was treated with a combination technique using the 308-nm excimer laser as a cleaning and sterilizing treatment following conventional preparation of the root canal.

Preliminary Investigations

All investigations were carried out with an excimer laser (EMG 102 by Lambda Physik, Acton, MA; MAX-10 by Technolas; Eximed by Summit Technology, Waltham, MA). The laser was filled with xenon and chloride and operated on a wavelength of 308 nm. The maximal primary energy was 30 to 150 mJ, pulse duration 10 to 60 nsec. The output energy was measured before and after each operation with a powermoter: joulmeter (Gentec ED 500). The laser beam was directed through a system of lenses and diaphragms that had been developed for this purpose (Liesenhoff et al, 1989a; Liesenhoff et al, 1990a; Liesenhoff et al, 1989b). By varying the distance of the sample to the described optical system, it was possible to irradiate with different energy densities.

Ablation Measurements

In these initial studies, we used freshly extracted, caries-free human teeth to measure the rate of enamel and dentin ablation. The teeth were stored in buffered formalin solution diluted in tap water and then embedded in plastic. The embedded specimens were then sectioned in an axial direction to produce slices of 0.5- to 1-mm-thick sections. Each section was individually measured with a micrometer gauge (accuracy: ±0.01 mm) and then assigned to either the dentin or enamel group. The number of samples per group was 60.

Within each group, the samples were randomly divided into 20 groups of three according to each position in the optical system. Each position was defined as the distance from the focus of the laser (n = 20). The rate of ablation was defined as the reduction of the sample thickness in the irradiated area per laser pulse. To determine the rate of ablation, we kept two parameters constant: (1) the thickness of the sample; and (2) the energy density (irradiated surface in defined distance to the focus of the laser beam). We then counted the number of pulses needed to perforate the sample. The moment of perforation and the size of the irradiated surface were determined by tracking on photosensitive paper. The size of the irradiated surface corresponded to the ablated area on the blackened photographic paper. The moment of sample perforation was set equal to the beginning of ablation on the blackened photographic paper, which was placed directly behind the sample. The measurements were repeated for each position and each sample. All measured data were plotted as rates of ablation at various energy densities.

Temperature Measurements

For the temperature measurements, the freshly extracted teeth were embedded in plastic and separated in half sagittally. A 0.5-mm-thick section was then separated from the pulpal and root canal side of the separated block to provide direct access to the pulpal chamber and the root canal space. To place a thermal probe inside the root canal and pulpal chamber, the root canal and pulpal chamber were enlarged by a dental drill, the thermal probe inserted, the surrounding lumen filled with a humid gel (Methocel), and the section was placed as a cover. This cover had a defined thickness of 0.5 to 1.0 mm. The thermal probe served a thermal microprobe without auto heat capacity (MTT 7615, accuracy = ± 0.1°C; Birke, Germany). The samples were then positioned in the ray path. The placed section (cover) was exposed at a defined distance (± 0.1 mm) to the focus and the pulpal chamber. This way it was possible to perforate the sample at defined distances to the thermal probe. The irradiation was performed until a stable maximum temperature was measured (plateau of registered curve).

Microscopic Evaluation of Irradiated Surfaces

All specimens were investigated macroscopically and with scanning and transmission electron microscopy (SEM and TEM). For SEM investigation, an enamel and dentin specimen was selected that had been exposed to defined numbers of pulses to evaluate changes in the surface structure according to the number of applied laser pulses. For the TEM investigations, dentin and enamel specimens were irradiated after embedding and trimming. This way it was possible to investigate the laser tissue effect on the surrounding tissue. To investigate the laser-tissue effect inside the root canals, a laser root canal preparation was performed on freshly extracted human teeth. The prepared teeth were sectioned axially to expose the root canal surfaces for direct visualization.

Effects on Bacteria

For these studies, we used a 308-nm excimer laser (Summit Technology, Waltham, MA) with a primary energy of about 65 mJ and a pulse duration of 60 nsec. The laser light was guided through an optical quartz glass fiber with a core diameter of 600 mm. The irradiation was performed with defined energy densities and number of pulses and a constant fiber suspension distance of 8 mm. Bacterial suspensions (bacteria in nutrient solution 1.0 to 6.0 × 10^6/mL) of *Staphylococcus aureus* (ATCC 25923), *Escherichia coli* (ATCC 25922), and *Enterococcus faecalis* (ATCC 29212) were used as the test organisms. The bacteria were incubated for about 6 hours and then adjusted to a concentration of 1.0 to 6.0 × 10^6/mL with nephelometry.

For irradiation, the bacterial suspensions were distributed into microtiter plates with 100 mL per portion. The setup was mounted on an oscillating table (frequency: 1,100/min). With a constant fiber suspension distance, the energy density and number of pulses were varied. After irradiation, the samples were diluted in sterile NaCl solution (0.9%) and spread on agar plates (Columbia-agar with 5% sheep blood). The agar plates were incubated for about 12 to 16 hours, and the colony-building units were counted. This way the dependence of bacterial growth on energy density and number of pulses could be investigated individually. Each series of measurements was performed with seven different energy densities and a variation from 0 to 2,000 pulses with a repetition rate of 20 Hz. For calculation, the number of surviving bacteria according to the number of applied pulses at a defined energy density were plotted as XY graphs, and the ED 90 (reduction of 90% bacteria) was calculated.

For all investigations, control groups were used that received the same treatment but no laser irradiation. To exclude a possible thermal effect on bacterial growth, temperature measurements were performed with a thermal probe (Keithley 870 digital thermometer type KTC probe) during irradiation. The temperatures were plotted according to the number of applied laser pulses.

In-Vitro Root Canal Preparation

The in-vitro root canal preparation was performed on freshly extracted human teeth that did not have any prior root canal treatment. After opening the pulpal chamber conventionally, the root canal preparation was performed with the 308-nm excimer laser only. The laser beam was guided through optical quartz glass fibers. The energy density was 6 to 9 J/cm^2, and the pulse duration was 60 nsec. The preparation was performed in a step-back technique with diameters of 100 to 900 mm and with continuous rinsing with saline solution. The prepared teeth were then processed for histologic examination as previously described.

In-Vivo Root Canal Treatment

Laser root canal treatment was performed on patients suffering from chronic apical periodontitis with different degrees of periapical osseous destruction. Two methods of endodontic treatment were performed. One group was treated with the 308-nm excimer laser only. The other group received conventional and 308-nm excimer laser treatment. All patients were examined clinically and radiologically before and after treatment. After trephination and exposure of the pulpal chamber, the root canal treatment was performed following determination of the preparation depth with radiography. The laser preparation was performed with a step-back technique starting with fibers of 100- to 200-mm diameter and ending with fibers of 600- to 900-mm diameter with continuous saline solution rinsing. The combined treatment was performed by hand instrumentation up to ISO size number 60 to 90 reamers followed by cleaning and sterilization by the laser applying about 5,000 laser pulses of 4 to 6 J/cm^2 with a pulse duration of 60 nsec at 20 Hz. The root canals were filled with Diaket (ESPE, Seefeld, Germany) and gutta-percha masterpoint.

Results of Investigations

Ablation of Dentin and Enamel

Irradiation of dentin and enamel with energy densities of less than 800 mJ/cm^2 did not result in ablation of tissue but rather in heat and carbonization. With energy densities of more than 800 mJ/cm^2, the threshold of ablation was passed, and with an increase in the energy density a maximum ablation of 0.9 mm/pulse for enamel and 3.2 mm/pulse for dentin was reached (Fig 12.1). The use of energy densities above 4 to 5 J/cm^2 did not increase the rate of ablation.

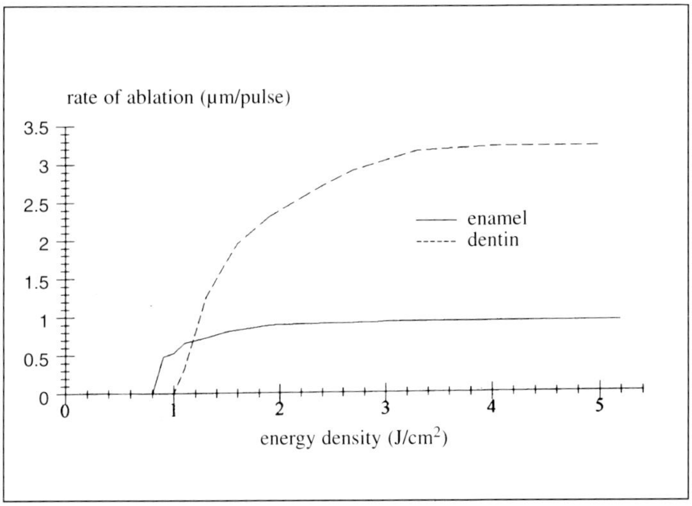

Fig 12.1 Plot of the rate of ablation depending on the energy density.

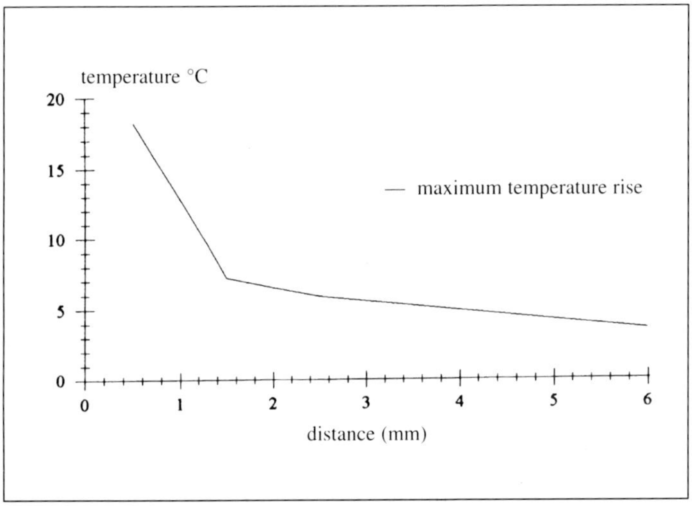

Fig 12.2 Plot of the maximum rise in temperature depending on the distance between the thermal probe and the location of ablation.

Change in Pulpal Chamber Temperature

Depending on the position of measurement (distance between temperature probe and location of ablation), the rise in temperature reached a characteristic value after application of about 5,000 to 8,000 laser pulses. For all measurements, a minimum of 10,000 pulses was applied. The analysis of the maximum rise in temperature (value of the stable maximum of the temperature curve) shows a steep rise in the values, which approaches linearily near the location of the thermal probe (Fig 12.2).

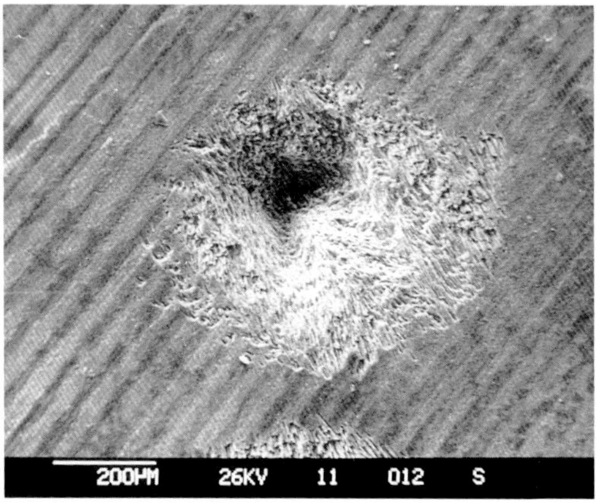

Fig 12.3 Enamel surface after irradiation with < 500 pulses.

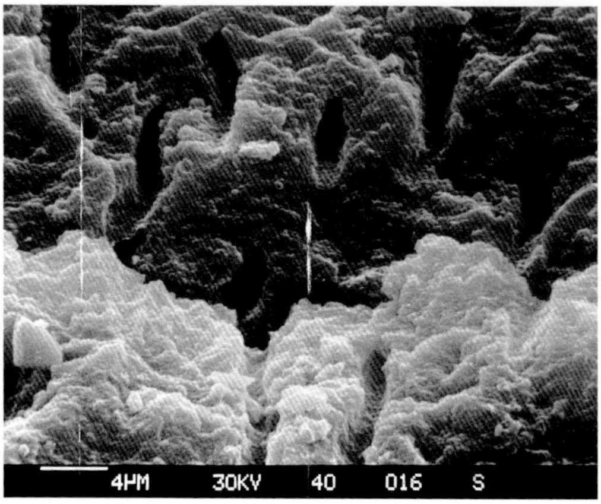

Fig 12.4 Dentin surface after irradiation with < 500 pulses.

Scanning Electron Microscopic Findings

The irradiated surfaces that appeared smooth but not shiny were investigated with SEM. Depending on the number of applied pulses, the morphologic structure appeared as roughness or craters. Enamel surfaces that had been irradiated with only a few pulses (< 500 pulses) were debrided from overlying structures. The enamel prisms were exposed, forming an ultrastructure similar to the etched surface of enamel (Fig 12.3). There was no sign of thermal or mechanical alteration of the surrounding tissue.

Dentin surfaces after exposure to 308-nm excimer laser irradiation appeared as being debrided from overlying tissue layers. There were no signs of thermal or mechanical alterations to that of the surrounding tissue. The ultrastructure of the irradiated surfaces corresponded to the natural tissue structure (Fig 12.4).

Transmission Electron Microscopic Findings

None of the specimens that had been irradiated with the 308-nm excimer laser with energy densities of 4 to 5 J/cm^2 showed any sign of alteration of the surrounding tissue. The microcrystalline structure remained intact adjacent to the location of ablation. When dental hard tissues were irradiated with the excimer laser with energy densities close to the threshold of ablation (1 to 3 J/cm^2), there were clear thermal alterations. The maximum depth of alteration was 1 mm.

Effects on Bacterial Growth

It was possible to demonstrate that bactericidal effects are attainable with irradiation with the 308-nm excimer laser at an energy density below the threshold of ablation. Irradiation of bacteria with a defined energy density of 0.8 J/cm^2 caused an 80% reduction, depending on the type of bacteria tested (Fig 12.5). A complete eradication of bacteria was achieved by applying 250 pulses. There was a rapid reduction in bacterial counts produced by in-

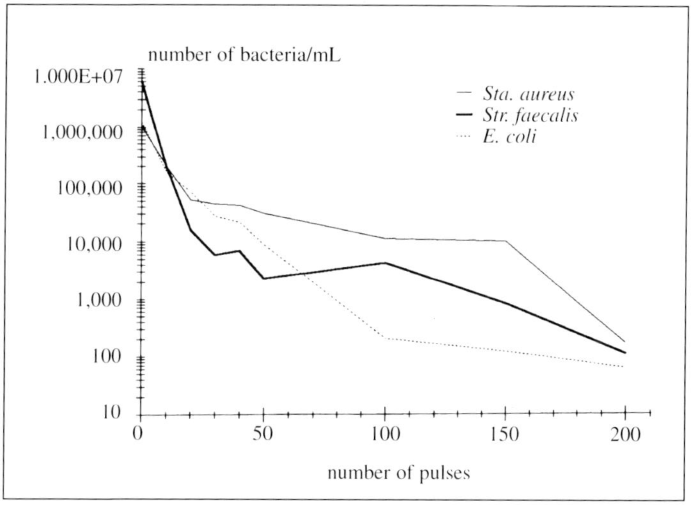

Fig 12.5 Killing curve of *Str. faecalis, E. coli, Sta. aureus* in semi-log relation.

creasing the number of laser pulses. This rapid reduction was also dependent on the energy density (Figs 12.6 and 12.7).

The investigation of the relationship between energy density and number of pulses necessary to gain a 90% reduction of bacteria was performed by plotting the iso curves of the ED90 according to the number of laser pulses and energy density. When using energy densities up to 1.2 J/cm^2, there was only a small change in the number of pulses needed to kill 90% of the bacteria. There was an obvious decrease in the number of pulses necessary to kill the same percentage of bacteria when applying energy densities between 1.2 and 1.8 J/cm^2. By applying energy densities greater than 1.8 J/cm^2, the decrease in the number of pulses needed to produce the same level of bacterial killing was only minimal (Fig 12.8).

The temperature measurement during irradiation showed a stable maximum of 13 K after 4,000 laser pulses with an energy density of 0.8 J/cm^2. The temperature interval was between 30.4°C (0 pulses) and 41.9°C (2,000 pulses) (Fig 12.9).

Root Canal Preparation

In-Vitro. In-vitro root canal preparation was performed on freshly extracted human molars, premolars, and anterior teeth. After opening the pulpal chamber in the conventional manner, the root canal preparation was performed. Because the 308-nm excimer laser ablates organic material much more easily than inorganic material, the entrance of the root canals (orifice) was found almost automatically. With continuous saline rinsing and use of a fiber with a core diameter of about 200 mm, the lower third of the root canal was reached with the first instrumentation. By varying the size of the optical fiber, all of the root canals were completely prepared with the excimer laser only. The most suitable energy density for root canal preparation was determined to be from 6 to 9 J/cm^2 at a repetition rate of 20 to 30 Hz. With these parameters, a smooth preparation of the

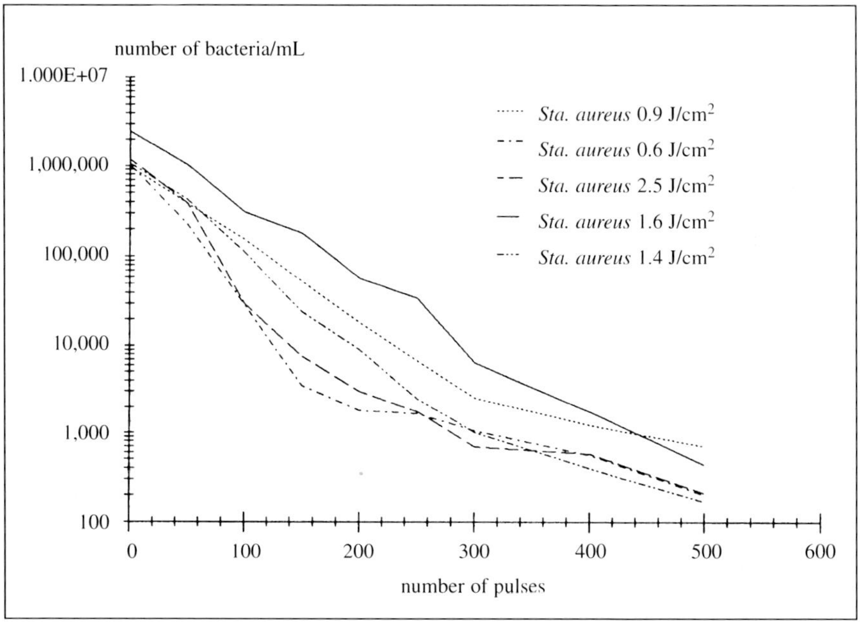

Fig 12.6 Killing curves of *Sta. aureus* at different energy densities as semi-log plot. The log relation between amount of microbial reduction and the number of applied pulses is demonstrated.

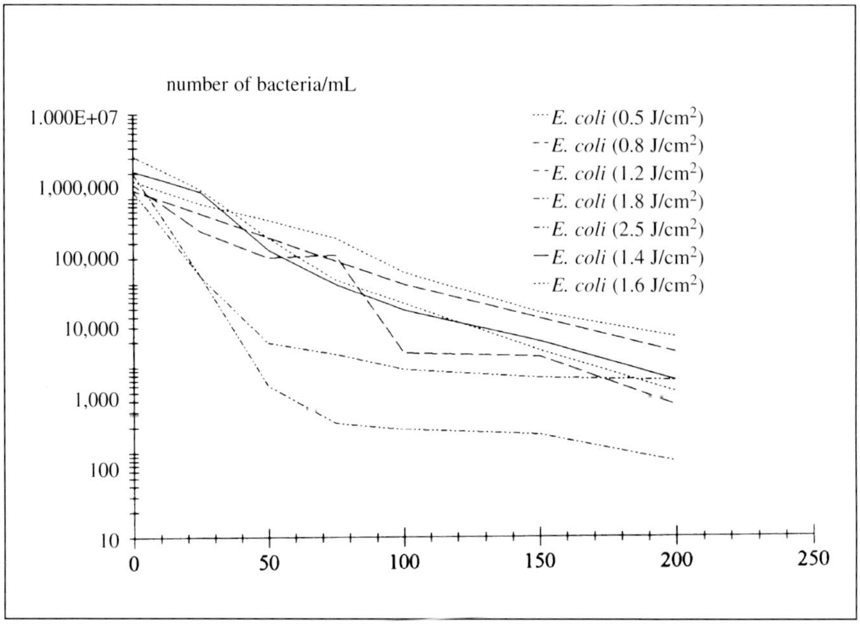

Fig 12.7 Killing curves of *E. coli* at different energy densities as semi-log plot. The log relation between the amount of microbial reduction and number of applied pulses is demonstrated.

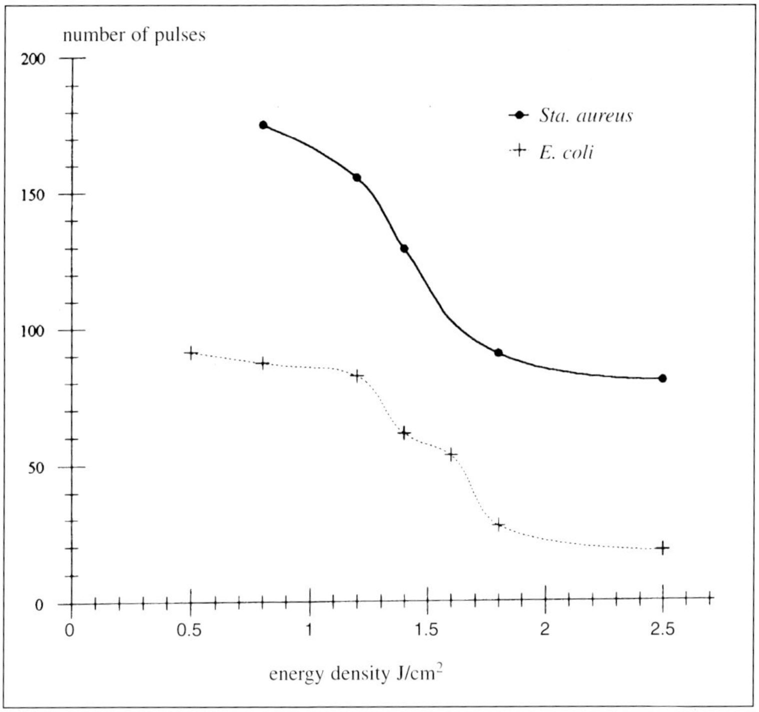

Fig 12.8 The iso-ED90 of *Sta. aureus* and *E. coli* as function of number of pulses and energy density. The temperature measurement during irradiation indicates a stable maximum of 13 K after 4,000 laser pulses with an energy density of 0.8 J/cm^2. The temperature interval was between 30.40°C (0 pulses) and 41.9°C (2,000 pulses).

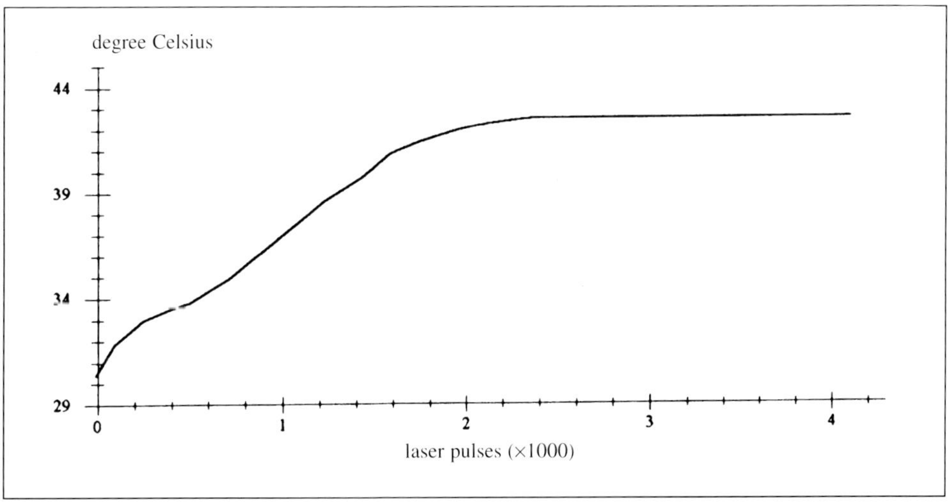

Fig 12.9 Plot of the temperature rise during irradiation of the bacterial suspension.

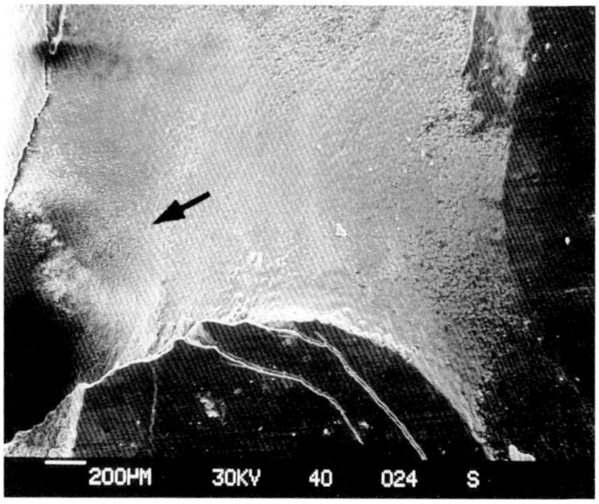

Fig 12.10 SEM of 308-nm excimer laser–prepared molar. The entrances of the root canals are free of pulpal and necrotic tissue (arrow).

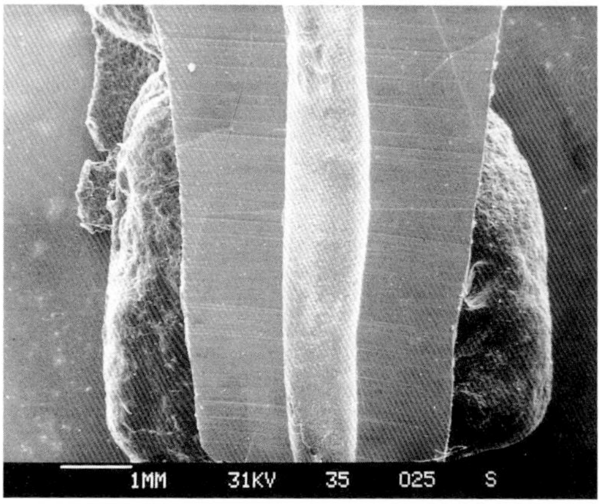

Fig 12.11 SEM of the apical third of a 308-nm excimer laser–prepared tooth. The root canal appears to retain its natural shape and is free of pulpal and necrotic tissue. All parts of the root canal have been completely debrided of soft tissue.

root canals was possible. Based on the SEM investigations of the prepared teeth, all root canals appeared to be free of soft tissue and debris (Figs 12.10 and 12.11). There was no smear layer detectable and there were no cases of straightening or overinstrumentation of the canals (see Fig 12.10). The root canals appeared to retain their natural shape, and the aberrant dentinal tubuli appeared to be open (Fig 12.12). There were no detectable thermal or mechanical alterations to the root canal walls, and the apical delta and the openings of the dentinal tubuli were completely debrided from pulpal and/or necrotic tissue remnants (Fig 12.13).

In-Vivo. Root canal treatments were performed on 45 patients suffering from chronic apical periodontitis. None of the teeth had prior root canal treatment. The degree of periapical infection varied for each case. The patients were divided into two groups. One group (n = 20) of patients was treated with the excimer laser only. The other group (n = 25) received a laser treatment after preparation. All root canals were filled directly after treatment with Diaket and a gutta-percha masterpoint. It was possible to prepare all root canals and to complete treatment of all cases in both groups. All patients responded well regardless of the method of treatment. There was no difference between the groups concerning postoperative complications or healing quality.

Because of the difference in the rate of ablation between dentin, pulpal, and necrotic tissue, the excimer laser was securely guided by the dentin walls of the root canal without producing a perforation of the canal wall. The entrances to the root canals were found almost automatically due to the described differences in ablation rate. Since most patients noticed a sensation that they described as a stick of a needle when reaching the apex, the laser treatments were performed with local anesthesia. For clinical application, it was preferable to work with a bundle of fibers (diameters: 200 to 900 mm) ready to use (Fig 12.14). The most convenient laser

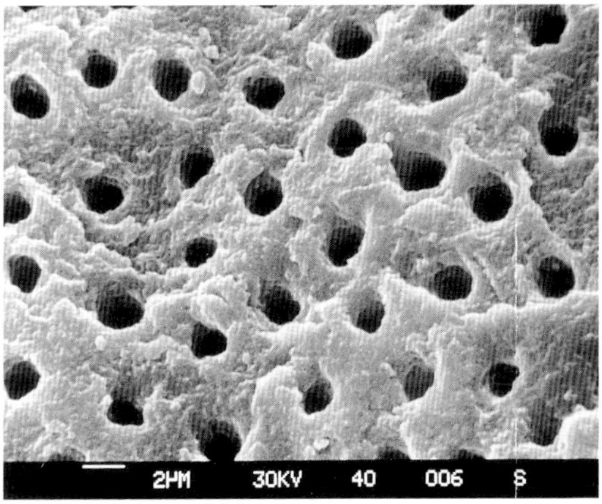

Fig 12.12 SEM close up of root canal wall after 308-nm excimer laser preparation. The entrances of the dentinal tubuli are open. No clogging or smear layer is detectable.

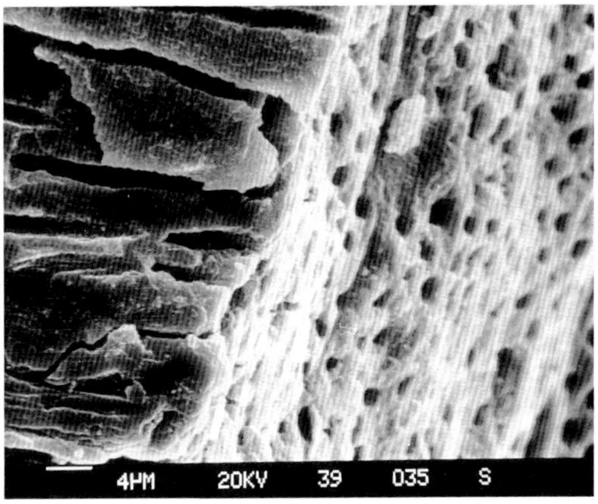

Fig 12.13 SEM of fractured root canal wall. The dentinal tubuli are free of soft tissue in their longitudinal course.

setting was an energy density of 6 to 9 J/cm^2 at a repetition rate of 20 to 30 Hz. If energy densities of more than 9 J/cm^2 were applied, the survival time of the optical fiber was clearly reduced. It was not possible to increase the preparation speed by raising the pulse repetition rate above 30 Hz.

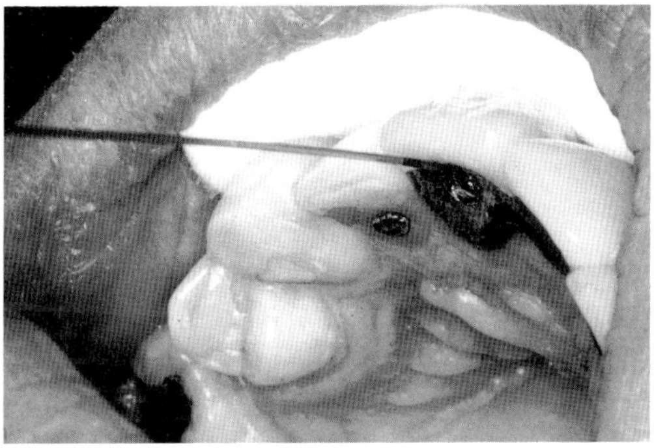

Fig 12.14 Optical fiber in upper front tooth. Postoperative control radiographs were obtained from all patients. The root canals appeared completely prepared to the level of the apex. The optical quartz glass fibers were flexible enough to be used for endodontic treatments on molars, premolars, and anterior teeth.

Discussion

The studies presented demonstrate that it is possible to remove dental hard and soft tissues in a controlled fashion with the excimer laser. This has also been the result of former investigations on excimer lasers in dentistry (Liesenhoff et al, 1989a, 1989b, 1989c, 1990a, 1990b, 1992). As reported by other research groups, the alteration of surrounding tissue due to 308-nm excimer laser irradiation is minimal (Frentzen and Koort, 1990; Murphy-Chutorian et al, 1986). Compared to all other existing laser systems that have been suggested or investigated for dental application (Nd:YAG, Ho:YAG, Er:YAG, and CO_2), the 308-nm excimer laser is the only system that offers precise ablation of tissue, fiber delivery, bactericidal effects, good transmission through water, and enamel surface conditioning (laser-etching) in one system.

The temperature elevations that were produced by the 308-nm excimer laser within the pulp chamber were 180°C maximum. This temperature rise should be tolerable for the living tooth (Zach et al, 1965; Serebro et al, 1987; Neiburger and Miserendino, 1988; Shoji et al, 1985; 1989; Stuben et al, 1964; Taylor et al, 1965) and remains far below the temperature rises caused by other laser systems (Serebro et al, 1987; Shoji et al, 1985, 1989). The described temperature rises were measured without any cooling system. Since the 308-nm excimer laser has good transmission through water, a continuous saline rinsing could prevent a rise in temperature.

The SEM and TEM investigations of the irradiated tissues demonstrated that it is possible to ablate dental hard and soft tissue without alterations in the surrounding tissue. The amount of ablation is dependent on the applied energy density and the beam size and quality. By using energy densities of more than 4 J/cm^2, maximum ablation can be achieved while the thermal side effects can be minimized. Contrary to CO_2 and YAG lasers, the excimer laser causes fewer thermal side effects when the energy density is raised. The maximal rates of ablation of about 1 mm/pulse for enamel and about 3.2 mm/pulse for dentin assure a high degree of precision.

The ultrastructural changes of the irradiated surfaces may provide a good retentive surface for filling materials (Frentzen and Koort, 1990; Liesenhoff et al, 1990a). The 308-nm excimer laser makes it possible to create retentive surfaces in dentin and enamel without ultrastructural changes in the underlying tissue layers. The SEM investigations of the root canal walls after laser preparation displayed openings of aberrant dentin tubuli free of a smear layer and of clogging by debris. Also, the aberrant dentinal tubuli were free of pulpal or necrotic tissue. This preparation quality allows oxygen and medicinal fluids to enter the dentin tubuli and the apical delta (Liesenhoff et al, 1989c, 1990b, 1992). This quality of preparation is not possible with conventional methods (Haikel and Alleman, 1988; El-Tagouri et al, 1988; Bolanos and Jensen, 1980; Petschelt, 1989).

The bactericidal effects of the 308-nm excimer laser have also been shown to be present at different energy densities. Since it is possible to achieve bactericidal effects even by applying the 308-nm excimer laser with energy densities far below the threshold of ablation, it is possible to influence bacterial growth in areas where the laser beam is out of focus (spot of maximum energy density). The disinfection of the apical delta and the periapical region seems to be one of the key roles for the good clinical results of the 308-nm excimer laser in root canal preparation.

The domain of the 308-nm excimer laser is the precise removal of tissue. All treatments that can be performed with conventional instruments, such as drills and root canal instruments, are not going to be replaced but rather significantly improved by the 308-nm excimer laser. The primary indications for the 308-nm excimer laser in dentistry are root canal treatments, periodontal treatments, and surface conditioning of dental hard tissues.

References

Adrian JC, Gross A. A new method of sterilization: the carbon dioxide laser. J Oral Pathol 1979;8:60–61.

Bende T, Seiler T, Wollensack J. Side effects in excimer corneal surgery. Graefs Arch Clin Exp Ophthalmol 1988;226:277–280.

Bolanos OR, Jensen JR. Scanning electron microscope comparisons of the efficacy of various methods of root canal preparation. J Endodontics 1980;6:815–822.

El-Tagouri H, Czonstkowsky M, Holstein F, Piesci N, Michanowicz AE. The effectiveness of canal finder system: a scanning electron microscopic investigation. J Endodontics 1988;14:194.

Frentzen M, Koort HJ. Lasers in dentistry–New possibilities with advancing laser technology. Int Dent J 1990; 40:323–332.

Haikel J, Alleman C. Effectiveness of four methods for preparing root canals: a scanning electron microscopic evaluation. J Endodontics 1988;14:340–345.

Hardee M, Miserendino LJ, Kos W. Evaluation of intracanal Nd-YAG laser irradiation (abstract). J Endodontics 1990;16:194.

Hardee M, Miserendino LJ, Kos W, Walia H. Evaluation of the antibacterial effects of intracanal Nd:YAG laser irradiation. J Endodontics, in press.

Hibst R, Keller U. Experimental studies of the application of the Er: YAG laser on dental hard substances. I. Measurement of the ablation rate. Laser Surg Med 1989;9:338–344.

Hooks TW, Adrian JC, Gross A, et al. Use of the carbon dioxide laser in sterilization of endodontic reamers. Oral Surg Oral Med Oral Pathol 1980;49:263–265.

Keller U, Hibst R. Zur ablativen Wirkung des Er:YAG Lasers auf Schmelz und Dentin. Dtsch Zahnaerztl Z 1989;44:600–602.

Keller U, Hibst R. Experimental studies of the application of the Er:YAG laser on dental hard substances. II. Light microscopic and SEM investigations. Laser Surg Med 1989;9:345–351.

Liesenhoff T, Bende T, Lenz H, Seiler T. Abtragen von Zahnhartsubstanzen mit Excimer-Laserstrahlen. Dtsch Zahnaerztl Z 1989a;44:426–430.

Liesenhoff T, Bende H, Lenz H, Seiler T. Grundlagen zur Anwendung des Excimer-Lasers in der Zahnheilkunde. Dtsch Zahnaerztl Z 1990a;45:14–16.

Liesenhoff T, Bende H, Lenz H, Seiler T. Untersuchungen zur Anwendbarkeit des Excimer-Lasers in der Zahnheilkunde. ZWR 1989b;98:328–331.

Liesenhoff TH, Lenz H, Seiler T. Wurzelkanalaufbereitung mit Excimer-Laserstrahlen. ZWR 1989c;98:328–331.

Liesenhoff TH, Lenz H, Seiler T. Root canal preparation with 308nm excimer laser under simultaneous control by spectral tissue identification. Innov Tech Biol Med 1990b;11:87–99.

Liesenhoff T. 308nm excimer-laser in endodontics. SPIE 1992;1643:68,380–385.

Mc Guff PE, Bell EJ. The effect of laser energy radiation on bacteria. Med Biol Illus 1966;16:191–193.

Melcer J. Die Vorteile des carbon dioxide Laserstrahls bei vorsaetzlich geplanter Replantation Implantation. Lasers Med Surg 1987;3:240–242.

Melcer J. Apport du laser carbon dioxide dans la sterilisation de certaines infections d'origine dentaire. Rev Stomatol Chir Maxillofac 1982;83:146–151.

Miserendino LJ. Sterilization of bacterially contaminated root apices by CO_2 laser irradiation (abstract). J Endodontics 1988;14:198.

Miserendino LJ, Pick RM, Kos W. In vitro sterilization of dental caries by CO_2 laser irradiation (abstract). Lasers Surg Med 1988;8:148.

Murphy-Chutorian D, Selzer PM, Kosek J, et al. The interaction between excimer laser energy and vascular tissue. Am Heart 1986;112:739–745.

Neiburger EJ, Miserendino L. Pulp chamber warming due to carbon dioxide-laser exposure. NY State Dent J 1988;54:25–27.

Petschelt A. Endodontie: Maschinell-manuell? Die Aufbereitung und Spnlung des Wurzelkanals. Dtsch Zahnaerztl Z 1989;44:407–413.

Serebro L, Segal T, Nordenberg D, Gorfil C, Barlev M. Examination of tooth pulp following laser beam irradiation. Laser Surg Med 1987;7:236.

Shoji S, Nakamura M, Horiuchi H. Histopathological changes in dental pulps irradiated by carbon dioxide-laser: a preliminary report on laser pulpotomy. J Endodontics 1985;9:379–384.

Shoji S, Horiuchi H. Histopathological changes of dental pulp after irradiation by argon, carbon dioxide or Nd-YAG laser in rats. In Yamamoto H, Atsumi K, Kuskari H (eds): Laser in Dentistry. Amsterdam: Elsevier-Verlag; 1989:253.

Staberg B. The carcinogenic effect of UVA irradiation. J Invest Dermatol 1983;81:517–519.

Stuben J, Hoppe WF. Experimentelle Untersuchungen uber die Veraenderungen der Pulpa nach normal- und hoechsttourigem Schleifen und Bohren im histologischen Bild. Dtsch Zahnaerztl Z 1964;19:601–611.

Taylor R, Shklar G, Roeber F. The effects of laser radiation on teeth, dental pulp and oral mucosa of experimental animals. Oral Surg 1965;19:786–795.

Trokel S, Srinivasan R, Braren B. Excimer laser surgery of the cornea. Am J Ophthalmol 1983;96:710.

Walsh JT, Flotte TJ, Deutsch TF. Er:YAG laser ablation of tissue: effect of pulse duration and tissue type on thermal damage. Laser Surg Med 1989;9:314–326.

Walsh JT, Deutsch TF. Er:YAG laser ablation of tissue: measurement of ablation rate. Laser Surg Med 1989; 9:326–337.

Zach L, Cohen G. Pulp response to externally applied heat. Oral Surg 1965;19:515–530.

Zakariasen KL, Dederich DN, Tulip J, et al. Bactericidal action of carbon dioxide laser radiation in experimental dental root canals. Can J Microbiol 1986;32:942–946.

Zakariasen K, Baron J, Cullinan J, et al. Temperature elevations occurring across carbon dioxide lased dentin (abstract). J Dent Res 1989;68:1143.

Chapter Thirteen

Clinical Applications of the Ho:YAG Laser

Harvey Passes

In dentistry, the Ho:YAG laser may prove to be the most versatile commercially available laser. Its unique characteristics offer an array of possibilities for clinical application; some of these possibilities are presently usable, while others are being researched with good results.

The Ho:YAG laser has been used in vascular surgery (Bass et al, 1989a, 1989b; Kopchock et al, 1990), neurosurgery (Black et al, 1990b, 1991a, 1991b, 1991c; Kopchock et al, 1991), arthroscopy (Black et al, 1990a; Dillingham et al, 1992; Fanton and Dillingham, 1990; Kopchock et al, 1991), ophthalmology (Hoskins et al, 1990), angioplasty (Geschwind et al, 1990; Haase et al, 1991; Lilge et al, 1989; White and Ramee, 1992; White et al, 1991), urology (Johnson et al, 1989; Johnson et al, 1992a, 1992b), otolaryngology (Oswald and Bingham, 1992; Shapshay et al, 1991a, 1991b), gastroenterology (Oz et al, 1989; Popp et al, 1989; Rubio, 1991), and orthopedics (Trauner et al, 1990; Vari et al, 1991). It has recently achieved clearance by the Food and Drug Administration (FDA) to be marketed for limited bone removal during dacryocystorhinostomy and in orthopedics for arthroscopy.

At present, the FDA has granted clearance for the marketing of the Ho:YAG laser for use on soft tissue in dentistry. According to the results of preliminary studies, it may also have good potential for use on hard tissue.

Characteristics of Holmium

The holmium laser combines characteristics of the Nd:YAG and the CO_2 lasers. The benefits of holmium to laser dentistry include its ability to be delivered accurately through a flexible bare quartz optic fiber almost anywhere in the mouth. Like a CO_2 laser, Ho:YAG can ablate soft tissue quickly. Similarly, holmium is highly absorbed into water and has a shallow depth of penetration. Compared to the CO_2 laser, the holmium laser offers better hemostasis and is safe and effective to use on bone and cartilage, as cleared by the FDA, for use in orthopedics and neurosurgery. Based on in-vitro studies, it has been theorized that holmium lasers may be safe and effective for use on hard tooth structures. Although not cleared for marketing in dentistry by the FDA at this time, Ho:YAG can ablate hard tissue such as carious enamel, dentin, bone, calcified arterial plaque, and cartilage (Mani, 1992).

Except for the CO_2 laser, and unlike visible wavelengths, the Ho:YAG laser relies solely on its high affinity and absorption characteristics for water to interact with tissue. It is this property that allows Ho:YAG to be absorbed by the water content of the tissue and then to convert its energy into heat with the subsequent ablation of the tissue. Similar to the CO_2 laser, this high absorptive affinity for water also results in a shallow depth of tissue penetration. Of particular interest is the fact that enamel and dentin contain significant amounts of water. The shallow depth of penetration by the Ho:YAG laser within these hard structures coupled with its high peak power produce a photodisruptive effect similar to ablation. This process is called *spallation* (Mani, 1992).

Other factors also make Ho:YAG a useful laser for dental applications. It incorporates solid-state, high peak–powered, free-running flash-lamp pumped, pulsed technology delivered through quartz fiberoptics; this is a virtually maintenance-free laser. It can interact with tissue under low power without the need for local anesthetic, and can control hemostasis similar to actions of the Nd:YAG laser. Unlike the Nd:YAG laser, which is well-absorbed by dark or pigmented tissue, holmium is absorbed well by either pigmented or white tissue. Holmium can be used with equal effectiveness in either the contact or noncontact mode on soft tissue.

The Physics of Holmium

The Ho:YAG laser has a wavelength of 2,090 nm and has an extinction depth of 0.3 mm in water. This characteristic allows holmium to ablate soft tissue rapidly. The holmium laser is a thulium and holmium-doped, chromium-sensitized YAG crystal, or THC:YAG. This combination of ions allows for a more effective and efficient transfer of energy. At present, the only current commercially available dental holmium laser is manufactured by Excel Quantronix (Hauppauge, NY). This system operates from 5 to 10 Hz and from 0.25 to 5.00 W. Its quartz optic fiber delivery is 400 μm in diameter, and the pulse width is 250 μsec.

Clinical Application

This dental laser is versatile. Its power and accurate delivery system make it ideal for soft tissue use. Use of this laser and maximizing the results require more technique than those with other wavelengths; thus, this laser may take longer to learn to use.

Lingual benign giant cell tumor.

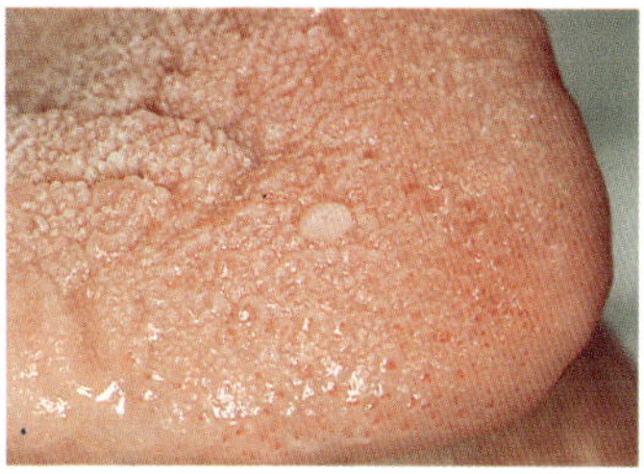

13.1a

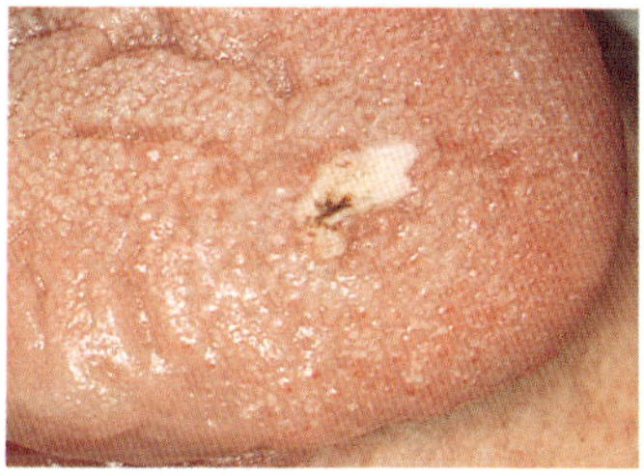

13.1b

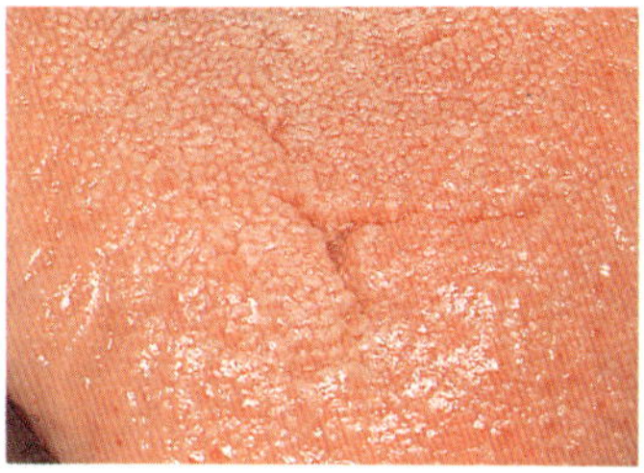

13.1c

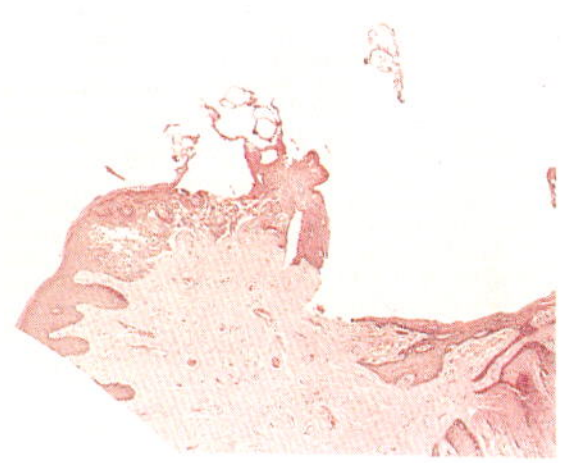

13.1d

Case 1. Excisional Biopsy of a Lingual Benign Giant Cell Tumor

A 57-year-old white woman sought treatment for the removal of a 4-mm pink ovoid raised lesion on the anterior dorsum of the tongue (Fig 13.1a). Clinical examination revealed no bleeding or any active infectious process from the lesion or to the surrounding tissue. On palpation, the lesion exhibited a firm consistency. Considering the location of this lesion, hard tissue testing and radiographic evaluation were not appropriate. The patient wanted the lesion removed because she was irritating it with her teeth. She noticed the lesion only a few weeks before her initial visit. Her medical history was noncontributory. There were no contraindications to treatment.

The objective was to remove the lesion and perform a biopsy. The patient expressed an interest in treatment with a laser. Alternate treatment plans were also discussed. After informed consent was given, excisional biopsy of this lesion was accomplished with the holmium laser. The rationale for use of the holmium laser was based on a number of factors. The laser would allow direct circumferential ablation of the surrounding tissue to the lesion, providing a clean biopsy specimen while maintaining effective hemostasis (Fig 13.1b). At a low power setting it would be possible to excise the lesion without the use of local anesthesia, but the patient desired a local anesthetic. Two percent lidocaine hydrochloride with 1:100,000 epinephrine was injected circumferentially to the lesion on the dorsum of the tongue. The holmium laser was used with a 400-µm quartz optic fiber. Excision of the lesion occurred at a power setting of 2.00 W at 10 pulses per sec with an exposure time of 1½ minutes. The tissue was undermined as the laser moved about 1 to 2 mm outside the border of the lesion. The surgical site remained visible at all times due to effective hemostasis. A tissue pickup secured the lesion as it was undermined and removed from the dorsum of the tongue and sent to the pathology laboratory for a diagnosis. There were no complications. Postoperative analgesia of 400 mg ibuprofen every 4 hours was instructed.

The prognosis for this excisional biopsy was excellent. That evening, the patient felt comfortable, experienced no bleeding or swelling, and was able to eat normally. She was seen 7 days later. The biopsy site appeared to be consistent with the surrounding tissue (Fig 13.1c). Clinically it was difficult to note that a biopsy had been performed, and the assessment of healing was satisfactory. The pathology report indicated that this lesion was a benign giant cell tumor of the tongue (Fig 13.1d).

Use of the holmium laser for excisional biopsy of this lesion offered an effective and less complicated service to the patient as well as for the clinician. The patient remained comfortable throughout and after the procedure. There was clear visibility during the procedure due to excellent hemostasis. The biopsy sample was of good quality, permitting a definitive diagnosis from the pathology laboratory. At low power settings, the holmium laser is an effective laser for excisional biopsy of a benign giant cell tumor of the tongue.

Traumatic fibroma.

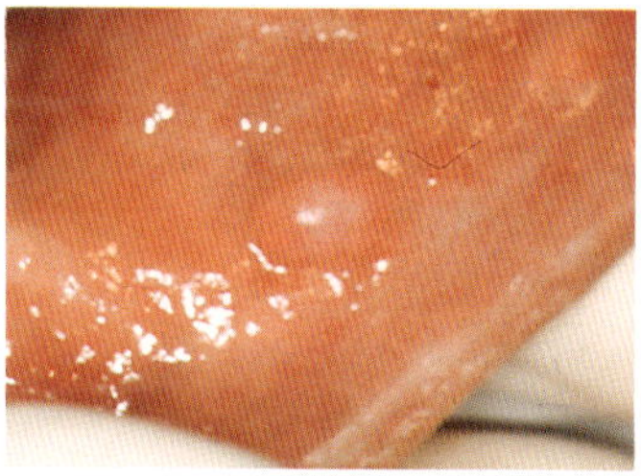

13.2a

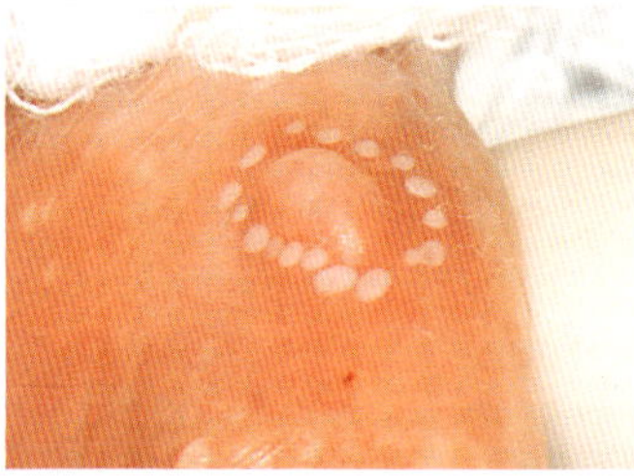

13.2b

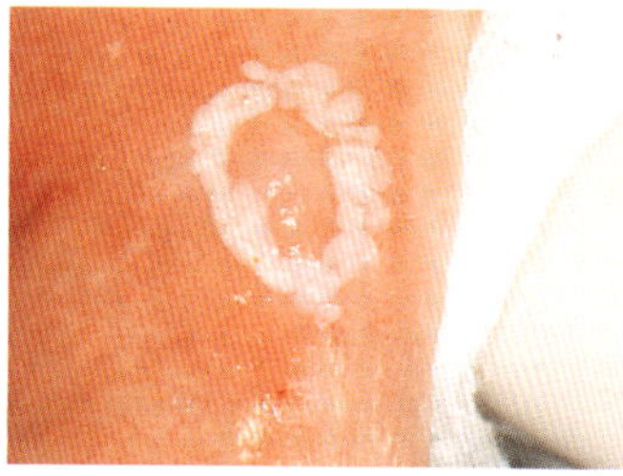

13.2c

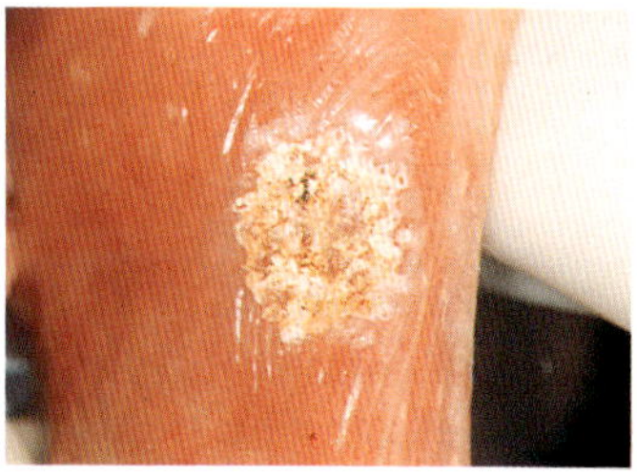

13.2d

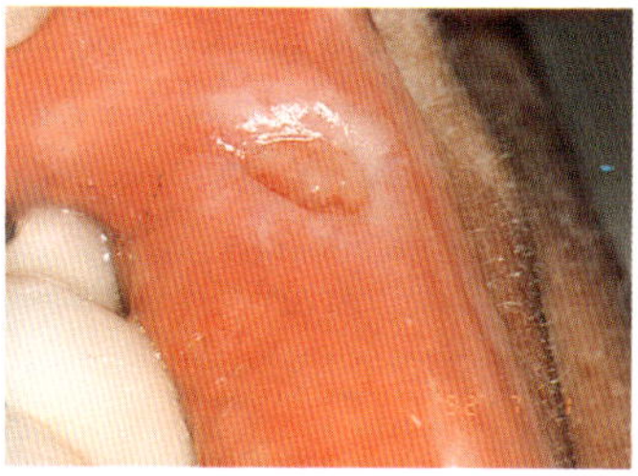

13.2e

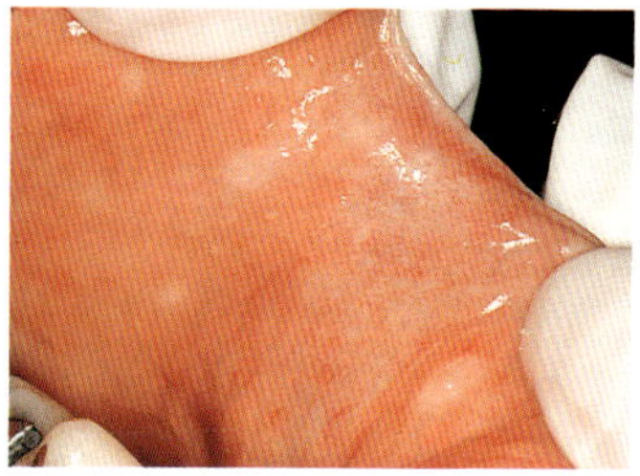

13.2f

Case 2. Excisional Biopsy of Traumatic Fibroma

A 75-year-old white woman sought treatment for the removal of a 4-mm diameter raised pink ovoid lesion on the internal labial mucosa of the left lip (Fig 13.2a). She explained that she had had this lesion for a number of years and would always irritate it or bite it accidentally. The patient wanted the lesion removed with a laser. She had undergone other forms of medical laser treatment and was satisfied with the outcomes. She actively sought a dentist who used a laser for this treatment.

Clinical examination revealed the lesion to be a firm, raised pink lesion with a broad, unpedunculated base. Tooth vitality, hard tissue, and radiographic examination were unnecessary due to the location of the lesion. Palpation was the only soft tissue test necessary. The lesion appeared to be a traumatically induced fibroma.

Because of the patient's desires, the only course of treatment indicated was a complete excisional biopsy. The patient's medical history was noncontributory and there were no contraindications to treatment. After informed consent was given, complete excisional biopsy of this lesion was accomplished.

The objective was to remove this lesion in the most comfortable manner possible with the least postoperative recovery time. The holmium laser was used due to its accurate delivery, rapid tissue ablation, shallow depth of penetration, and effective hemostasis. The laser was first used at an average power of 500 mJ at 5 pulses per sec for about 3 sec to circumscribe the lesion. It was then increased to an average power of 3.00 W, at 10 pulses per sec, and an exposure time of 3 min to excise the lesion. The fiberoptic beam diameter was 400 μm.

The treatment sequence was as follows. Although the patient was told that a local anesthetic would not be necessary, she requested it. Two percent lidocaine hydrochloride with 1:100,000 epinephrine was infiltrated around the lesion. This made the raised lesion stand out even more, which proved to be helpful during the procedure. In the noncontact mode, 2 mm from the tissue surface, the holmium beam was delivered circumferentially to the lesion (Fig 13.2b). This was with the average power of 500 mJ, 5 pulses per sec, for about 2 sec. This created a blanching effect or white dots around the border of the lesion, which helped to maintain a perspective on the tissue. Then the average power was raised to 3.00 W, at 10 pulses per sec, with an exposure time of 3 min. The dots were connected (Fig 13.2c) and the lesion was then undermined and removed with a tissue pickup. The remaining biopsy site was clearly visible with good hemostasis. The site was yellowish with a rough texture (Fig 13.2d). The biopsy sample was sent to the pathology laboratory for evaluation and diagnosis.

The patient remained comfortable immediately after the surgery and was instructed to take 400 mg ibuprofen every 4 hours. That night, she was comfortable and was not bleeding. She was advised to try to avoid traumatizing the area during the healing period. Three days after the surgery, the patient called to say that she was suddenly experiencing some sharp discomfort. This was probably due to the slightly longer exposure time of the laser on the tissue. Her prescription was changed to diflunisal, 500 mg every 8 to 10 hours, with a loading dose of 1,000 mg. She was not able to return until 12 days after surgery (Fig 13.2e). The clinical appearance was of a slightly yellow-pink–looking concavity that was healing via secondary intention. The previous sharp discomfort had disappeared 4 days after surgery. The patient did not return until 33 days after surgery. The biopsy site had blended well with the adjacent tissue. The concavity seen on the twelfth day had disappeared (Fig 13.2f). The patient remained satisfied with laser treatment.

The use of the holmium laser for excisional biopsy of a traumatically induced fibroma of the internal labial mucosa is effective if used under low power with the shortest exposure time.

Multiple epulides fissurata.

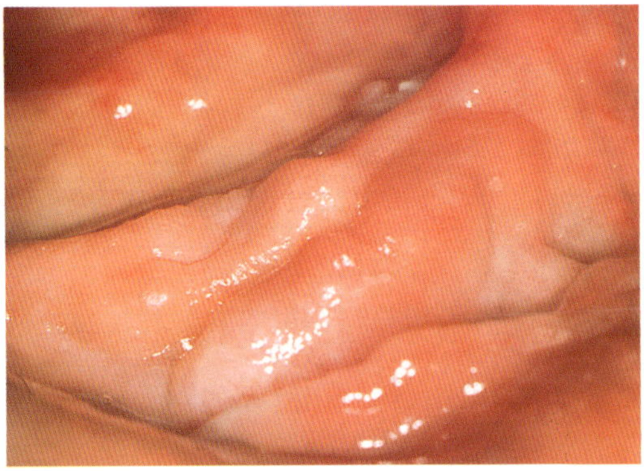

13.3a

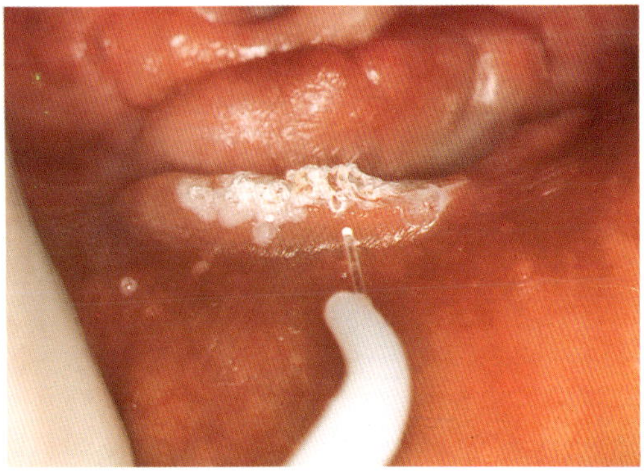

13.3b

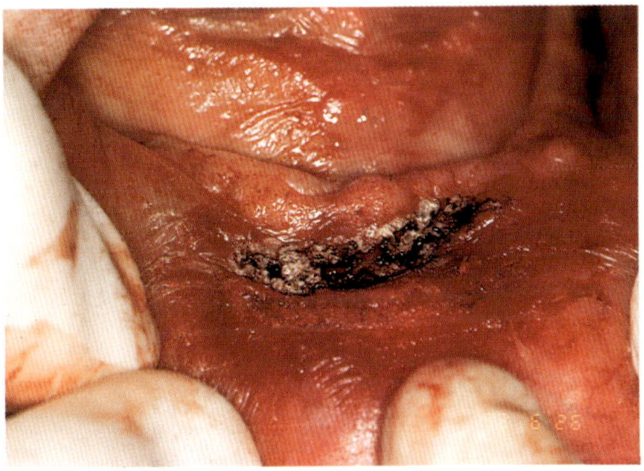

13.3c

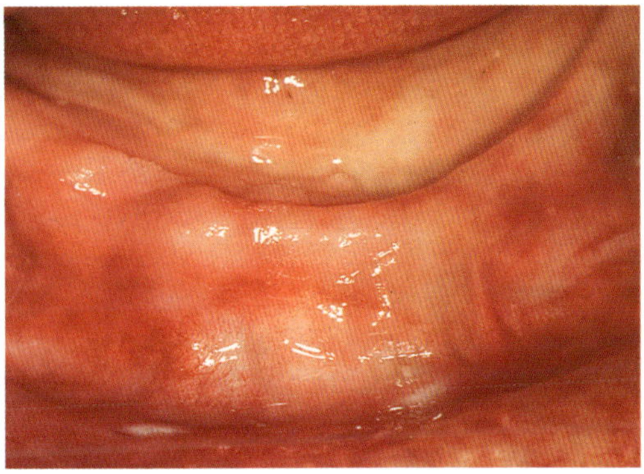

13.3d

Case 3. Removal of Multiple Epulides Fissurata

A 62-year-old white woman who had worn full upper and lower dentures for the past 10 years complained of an ill-fitting lower denture. Clinical examination revealed that anterior to the mandibular ridge were two epulides fissurata separated by 4 mm of folded mucosa (Fig 13.3a). The anterior lesion on the lingual aspect of the lip measured 2-mm wide and 2-mm thick by 12-mm long. The posterior lesion measured 5 mm vertically by 4 mm labially and 10 mm long. It was connected to the underlying tissue by a dense base. The patient's complaint focused on her difficulty in eating due to the "bumps" under her denture. She wanted them removed so that her denture would feel comfortable again.

Clinical assessment involved soft tissue examination and palpation. A panorex radiograph showed no bony involvement by these lesions. Any other hard tissue and tooth studies were unnecessary considering the edentulous nature of the case.

The treatment plan included removal of these lesions and relining the lower denture with an interim tissue conditioner–lining material with the subsequent relining of a suitable laboratory-processed acrylic denture lining. Alternate treatment plans were offered to the patient, including excision with the laser. The thickness of the lesions indicated that a great deal of traditional blade surgery and suturing would be necessary for their removal. This conventional treatment plan discussed with the patient included at least one or two individual surgical procedures. The patient was presented with the following options: (1) traditional excisional biopsy (scalpel) including multiple suturing and postoperative care; (2) electrosurgery; (3) laser ablation; or (4) a combination of options *1* and *3* as part of a case study involving multiple wavelengths.

The alternatives were described to the patient. It was explained that traditional excisional biopsy with a scalpel involved possible multiple operative and postoperative visits. These multiple lesions could produce postoperative scarring and fibrosis of the surgical site, and abundant sutures could also produce inflammation. The traditional blade technique could cause possible loss of the vestibular space and potential swelling and pain. Deep zones of thermal injury and necrosis could occur with electrosurgery. Laser ablation may allow for fewer operative and postoperative visits and minimal pain with diminished swelling of the surgical site. Hemostasis without suturing would not affect the vestibular space. Based on the information presented, the patient selected laser treatment. She also consented to be part of a study with different lasers. The patient's medical history was noncontributory, and there were no contraindications to treatment. The plan was to fully ablate the anterior lesion and to excise with a scalpel and submit the posterior lesion to the pathology laboratory for a diagnosis as part of treatment and another study.

The holmium laser within the Duopulse 2000, supplied by Excel Technology (Hauppauge, NY), was used. This procedure seemed ideal for the holmium laser due to the laser's unique operating characteristics. An average power of 3.00 W at 10 pulses per second with a quartz fiberoptic beam diameter of 400 μm was used. High-speed evacuation is always used during a laser procedure.

The treatment began without local anesthesia until the patient said that she felt a slight tingling feeling. Two carpules of 2% lidocaine hydrochloride with 1:100,000 epinephrine was infiltrated within the surgical sites. The anterior lesion was completely ablated at first in the noncontact mode and then, for more rapid ablation, in the contact mode. Clinically, it was determined that the procedure was completed when the base of the lesion was level with the adjacent unaffected tissue. No bleeding was observed during the removal of the anterior lesion (Fig 13.3b). There was clear visibility of the surgical site at all times. The resultant immediate postoperative site had a yellow crusty appearance. The second posterior lesion was part of another study. While this would have been an appropriate application for the holmium laser, for research purposes this tissue was removed with a no. 15 blade, and the tissue specimen was sent to the pathology laboratory. This procedure caused copious bleeding that was not controlled with suturing. The holmium laser was used to induce hemostasis. This was accomplished in the noncontact mode at 3.00 W and 10 pulses per second (Fig 13.3c). A soft interim tissue conditioner was placed.

The laser removal of the first anterior lesion was much less traumatic to the patient than the conventional surgical removal of the more posterior lesion. To control bleeding during the conventional procedure of the posterior lesion, a gentle stream of air was applied concomitant to the holmium laser in the noncontact mode. This technique provided good hemostasis.

Traditional postoperative surgical instructions were given. This included ice packs and 1,000 mg acetaminophen as needed. That evening, the patient was comfortable and had taken the analgesic as a preventive measure. Unfortunately, she was not able to return to the clinic for 30 days. When she returned, examination of the surgical site revealed that complete healing had occurred (Fig 13.3d). A more permanent reline was performed.

There were no side effects to treatment. It was assessed that complete removal of multiple epulides fissurata at 3.00 W and 10 pulses per second with the holmium laser is an acceptable technique. The use of quartz fiberoptic delivery, in the contact and noncontact mode, allows for accurate placement of the holmium laser beam to the surgical tissue site. Clinically, its effect on tissue appears to simulate the CO_2 laser in both speed and soft tissue effects. It was interesting to note that when holmium is used to control bleeding from an open wound, the resultant appearance of the site is black. If the tissue is ablated from the beginning with the holmium laser, its appearance is more yellow-pink, which is more esthetic.

Although we did not view the results at 7, 14, and 21 days after surgery, it was still possible to evaluate the results at 30 days. The clinical appearance of the tissue was satisfactory (Passes et al, 1992b).

A Laser for All Reasons

Fortunately, industry has responded to the interest that the dental profession has shown for laser applications. Research and development have produced many different types of lasers for use in dentistry. Naturally, no one laser is able to completely perform all of the procedures required by our patients.

The 2,090-nm-wavelength laser is useful for soft tissue applications as well as for potential hard tissue applications. Wherever rapid soft tissue reduction is needed, the holmium laser performs well. Whenever visibility during a surgical procedure is needed, the holmium laser produces excellent hemostasis. What makes this laser so useful is that it can produce the same desired effects as both the Nd:YAG and CO_2 lasers. Its fiberoptic delivery system assures accurate application to the target tissue. During placement of a composite, it provides rapid hemostasis if the tissue happens to bleed into the cavity preparation. It enables delicate sculpting of the gingival tissue for cosmetic laminate veneers without bleeding. It is most effective in exposing implants and allowing for an implant post impression the same day without bleeding (Passes et al, 1992a). The general practitioner usually avoids soft tissue procedures near the floor of the mouth, the tongue, or on the buccal mucosa because of the potential bleeding problems that could occur. The holmium laser allows for rapid frenectomies, biopsies, operculectomies, and other soft tissue procedures that have previously been considered forbidden areas for treatment by general practitioners.

Use on Hard Tissue

The future for this laser is very bright. Our colleagues in medicine have been researching the use of the holmium laser on bone and cartilage. Some procedures have already gained FDA clearance for marketing in medicine. The potential for use in apicoectomies is intriguing. In the future, it may be possible to gain access to periapical lesions with a fiber and ablate the tissue. The holmium laser might then be able to ablate the root apex and heat-seal the tip, all without laying back a flap. Certainly, a flap could still be performed while using holmium to continue the procedure with minimal injury to the adjacent tissue. Research is currently being performed to evaluate the use of this laser on decayed or healthy enamel and dentin. Work is also being done with this laser in the root canal to expedite and offer sterilization in some endodontic procedures. The holmium laser may also have the ability to sculpt bone for difficult periodontal osseous procedures.

Acknowledgments

Special thanks to Jeff Manni of JGM Associates, Margaret Morrissey and Rama Rao of Excel Quantronix, and Paul S. Kaufman, Barry Weinberg, and Lewis Gilmore of the Jamaica Hospital's Department of Dentistry.

References

Bass LS et al. The THC laser: a new tool for microvascular anastomosis. Laser surgery advanced characterization, therapeutics and systems. Proc SPIE 1989a; 1066:111–114.

Bass LS et al. Sutureless microvascular anastomosis using the THC:YAG laser: a preliminary report. Microsurgery 1989b;10:189–193.

Black et al. Arthroscopy using the pulsed Ho:YAG laser. Clin Laser Mon 1990a;Apr:55–57.

Black et al. Anterior cervical discectomy using Ho:YAG laser. Surg Forum 1990b;41:527–530.

Black et al. Percutaneous lumbar discectomy using holmium:YAG laser. Lasers Surg Med Suppl 1991;3:54.

Black et al. Percutaneous lumbar discectomy using Ho:YAG laser. Lasers in orthopedic, dental, and veterinary medicine. Proc SPIE 1991;1424:20–22.

Black et al. Anterior cervical discectomy using Ho:YAG laser. Lasers Surg Med Suppl 1991;3:54.

Brillhart AT. Arthroscopic laser surgery: the Ho:YAG laser and its use. Am J Arthroscopy 1991;1:7–11.

Dillingham MF, Fanton GS, Perkash R. The use of the Ho:YAG laser in operative knee arthroscopy: a retrospectve study comparing postoperative recovery rates of patients with lateral retinacular release surgery using the Ho:YAG laser vs conventional instruments. Am J Sports Med.

Fanton FS, Dillingham MF. Arthroscopic menisectomy using the Ho:YAG laser: a double blind study. Presented at the Arthroscopy Association of North America Annual Meeting, 1990.

Geschwind HJ et al. Percutaneous coronary angioplasty with a mid-infrared laser and a new multifiber catheter. Lancet 1990, July.

Haase KK et al. Potential use of holmium lasers for angioplasty: evaluation of a new solid state laser for ablation of atherosclerotic plaque. Lasers Surg Med 1991; 11:232–237.

Hoskins HD, Iwach AG, Drake MV. Subconjunctival THC:YAG laser limbal sclerostomy ab externo in the rabbit. Ophthalmic Surg 1990;589–592.

Johnson JP et al. THC:YAG, ultrasonic and electrohydraulic gallstone lipotriptors. Laser surgery: advanced characterization, therapeutics and systems. Proc SPIE 1989;1066:141–144.

Johnson DE, Cromeens DM, Price RE. Transurethral incision of the prostate using the holmium:YAG laser. Lasers Surg Med 1992;12:364–369.

Johnson DE, Cromeens DM, Price RE. Use of the Ho:YAG laser in urology. Lasers Surg Med 1992;12: 353–363.

Kopchock GE et al. Holmium:YAG laser ablation of vascular tissue. Lasers Surg Med 1990;10:405–413.

Kopchock GE et al. Holmium:YAG laser of human intervertebral disc: preliminary evaluation. Lasers Surg Med Suppl 1991;3:54.

Lilge L, Radtke W, Nishioka N. Pulsed holmium laser ablation of cardiac valves. Lasers Surg Med 1989;9: 458–464.

Mani GJ. Holmium Laser in Dental Applications of Advanced Lasers. GJM Associates Inc; 1992:11–13.

Oswald VH, Bingham BJ. A pilot study of the holmium:YAG laser in nasal turbinate and tonsil surgery. J Clin Med Surg 1992;10:211–216.

Oz MC et al. In vitro comparison of the THC:YAG and argon ion lasers for welding billiary tissue. Lasers Surg Med 1989;9:248–253.

Passes H, Kaufman PS, Weinberg B. Preliminary study: multiwavelength exposure of titanium implants in vitro. Presented at the International Academy of Laser Dentistry, second annual meeting, Honolulu, HI, 1992a.

Passes H, Kaufman PS, Weinberg B. Case study: the removal of multiple epulides fissurata with the holmium laser. Presented at the International Academy of Laser Dentistry, second annual meeting, Honolulu, HI, 1992b.

Popp HW et al. Welding of gallbladder tissue with a pulsed 2.15 micron THC:YAG laser. Lasers Surg Med 1989;9:155–159.

Rubio PA. Endoscopic cholecystectomy with Ho:YAG laser: preliminary report. J Clin Laser Med Surg 1991;Apr:127–128.

Shapshay SM et al. Holmium:YAG laser-assisted endoscopic sinus surgery: laboratory experience. Laryngoscope 1991;101:142–149.

Shapshay SM et al. Holmium:YAG laser-assisted endoscopic sinus surgery: clinical experience. Presented at the 94th Meeting of American Laryngology, Rhinology, and Otology Society, 1991.

Trauner K, Nishioka N, Patel D. Pulsed Ho:YAG laser ablation of fibrocartilage and articular cartilage. Am J Sports Med 1990;18:316–321.

Vari SG, Shi WQ, Fishbein MC, Grundfest WS. Ablation study of knee structure tissues with a Ho:YAG laser (abstract). Lasers Surg Med 1991;suppl 3:205.

White CJ, Ramee SR. Holmium:YAG coronary laser angioplasty (HOLCA). J Clin Laser Med Surg 1992;9: 459–466.

White CJ et al. Recanalization of arterial occlusions with a lensed fiber and a Ho:YAG laser. Lasers Surg Med 1991;11:250–256.

Chapter Fourteen

Clinical Applications of the Nd:YAG Laser

Alan Goldstein, Joel M. White, and Robert M. Pick

In 1977, Adrian and associates studied the effects of the Nd:YAG laser on the dental pulps of rhesus monkeys. While the report was preliminary in nature, the investigators expressed their optimism about the future of this laser (Adrian et al, 1971; Adrian, 1977). Hard tissue studies continued (Yamamoto and Ooya, 1974; Yamamoto and Sato, 1980; Winkler et al, 1973; Liberman et al, 1984) to suggest the positive effects that Nd:YAG as well as CO_2 lasers could have on hard tissues. In May 1990, the Food and Drug Administration approved the 510K application of the dLase 300 (Sunrise Technologies, Fremont, CA), which allowed American Dental Laser (Birmingham, MI) to market a free-running, pulsed neodymium:YAG laser for intraoral soft tissue surgical applications. Since then, several manufacturers of Nd:YAG lasers have introduced various systems into the marketplace.

Much of the literature on the Nd:YAG laser concerns itself with the capacity of the laser to improve the ability to perform soft tissue procedures. Initially the Nd:YAG was used for the excision of gross pathologic conditions (Ohyama et al, 1985), but more recently, with the development of the fiberoptic, direct contact delivery system, one can not only cut, but sterilize and seal with very low power. The ability to perform procedures at very low power settings is a unique and positive feature of the free-running, pulsed Nd:YAG laser since the aim should always be to use the smallest amount of energy to achieve therapeutic goals.

With the development of the fiberoptic contact delivery system and related surgical technique, the Nd:YAG laser has been used in the medical-surgical environment for many soft tissue–cutting applications, including procedures, such as liver resection, mastectomy, and hemorrhoidectomy, that involve highly vascular tissues (Iwasaki et al, 1985; Washida et al, 1984; Joffe 1986; Joffe et al, 1986).

Research specific to Nd:YAG laser usage in dentistry has investigated the removal of carious lesions along with lack of damage to surrounding tooth enamel and minimal associated discomfort (Myers and Myers, 1985a; 1985b). Theoretically, most soft tissues encountered in dental surgery can also be cut or excised with the laser with the fiberoptic contact delivery system. The interaction of laser wavelength and energy density with tissue at the tip of the fiberoptic contact delivery system allows simultaneous cutting and coagulation of tissue. The contact fiber laser handpiece is used much like an electrosurgical pencil and can be used in and around the dentition where access is difficult with the scalpel.

A particularly exciting conclusion was reached in a study done by Myers and Myers, which suggested that carious lesions that had not yet penetrated the dentino-enamel junction could be removed and the area sterilized using a free-running, pulsed Nd:YAG laser (Myers and Myers, 1985a). More recent studies by White and associates continue to explore this feature of the Nd:YAG laser. Additionally, patients who received caries removal and restoration were evaluated 3 years after treatment and the restorations were intact and servicable with healthy pulps (White et al, 1993).

Laser investigations have also been proceeding in the field of endodontics (Dederich et al, 1984; Dederich et al, 1985; Zakariasen et al, 1985; Bahcall et al, 1993), where it is being clearly demonstrated that the Nd:YAG laser has the potential to sterilize the root canal (Hardee et al, 1990) and seal the dentinal walls (Miserendino et al, 1990; Miserendino et al, 1992). The Laser 35, a water-and-air–cooled, free-running pulsed Nd:YAG laser is said to have endodontic applications because of its capacity to utilize the photoacoustic (shock wave) effect (Miserendino and Miserendino, 1992). The air-and-water coolant reduces the Nd:YAG laser energy at the tip of the fiber but also reduces potential thermal effects (Miserendino and Rizoiu, 1993).

Nd:YAG Laser Physics

The active medium in the Nd:YAG laser is an yttrium-aluminum-garnet host crystal uniformly doped with small amounts of the element neodymium (Nd). It is the dopant ions, in this case the neodymium, that impart the emission wavelength characteristics of each individual solid-state laser. To visualize this, imagine a rod the size of a cigarette, which is the YAG (or host crystal), and then imagine a small amount of neodymium impregnated into the surface of the crystal. When laser emission occurs, it is at 1,064 nm on the electromagnetic spectrum. Other wavelengths exist with Nd:YAG, but are not typically used in dentistry.

One thousand sixty-four nanometers lies in the infrared part of the electromagnetic spectrum. It is very important to note that it is nonionizing in character and therefore nonmutagenic. This wavelength is invisible and therefore we always have an additional laser beam or white light aiming beam as an integral part of the system; the He:Ne beam is red and therefore acts as the aiming beam. To the best of our knowledge, it does not vary the therapeutics of treatment, although there are reports of biostimulation from the low power aiming beam.

Tissue Effects

When striking biologic tissues, dental lasers act by photothermal effects. The laser energy is absorbed by tissue and it is this absorbance that allows surgical excision and coagulation of tissue. The photothermal effect occurs when laser light (laser energy) is absorbed by tissue and converted into heat. Other possible laser-tissue interactions are transmission and reflection. Although often erroneously stated, transmission of photons through tissue does not cause detrimental effects. The body is relatively translucent to any form of electromagnetic radiation and laser light can pass through oral tissues without damaging effects. It is only when transmitted and reflected laser light is absorbed by adjacent tissue that a potential detrimental interaction can occur. Often the Nd:YAG laser light energy diminishes rapidly when reflected and transmitted in oral tissues and the clinical evidence indicates that this wavelength does not cause deep photothermal effects even though it is transmitted through water.

When the laser energy is absorbed, the temperature of the tissue rises. If sufficient energy is applied, the water component of the tissue vaporizes, causing tissue ablation. Neodymium:YAG lasers have a particular affinity for melanin (or other dark pigments); therefore, this laser works more efficiently when the energy is applied in the presence of a pigment. This is the reason that hemostasis occurs with this wavelength. Continuous wave as well as some pulsed Nd:YAG lasers have special kinds of tips at the distal end of their delivery systems that improve the absorption of energy at the point of contact and that lessen the amount of penetration.

Variables That Affect How Lasers Work

Laser variables include wavelength, pulse duration, energy per pulse, and delivery system. The Nd:YAG laser is located at 1,064 nm on the electromagnetic spectrum. Among the Nd:YAG lasers, one must distinguish between continuous or pulsed laser beams. Continuous beam means that there is no variation in the amount of laser energy. The laser is either on or off like a light bulb. Today, manufacturers are interrupting the beam and achieving duty cycles of 50% (on only half of the time). For these continuous or interrupted pulse lasers, the peak power, the average power, and the total power are all the same magnitude.

Pulsed lasers operate much differently. Peak powers are orders of magnitude higher than average powers. There are very high spikes with peak power being 1,000 times higher than the average power, and relatively long rest periods. Pulse widths (the amount of time for each pulse) vary from 90 to 800 μsec in different pulsed Nd:YAG lasers and are an important component of this technology (see Chapter 2). The short duration allows for a long resting time, which sometimes obviates the need for local anesthesia. The number of pulses per second is one of the crucial variables in pulsed Nd:YAG lasers. With a high repetition rate (from 10 to 100 Hz in different devices), one can achieve smoother cutting at a very low power setting because the peak power in each pulse can be very high. A good analogy is that laser pulses are like boxers. A laser can have high energy per pulse (200 to 300 mJ/pulse) and remove large amounts of tissue, like the knockout punch. Or a laser can have many punches of low energies (30 to 50 mJ/pulse), like the rabbit punches of a boxer. The clinical implications of this are that the practitioner has a range of choices between high power or high pulse rate, and depending on the type of tissue one is working on, these options are helpful. Histologic evaluation and temperature measurements during the cutting process indicate that the laser operator can increase either power or repetition rate but not both at the same time (White et al, 1992).

Contact and Noncontact Modes

There are two modes of delivery of lasers in dentistry today: first and most popular is the contact mode used with most fiberoptic-delivered lasers (neodymium, argon and Ho-Nd). The second type of delivery is line of sight, point and shoot, noncontact delivery by articulated arm, or waveguide (CO_2 and erbium). In contact delivery, the fiber tip is placed directly on the tissue to be removed and therefore reduces reflection with site-specific delivery. Fibers come in different widths with the quartz delivery systems. Most of the manufacturers offer quartz diameters ranging from 100 to 600 μm. A smaller diameter means higher energy density, faster cutting, and more heat. With larger diameters, more energy is needed to cover a broader area to work more quickly. Thus, variations of diameters offer endodontic and periodontic access. The final variable is the total power a device emits. In the high-pulse-rate devices, this is a less important variable since the amount of power per pulse (measured in millijoules) is more significant. But total power still must be noted. The ranges are from maximums of 3 to 35 W and for the sake of completeness, the range in pulse rates are from 10 to 100 Hz. The individual practitioner must be knowledgeable of the type of delivery system, power, and repetition ranges for each laser device. It is our clinical experience that for intraoral soft tissue excision, powers need not be higher then 6 W and repetition rates no higher than 100 Hz, and never both at the same time.

Advantages of Nd:YAG Lasers

The fiberoptic contact delivery system offers dentistry a technology that utilizes our already-learned digital skills, and while we clearly have to learn how to use this new form of energy (light energy vs mechanical) the contact delivery system feels more comfortable. The relationship between hemostasis and surgical precision in one instrument is one of the main advantages of Nd:YAG lasers. It is a great advantage to be able to cut and cauterize at the same time.

Patient comfort is another advantage of the Nd:YAG. Our patients have been very comfortable during laser soft tissue surgery. Another reason for the popularity of the laser with patients, and dentists, is that given the concern about bleeding and sterility, any technology that decreases bleeding is welcome. Patients truly appreciate this quality, and dentists are afforded greater peace of mind.

All demographics point to an aging population. What logically follows is that this population is taking more medications than ever before, and these medications may have some effect on oral tissues. One of the common side effects that we are seeing with some heart medications is gingival hyperplasia; consider nifedipine or cyclosporin to name a few. The pulsed Nd:YAG laser not only allows the easy removal of the redundant tissue without bleeding or pain, but also obviates the need for other medications and another round of potential drug interactions.

Scientific Basis for the Pulsed Nd:YAG Laser in Dentistry

The pulsed fiberoptic laser has entered dentistry with sound laboratory and clinical science to support its safety and effectiveness. The bottom line for the practitioner is: Can the treatment objective be accomplished and does this technology offer any advantages over existing methods? We are now performing procedures that we would have never envisioned before the emergence of the pulsed fiberoptic delivered Nd:YAG laser. For the most part, these procedures are performed earlier in the disease process and are less invasive and less costly then alternative therapies. The pulsed fiberoptic delivered Nd:YAG laser is the only device that has specific indications for use for cutting and coagulation of intraoral soft tissue, including the epithelial lining of the free marginal gingiva. To our knowledge, the only laser device that has emerged on the marketplace supported by clinical testing for pocket depth reduction is the pulsed fiberoptic delivered Nd:YAG laser.

The clinical study of White et al (1991) provides the basis for most applications of laser devices in dentistry today. The study, completed at a university under well-controlled conditions, compared traditional techniques to those completed with the pulsed Nd:YAG laser. Other study methods have been used with lasers, such as case reports and case summaries, but for laser dentistry to continue to grow and develop, more clinical studies of all types of lasers are needed.

The study by White et al was designed to evaluate the Nd:YAG laser's soft tissue cutting abilities in comparison with conventional soft tissue excision by knife. The study's primary goal was to determine if the laser could be used to perform gingivectomy, curettage, excision, gingivoplasty, fibrotomy, and frenectomy while reducing or even eliminating bleeding of the cut surfaces, without the use of anesthesia as required in conventional surgery. A secondary goal was to compare the surgical prognosis to actual healing in both laser and traditional surgery.

Two surgery sites in 29 randomly selected patients were treated, and an additional 41 patients were exclusively treated with the Nd:YAG laser. The number of procedures performed was as follows: gingivectomy, 19; gingivoplasty, 11; gingival curettage, 10; frenectomy, 2; tissue excision, 13; distal wedge, 2; and pocket elimination with restoration, 13. The surgical technique was then evaluated for periodontal pocket depths (Fig 14.1), bleeding (Fig 14.2), degree of pain perceived (Fig 14.3), inflammation, procedure time, and anesthesia. The prognosis was estimated at surgery and compared to actual healing 1 week and 1 month after surgery. In 11 cases, the specimens were examined histologically (Fig 14.4).

No significant differences were observed between laser and scalpel surgery in pocket depth reduction, postoperative pain, postoperative inflammation, and treatment time. However, operative and postoperative bleeding with laser surgery were significantly less than that with conventional surgery. While scalpel surgery requires anesthesia, most patients who underwent laser treatment had minimal pain without anesthesia.

The study examined the use of the Nd:YAG laser for soft tissue reduction, including excessive periodontal pocket depth, inadequate remaining tooth structure above the gingiva for restorations, and excessive tissue preventing accurate impression of tooth structure. Soft tissue procedures included elongation of clinical crowns, gingivectomies, gingivoplastics, gingival curettage, preparation of tissues for impressions, and the control of bleeding around the gingival margin. While these procedures have been performed successfully with the carbon dioxide laser (Pick et al, 1985; Pick and Pecaro, 1987; Pogrel, 1989), the Nd:YAG laser offers an additional advantage over the scalpel and

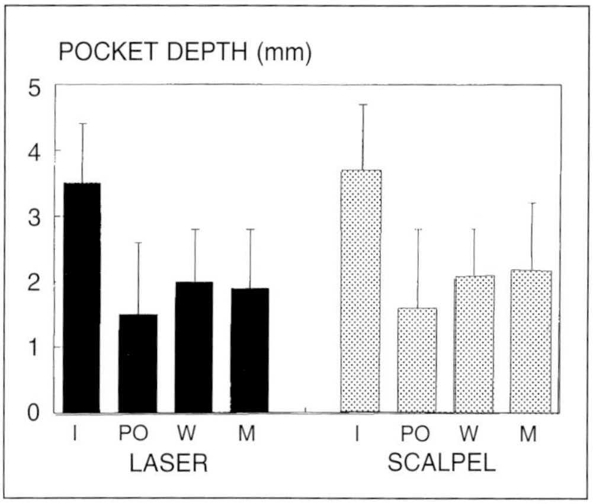

Fig 14.1 Comparison of pocket depth reduction in millimeters between laser and scalpel surgeries (I = initial pocket depth, PO = immediate postoperative pocket depth, W = pocket depth at 1 week, M = pocket depth at 1 month).

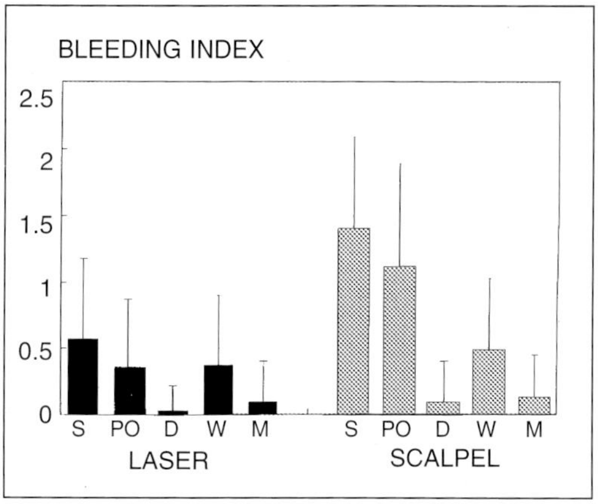

Fig 14.2 Bleeding index (0 = none, 1 = mild, 2 = moderate, 3 = severe) over time (S = during surgery, PO = immediately postoperative, D = 24 hours after surgery, W = 1 week after surgery, M = 1 month after surgery) of laser and scalpel surgical techniques.

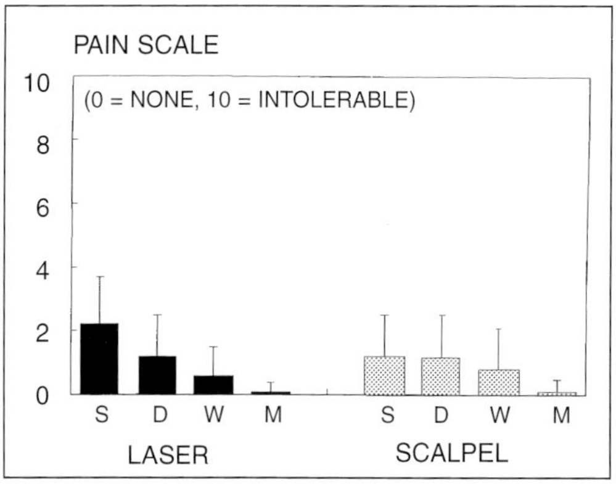

Fig 14.3 Patients' perception of pain measured on the visual analogue scale (0 to 10) for laser and scalpel surgeries over time (S = during surgery, D = 24 hours after surgery, W = 1 week after surgery, M = 1 month after surgery).

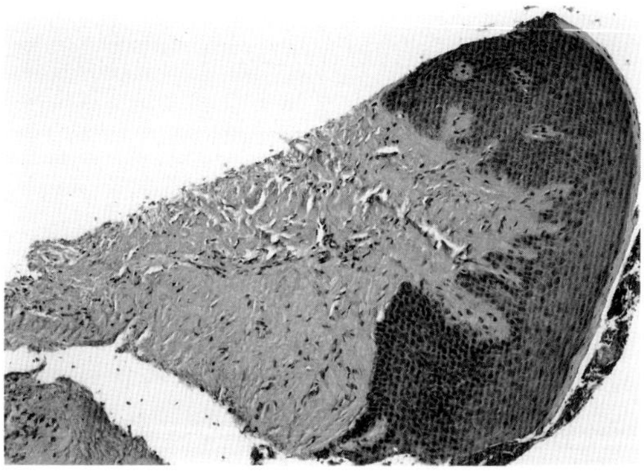

Fig 14.4 Representative histologic specimen obtained from patient undergoing laser gingivectomy. Note small area of thermal coagulation at superior border (original magnification × 33).

other lasers. Because of its site-specific delivery system, it allows the dentist to remove as little as 320 µm of tissue with less bleeding and a decreased requirement for anesthesia. These results indicate that the Nd:YAG laser can be used successfully for intraoral soft tissue applications and that, compared to scalpel surgery, it is well tolerated without anesthesia, and minimal bleeding occurs. This study demonstrates the Nd:YAG laser's safety and effectiveness for intraoral soft tissue surgery.

Case 1. Gingivectomy/Gingivoplasty/Frenectomy

This case study demonstrates the versatility of a free-running, pulsed Nd:YAG laser that has the capacity to operate at high repetition rates. A gingivectomy/gingivoplasty was performed on very delicate sulcular epithelium and, by changing the pulse rate and power settings, a frenectomy was performed on fibrous tissue.

A 35-year-old hispanic woman had for many years desired cosmetic improvement for her "very short teeth" (Fig 14.5a). Both central incisors appeared box-like because of the position of the gingiva, which was approximately 3-mm incisal to the cementoenamel junction. On closer examination, it was clear that it was not only the central incisors, but all six anterior teeth that were involved. The gingiva of these teeth hid the subtle contours of the apical third of all six maxillary anterior teeth. The midline frenum, which was located in a visually obtrusive position, detracted from the ultimate esthetic effect desired.

Diagnostics revealed vital and healthy teeth. Readings on the pulptester were within normal limits, there was good gingival color and texture with pocket depths of 3 mm, and normal radiographs. The treatment plan included a gingivectomy/gingivoplasty on teeth numbers 6 through 11, as well as a midline frenectomy. No contraindications were present. Chosen was a free-running, pulsed Nd:YAG laser, based on its capacity to cut and sculpt soft tissue precisely and at the same time provide excellent hemostasis. The patient was offered the option of traditional surgery and she chose the laser surgery, based on our comfort with this modality. The treatment objective was to reduce the gingiva 3 mm and bevel the gingival margin and therefore improve esthetics. A midline maxillary frenectomy was also performed.

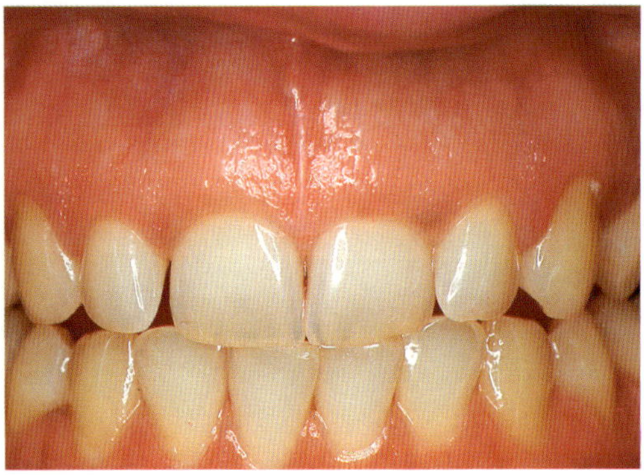

14.5a

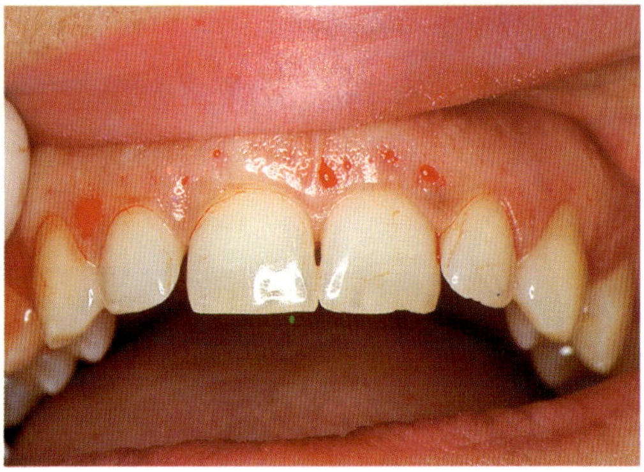

14.5b

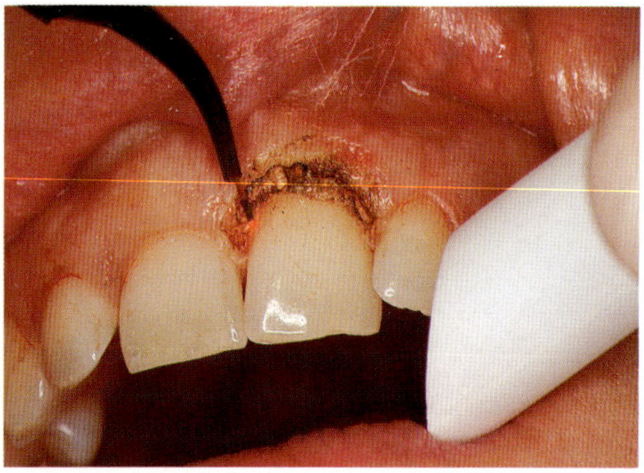

14.5c

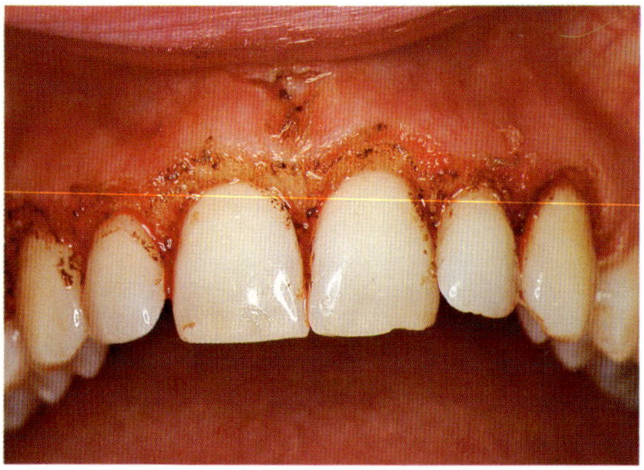

14.5d

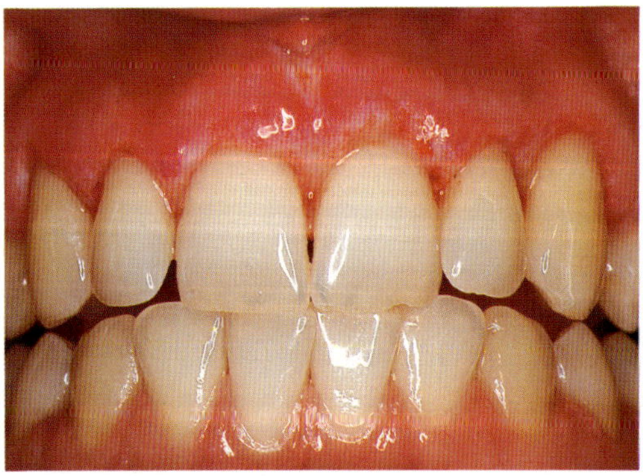

14.5e

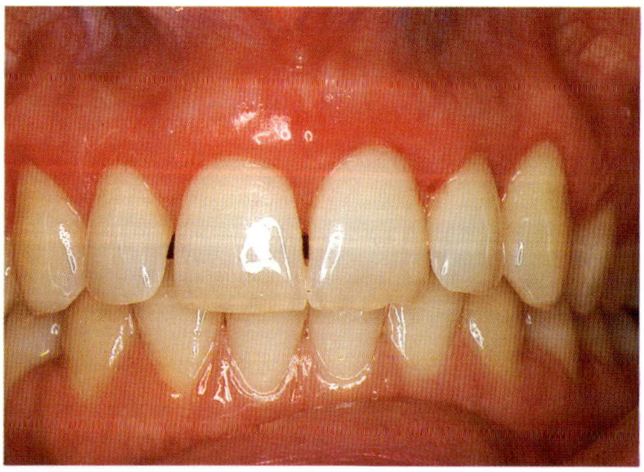

14.5f

The bleeding points located the gingival attachment and therefore provided an accurate guide in the surgery (Fig 14.5b).

A free-running, pulsed Nd:YAG laser, operating at 1,064 nm was set at 50 Hz, 60 mJ/Hz, and 3 W total power. The beam diameter was 300 μm, which was the diameter of the fiberoptic delivery system. The exposure time was approximately 1 minute per tooth. For the frenectomy, the settings were 20 Hz, 100 mJ/Hz, total power 2 W with a 300-μm beam diameter. Lidocaine with 1:100,000 epinephrine was infiltrated in the area. The gingiva was thinned slightly with a no. 5 round diamond bur in a high-speed handpiece, and the frenectomy was performed (Figs 14.5c and d). Excellent hemostasis was achieved. The procedure was completed in 40 minutes after which the patient was given postoperative instructions. The surgical site was very clean and a very uneventful postoperative course was anticipated (Fig 14.5d). That evening, the patient reported slight sensitivity, but no bleeding or swelling, and she did not require acetaminophen.

The healing process at 7 and 21 days is shown in Figs 14.5e and f. No side effects were observed. The gingiva subsequently returned to complete health, the frenum healed in a more superior position, and everyone was very satisfied with the treatment results.

Case 2. Coagulation of a Graft Donor Site

This case demonstrates the ability of a pulsed Nd:YAG laser (Laser-35, Medical Laser Technologies Inc, San Clemente, CA), which operates with an air-and-water spray, to effectively coagulate an active bleeding site. Traditionally, when soft tissue grafts are performed, a wound is created on the palate that must heal by secondary intention. This leaves an area that bleeds actively, is nearly impossible to suture, and frequently causes postoperative pain and discomfort for up to 10 days. Because the Nd:YAG wavelength is preferentially absorbed by pigmented tissue and is not affected by water, sites of active bleeding can be coagulated easily. Because of the versatility of this laser, effective coagulation is achieved with air spray without water, which not only clears away the bleeding but also provides better visibility during the procedure.

In this case, the patient was a 17-year-old caucasian boy who required a soft tissue graft on the facial surface of tooth numbers 24 and 25 due to active recession. The procedure was performed with lidocaine with 1:100,000 epinephrine. A Pacquet knife was used to dissect the donor tissue from the palate, leaving a bleeding wound (Fig 14.6a). The Laser-35 was selected for this procedure because of its

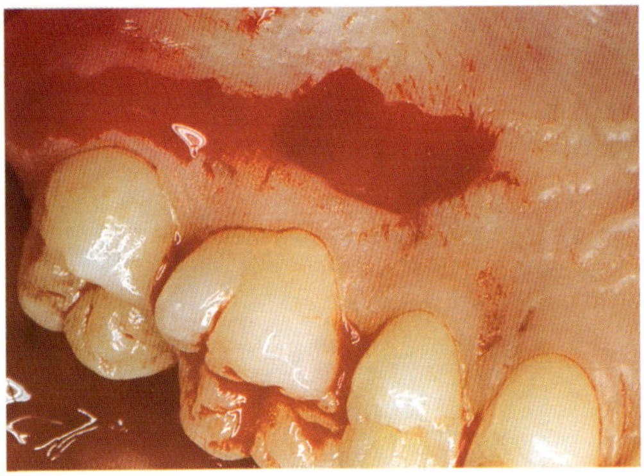

14.6a

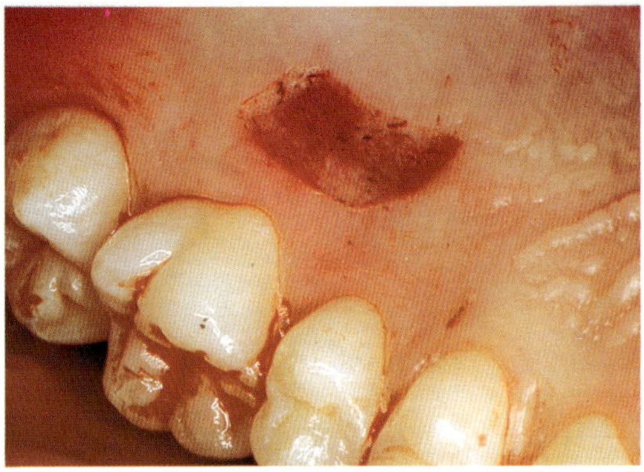

14.6b

ability to provide an air-and-water spray. The laser was set at an indicated power of 3 W and an air setting of 4 psi. The water spray was not used. A 300-μm fiber was brought into contact with the bleeding tissue and the wound was easily coagulated by using sweeping motions across the entire wound (Fig 14.6b). The patient experienced no bleeding after surgery. There was little pain the first night, and further recovery was uneventful.

Case 3. Maxillary Midline Frenectomy

The frenectomy is usually performed with a scalpel, which usually causes copious bleeding, requires suturing of the mucosa, and is accompanied by considerable swelling and postoperative pain. Afterward, the sutures, which may be partially buried, must be removed from the soft, nonkeratinized mucosa, making removal difficult and painful for the patient. The Nd:YAG laser effectively helps perform frenectomy without suturing and with minimal swelling and a better postoperative course with little discomfort.

The patient in this case was a 16-year-old caucasian boy with an aberrant and heavy frenum pull on the papilla between the two central incisors (Fig 14.7a). When the frenum was stretched, the papilla was pulled out and away from the respective teeth. In addition, the frenum was thick with fiber insertions extending to the palate.

The area was infiltrated with lidocaine and with 1:100,000 epinephrine. The Laser-35 was used with a 300-μm fiber, without air-and-water spray. We have found that when thicker tissue must be removed, or when an area requires vaporization such as in frenectomy, the water

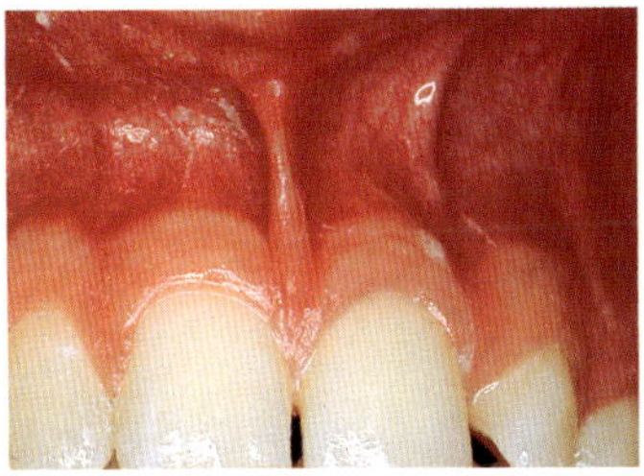

14.7a

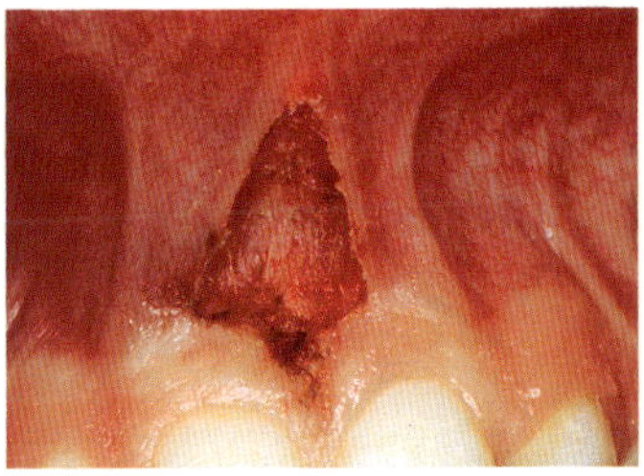

14.7b

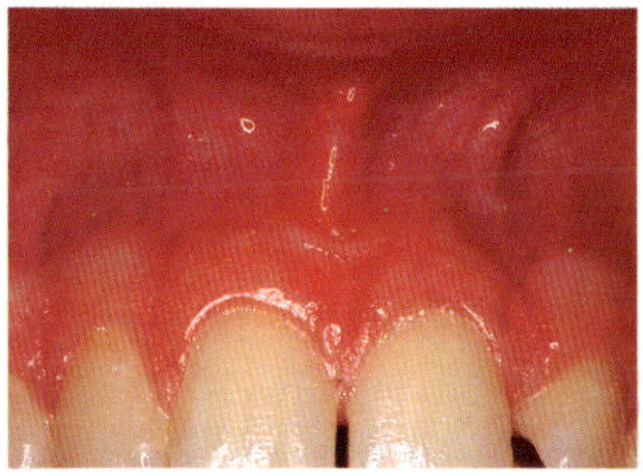

14.7c

spray impedes tissue removal and requires the use of much higher power settings. In this case, the laser output was set at 3 W. For this procedure, the lip is grasped and stretched out and forward to place maximum tension on the frenum. The fiber is then brought to the greatest concavity of the frenum, the laser is activated, and the frenum is easily vaporized. This releases the pull of the frenum on the papilla and reduces the bulk of the frenum. The procedure is accomplished with no bleeding, and sutures are not required (Fig 14.7b). After surgery, the patient reported no swelling, bleeding, and most impressively, no pain. The appearance eight weeks after surgery is shown in Fig 14.7c.

Case 4. Excisional Biopsy of a Pyogenic Granuloma

This particular case demonstrates the ability of an Nd:YAG laser to effectively perform a biopsy of a relatively large intraoral tumor. On initial examination it appeared that the lesion was broad-based, covering a large area (Fig 14.8a). On closer inspection, the lesion was found to be on a stalk, but had enlarged, tightly juxtaposing the tissue. The lesion also appeared vascular in nature, since each time the lesion was pulled away from its base, bleeding occurred (Fig 14.8b). Because the Nd:YAG laser operates via fiber delivery, which can touch the tissue, it became the laser of choice for removal of this lesion. A CO_2 laser would not have been able to get under the lesion without vaporization of adjacent tissue and would possibly cause damage to the tooth. Argon or Ho:YAG lasers would also have been applicable in this case. If done conventionally, this lesion would be removed with a scalpel, and sutures would be needed to control the bleeding. Suturing these types of wounds can be difficult since there is a base without approximating margins.

This patient was a 7½-year-old caucasian boy with a noncontributory medical history. The lesion was located on the left side of the palate with the stalk emanating between the central and lateral incisors. Be-

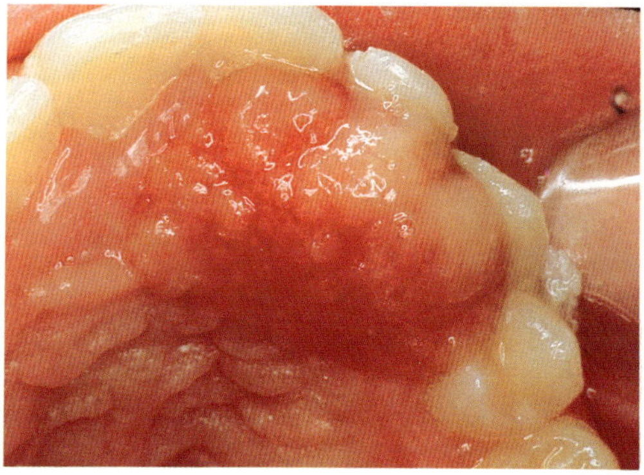

14.8a

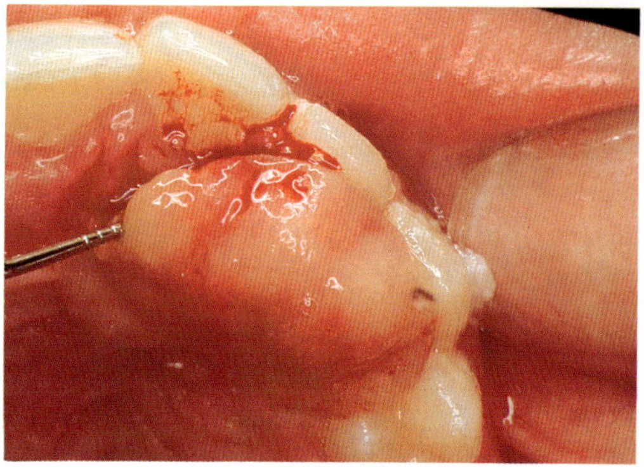

14.8b

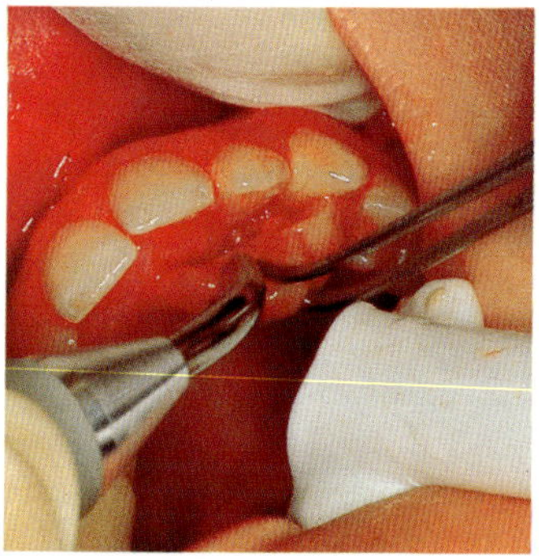

14.8c

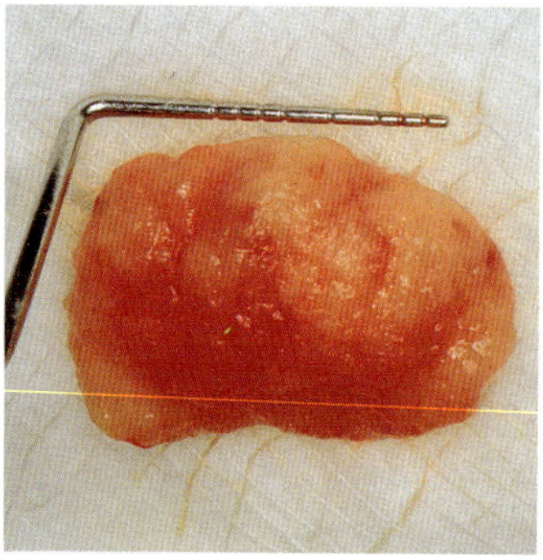

14.8d

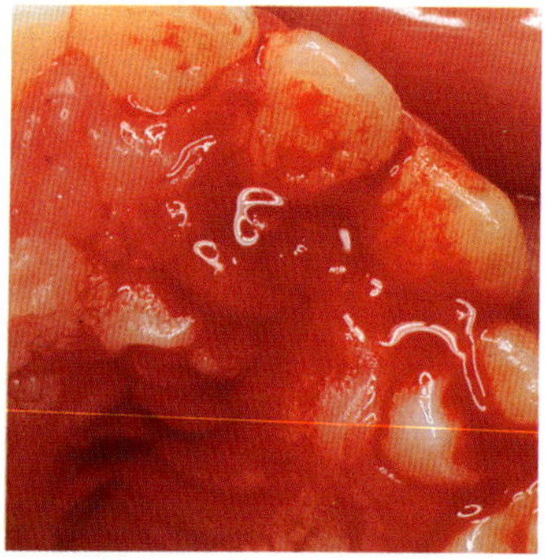

14.8e

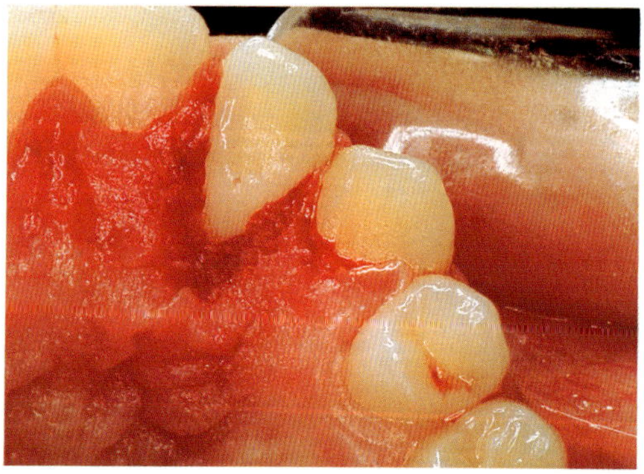

14.8f

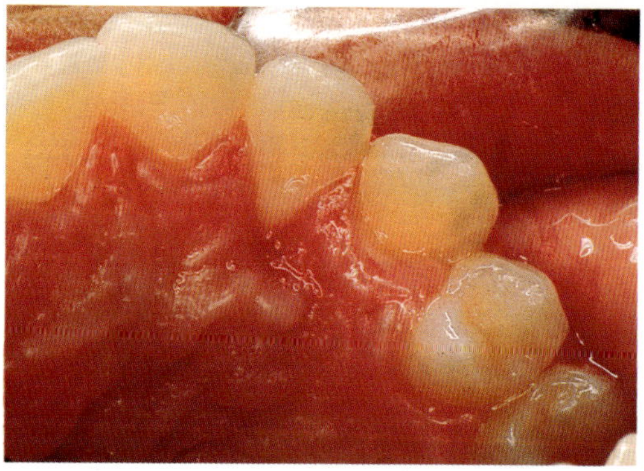

14.8g

cause of the bleeding nature of this lesion and its approximation to tooth structure, an Nd:YAG laser (Laser-35) was used. The laser was set at 6 W with automatic air-and-water spray settings. With air-and-water spray, the laser's penetration depth can be controlled to avoid damage to tooth structure, and active bleeding is flushed away, affording better visibility. The surgical site was infiltrated with lidocaine and 1:100,000 epinephrine. The lesion was grasped at one edge with a tissue pickup and maximum tension placed outward from the base. The fiber was brought to the base of the stalk, and the lesion was undermined and freed from its base (Fig 14.8c and d). The procedure lasted less than 2 minutes. Once the lesion was removed, there was active bleeding from the wound (Fig 14.8e). The laser was then reset to 3 W without air-and-water spray to achieve coagulation (Fig 14.8f). The patient recovered without complications. There was no swelling, scarring, or pain (Fig 14.8g) 6 weeks following surgery.

Case 5. Excisional Biopsy of Hemangioma

This case illustrates the ability of the Nd:YAG laser to effectively biopsy a hemangioma without hemorrhage, postoperative bleeding, or sutures. In addition, there is no damage to adjacent tooth structure with this method.

The patient was a 3-year-old caucasian boy with no contributory medical findings. A red lesion measuring 3 mm × 3 mm was present on the interproximal facial gingiva between the mandibular right canine and first primary molar (Fig 14.9a). Blood was expressed from the lesion when it was compressed (Fig 14.9b). Because the mesial extent of the lesion was in contact with the canine, an Nd:YAG laser with air-and-water spray was used. In this example, the fiber is used to undermine the lesion and aid in the excision. This case also illustrates the ability of the Nd:YAG laser to excise tissue without damage to the adjacent canine tooth. A Laser-35 operating at 1,064 nm was used with automatic air-and-water spray. Power output was set at 6 W. The area was infiltrated with lidocaine and 1:100,000 epinephrine. The biopsy was performed with the technique as described in Chapter 8. On completion of the biopsy, there was complete coagulation (Fig 14.9c). The area appeared normal 6 weeks after surgery (Fig 14.9d).

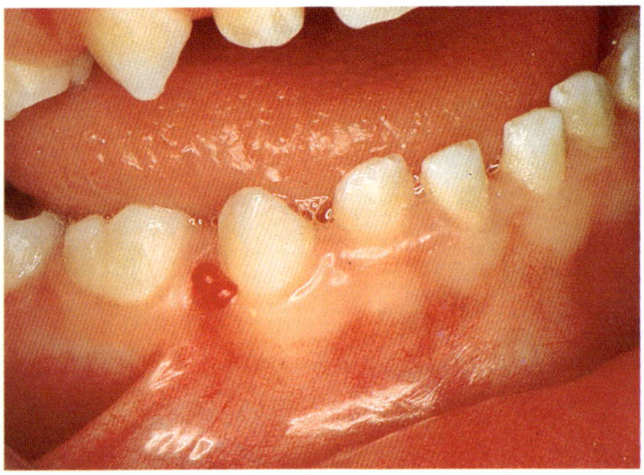

14.9a

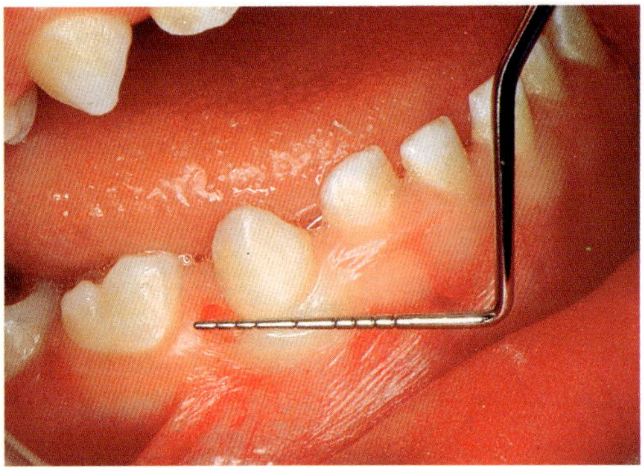

14.9b

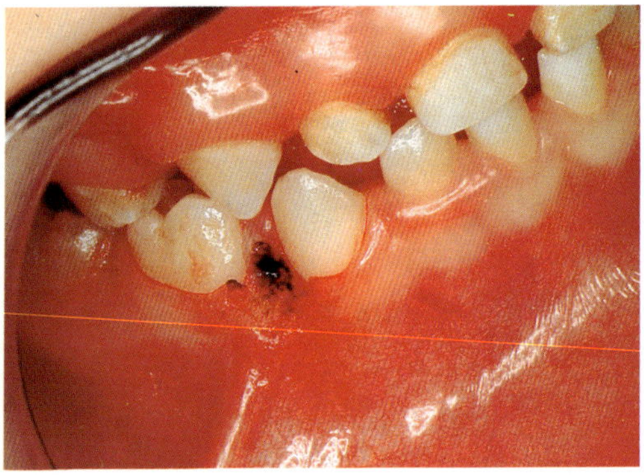

14.9c

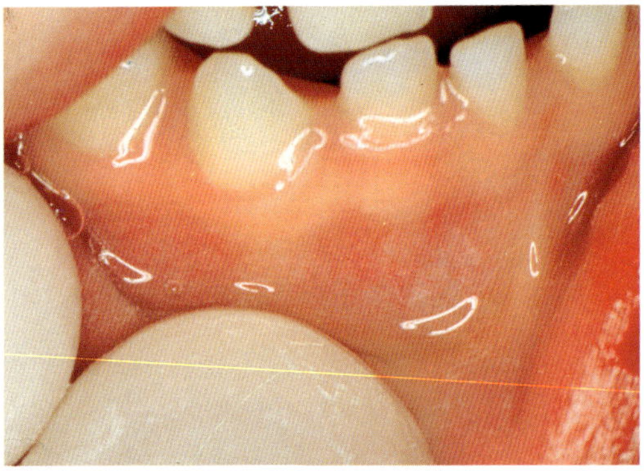

14.9d

The Nd:YAG Laser in Periodontal Therapy

Nd:YAG lasers can be used in periodontics for a number of procedures. For gingivectomies, gingivoplasties, soft tissue crown lengthenings, and minor soft tissue recontouring, the Nd:YAG laser can be very efficacious.

For most Nd:YAG lasers, regardless of power settings, the bare fiber should never be placed at the base of a sulcus or pocket (Fig 14.10). When conditions exist that require submarginal incisions, extensive osseous surgery, or removal of bone, use of the laser is not advised because of its inability to efficiently ablate osseous tissue and its tendency to overheat the osseous tissues with deep penetration causing possible bony sequestrations. The Nd:YAG laser, however, can be highly effective for gingivectomies. When a gingivectomy is performed, the fiber tip is brought in contact at the depth at which the tissue is to be removed. This depth measurement is accomplished either with a pocket marker or the pseudopocket is measured with a periodontal probe and that measurement is transferred to the external tissue surface. The laser is then activated and the fiber is dragged in either direction at the specific depth as the tis-

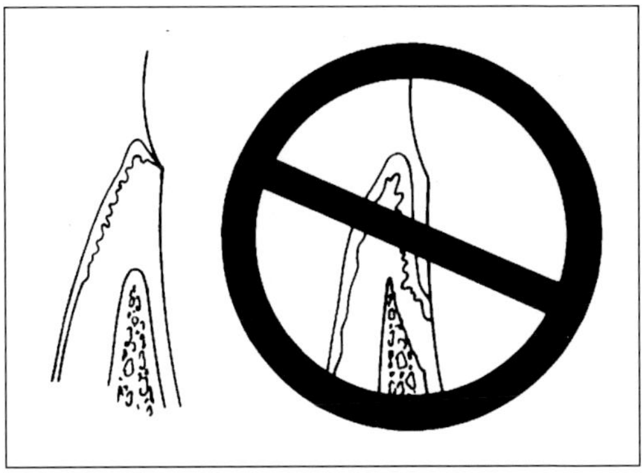

Fig 14.10 The bare fiber should not be placed at the base of a sulcus.

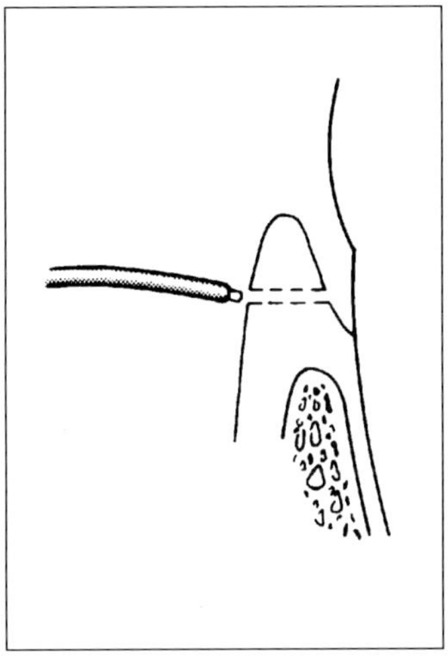

Fig 14.11 The fiber is pulled at a specific depth to remove tissue.

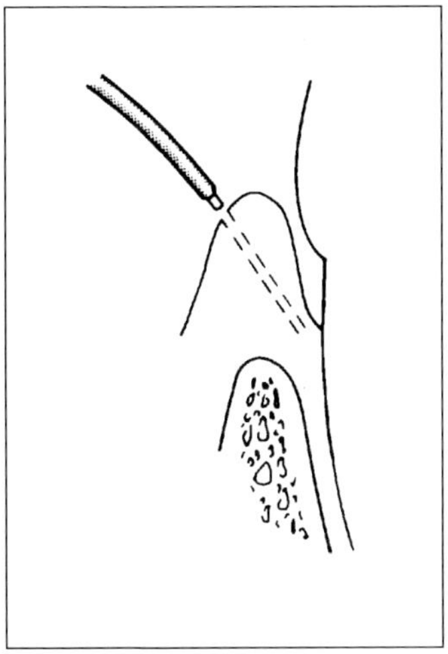

Fig 14.12 Internally beveled gingivectomy performed with a laser.

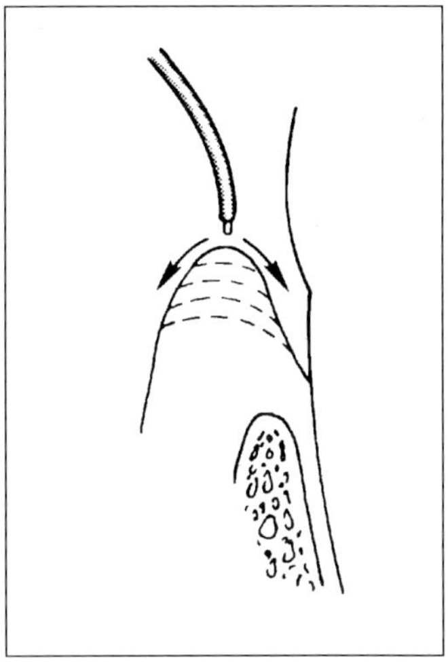

Fig 14.13 Gingivoplasty as performed with a laser.

sue is removed (Fig 14.11). Because of the hemorrhage-free nature of the wound, one can continually operate and recontour as necessary without aspirating blood in the field.

This technique applies to soft tissue crown lengthening. When there is excessive tissue covering a clinical crown and the clinical crown is shorter than the anatomic crown, the tissue can be removed with this technique. It is important to note that if the clinical crown and anatomic crown are equal and crown lengthening is necessary, then conventional crown lengthening via submarginal incisions and osseous recontouring must be performed.

The fiber can also be used to perform the classic externally beveled gingivectomy (see Fig 14.11) or can be adjusted to perform an internally beveled gingivectomy removing the epithelial lining at the tissue margin (Fig 14.12). The technique used with an Nd:YAG laser is similar to removing the tissue with a scalpel. The tissue is actually cut rather than vaporized as with other wavelengths such as with the CO_2 laser.

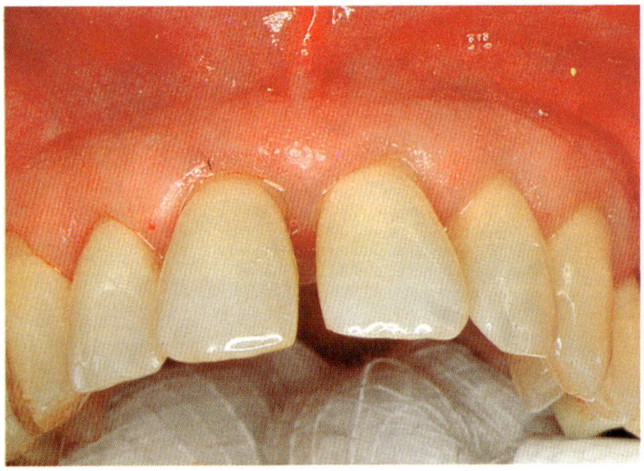

14.14a

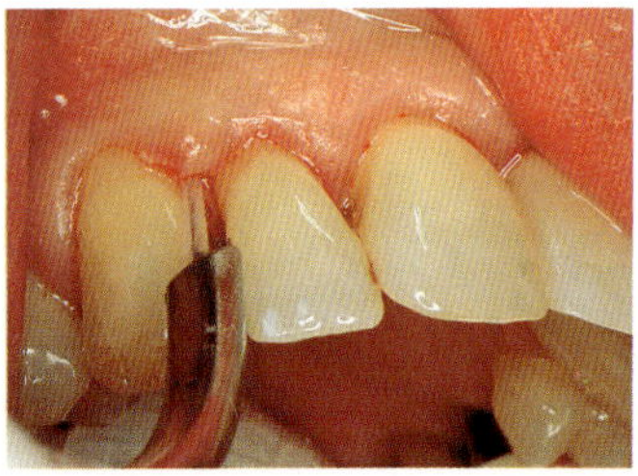

14.14b

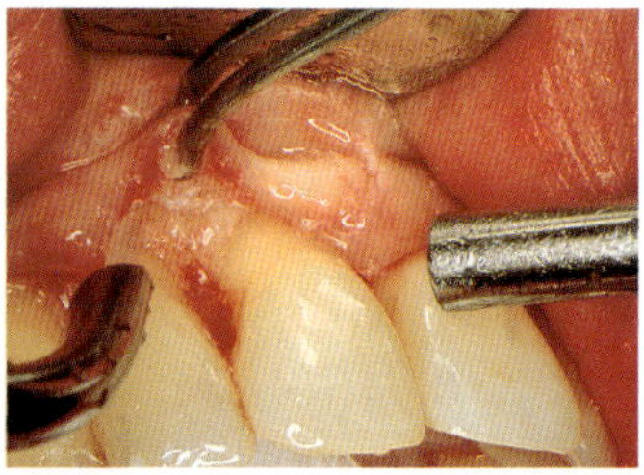

14.14c

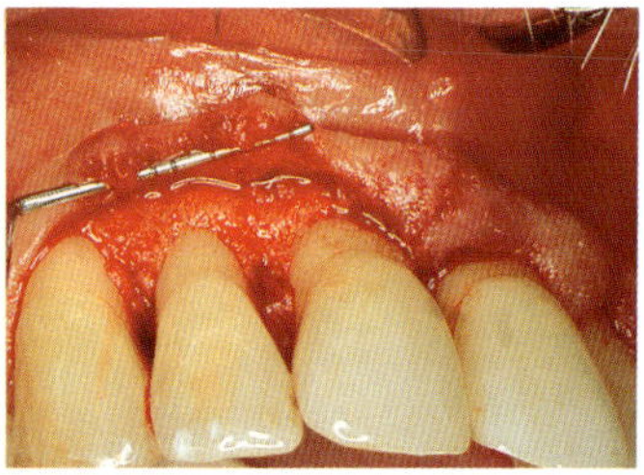

14.14d

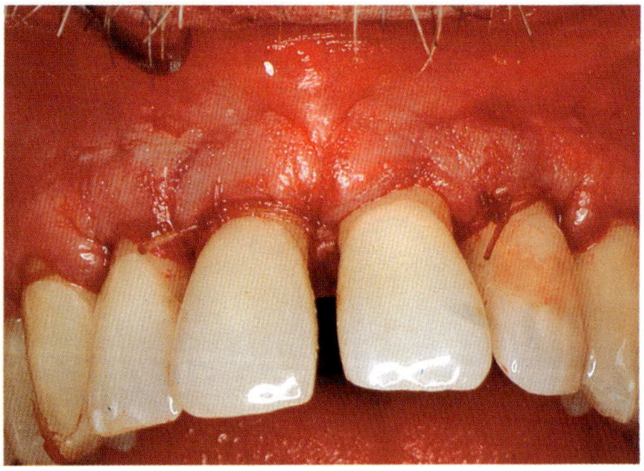

14.14e

The Nd:YAG laser can also be used to reshape tissue and perform gingivoplasties. The laser is brought in contact with the tissue to be operated on and, by moving the tip across the tissue surface in an up-and-back direction, the tissue is vaporized; hence, the gingivoplasty is performed (Fig 14.13). After lasing, the area is completely coagulated, leaving a surface that will heal uneventfully with no postoperative pain for the patient.

In the past, the use of lasers in actual periodontal flap therapy has been very limited (Pick, 1993). With use of an Nd:YAG laser with air-and-water cooling, periodontal flap therapy has been accomplished recently. The procedure has only been performed with sulcular incisions and used only for Widman-type flaps, where conservative therapy that also preserves esthetics was the goal.

The patient is anesthetized with lidocaine with 1:100,000 epinephrine (Fig 14.14a). A Laser-35 Nd:YAG laser was used at a power setting of 9 W, pulsed, with automatic air-and-water spray. The area requiring surgery was the maxillary anterior sextant (Fig 14.14b). Probing depths were from 3 to 6 mm, with the deeper probings used for the interproximal measurements. Radiographs of the area revealed mild-to-moderate horizontal bone loss. The area had been previously scaled and root planed with local anesthesia. Each scaling visit was associated with oral hygiene instruction. There was resolution of active bleeding and inflammation, but not of probing depths.

The surgery is initiated from either end of the sextant. The fiber is inserted using a split dissection technique and the laser is activated (Fig 14.14c). The tip is then dragged, using sweeping motions to prevent accumulation of tissue debris at the tip. A tissue pickup is used to grasp the tissue margin at the operative site, and by using a technique very similar to traction-countertraction, the flap is easily elevated away from the underlying bone (Fig 14.14d). Once this has been accomplished, the laser can be used to help degranulate the area for scaling of root surfaces and necessary bony changes made depending on the case. Sutures are then used to close the flap (Fig 14.14e).

Clearly, dentistry will witness a proliferation of lasers over the next few years, allowing the professional to practice a superior, precise, and exacting type of dentistry. As research progresses and clinical experience increases, the possibilities of laser uses in dentistry will continue to expand as well. With fiber technology lasers and future research with biomaterials, it is not inconceivable to use the laser for incisions, accomplish flap reflection, and clean out or degranulate the area with the laser. The flap reflection can be laser-welded to position, thus eliminating sutures and allowing for exact flap placement.

Acknowledgments

We would like to thank the clinical investigators Rahmat Barkhordar, Grayson Marshall Jr., Renaldo Parisi, Paul Atkinson, George Denes, Doug Van Thorre, and Dean McDaniel for their expertise and commitment to this investigation. We acknowledge the combined efforts of American Dental Laser and Sunrise Technologies and thank John Sulewski for editorial assistance in preparation of this manuscript.

References

Adrian JC, Bernier J, Sprague WG. Laser and the dental pulp. J Am Dent Assoc 1971;83:113–117.

Adrian JC. Pulp effect of neodymium laser, a preliminary report. Oral Surg Oral Med Oral Pathol 1977;44:301–305.

Bahcall JK, Miserendino LJ, Walia H, Belardi DW. Scanning electron microscopic comparison of canal preparation with Nd:YAG laser and hand instrumentation: A preliminary study. Gen Dent 1993;41:45–47.

Dederich DN, Zakariasen KL, Tulip J. Scanning electron microscopic analysis of canal wall dentin following neodymium-yttrium-aluminum-garnet laser irradiation. J Endodontics 1984;10:428–431.

Dederich DN, Zakariasen KL, Tulip J. S.E.M. analysis of dyed canal dentin following Nd:YAG laser irradiation (abstract). J Dent Res 1985;64:239.

Hardee M, Miserendino LJ, Kos W. Evaluation of intracanal Nd-YAG laser irradiation (abstract). J Endodontics 1990;16:194.

Iwasaki M, Sasaka M, Konishi T, Maruyama Y, Wada T. Nd:YAG laser for general surgery. Lasers Surg Med 1985;5:429–438.

Joffe, SN. Contact neodymium:YAG laser surgery in gastroenterology: A preliminary report. Lasers Surg Med 1986;6:470–472.

Joffe, SN, Bracket KA, Sankar MY, Daikuzono N. Resection of the liver with the Nd:YAG laser. Surg Gynecol Obstet 1986;163:437–442.

Liberman R, Segal TH, Nordenberg D, Serebro LI. Adhesion of composite materials to enamel: comparison between the use of acid and lasing as pretreatment. Lasers Surg Med 1984;4:323–327.

Miserendino LJ. A histologic evaluation of pulsed Nd:YAG laser for conventional endodontic treatment. Presented at the International Society of Laser Dentistry Meeting; Paris, France; 1990.

Miserendino LJ, Miserendino CA. Removal of foreign objects from the root canal: Effects on endodontic retreatment (abstract). Presented at the International Society for Lasers in Dentistry Meeting; Salt Lake City, UT; Aug 1992.

Miserendino LJ, Rizoiu I, Levy G. Effects of Nd:YAG irradiation on the permeability of root canal wall dentin (abstract). Presented at the International Society for Lasers in Dentistry Meeting; Salt Lake City, UT; Aug 1992.

Miserendino LJ, Rizoiu IM. Interaction du Laser Nd:YAG et de la dentine canalaire lors du traitement endodontique. ENDO Rev Fr Endodontie 1993;12:23–28.

Myers TD, Myers WD. The use of a laser for debridement of incipient caries. J Prosthet Dent 1985a;53:776–779.

Myers TD, Myers WD. In vivo caries removal utilizing the YAG laser. J Mich Dent Assoc 1985b;68:66–69.

Ohyama M, Katduda K, Nobori T, et al. Treatment of head and neck tumors by contact Nd:YAG laser surgery. Auris Nasus Larynx 1985;12:138–142.

Pick RM, Pecaro BC, Silberman CJ. The laser gingivectomy. The use of the CO_2 laser for the removal of phenytoin hyperplasia. J Periodontol 1985 (Aug): 492–496.

Pick RM, Pecaro BC. Use of the CO_2 laser in soft tissue dental surgery. Lasers Surg Med 1987;7:207–213.

Pick RM. Using lasers in clinical dental practice. J Am Dent Assoc 1993;124:37–47.

Pogrel MA. The carbon dioxide laser in soft tissue preprosthetic surgery. J Prosthet Dent 1989;61:203–208.

Washida H, Tsugaya M, Hirao N, Hachisuka Y. Experience using the laser rod in urological surgery (abstract). Hinyokika (Jpn) 1984;30:891–896.

White JM, Goodis HE, Setcos JC, et al. Effects of pulsed Nd:YAG laser energy on human teeth: A three-year follow-up study. J Am Dent Assoc 1993;124: 45–50.

White JM, Goodis HE, Kudler JJ, Tran KT. Thermal laser effects on intraoral soft tissue, teeth and bone in vitro. Third International Congress on Lasers in Dentistry. Salt Lake City: University of Utah Printing Services; 1992:189–190.

White JM, Goodis HE, Rose CM. Use of the pulsed Nd:YAG laser for intraoral soft tissue surgery. Lasers Surg Med 1991;11:455–461.

White JM, Goodis HE, Marshall GW, Marshall SJ. Identification of the physical modification threshold of dentin induced by neodymium and holmium YAG lasers using scanning electron microscopy. Scan Microsc 1993;7:239–246.

White JM, Goodis HE, Daniels TE. Effects of Nd:YAG laser on pulps of extracted teeth. Lasers Life Sci 1991;4:191–200.

Winkler S, Flynn KL, Miller WA. Neodymium laser fusion of restorative materials to tooth structure, a preliminary report. NY State Dent J 1973;39:614–618.

Yamamoto H, Ooya K. Potential of yttrium-aluminum-garnet laser in caries prevention. J Oral Pathol 1974; 3:7–15.

Yamamoto H, Sato K. Prevention of dental caries by Nd:YAG laser irradiation. J Dent Res 1980;59:2171.

Zakariasen KL, Dederich DN, Tulip J. Nd:YAG laser fusion of dentin plugs in root canals (abstract). J Dent Res 1985;64:239.

Chapter Fifteen

Clinical Applications of Argon Laser in Restorative Dentistry

Richard Blankenau, W. Patrick Kelsey, and V. Kim Kutsch

The argon laser is unique in its ability to be used for a number of nonsurgical applications in restorative dentistry. The earliest applications of argon lasers in restorative dentistry involved illumination of teeth for the detection of decay (Alfano and Yao, 1981; Bjelkhagen et al, 1982). Since the early 1980s, additional research in dentistry has focused on the photopolymerization of composite resins (Benedicenti et al, 1984, 1986; DeMichelis et al, 1986; Kelsey et al, 1989; Powell et al, 1989; Severin and Manquin, 1989; Blankenau et al, 1991a, 1991b; Potts and Petrou, 1991). The Food and Drug Administration (FDA) granted marketing clearance for the use of the argon laser in dentistry in 1991, and since that time the argon laser has been used for a variety of hard and soft tissue applications.

The principal reason for the interest in this source of light is that its specific wavelength parallels the requirements for the initiation of polymerization of the growing family of light-activated restorative materials (Kelsey et al, 1989). These include restorative resins, bases and liners, cements, pit and fissure sealants, and light-activated impression materials. Preventive dental treatments have also been described as potential areas of interest for the argon laser.

Argon Laser Interaction with Restorative Materials

Currently, photoactivated dental resins employ a diketone, such as camphoroquinone, and a tertiary amine reducing agent to initiate polymerization (American Dental Association, 1985; Craig, 1984). This photoinitiator system is sensitive to light in the blue region of the visible spectrum with broad peak activity in the 480-nm region (Cook, 1982). When exposed to light of this wavelength, free radicals are formed that induce the polymerization reaction. Current visible light units use a tungsten-halogen bulb as the light source and a filter to reduce the output of undesired wavelengths. The argon laser's monochromatic wavelengths of 488 nm and 514.5 nm have been shown to be effective in the initiation of polymerization of dental resins. Studies by Blankenau et al have demonstrated that the argon laser can be used to polymerize both hybrid and microfilled composite resins with an enhancement of the physical properties of the polymerized restorative material following argon laser exposure compared to conventional visible light curing. This tendency was more pronounced for the microfilled materials and appeared to be related to the fact that the argon laser was associated with a greater degree of resin polymerization (Blankenau et al, 1989a).

Additional research has shown that when argon laser energy is used with dentin bonding materials, adhesion to dentin will rival or exceed that which is obtainable with conventional visible light sources (Blankenau et al, 1989b). The attachment of pit and fissure sealants to the enamel of teeth was also significantly improved with argon laser polymerization compared to visible light curing and the microleakage associated with these sealants was significantly reduced. It has also been demonstrated that the enhanced physical properties, the improved adhesion, and the reduced microleakage can be achieved with significantly reduced exposure time. Argon laser polymerization requires a 10-second cure cycle while visible light activation usually takes approximately 40 seconds (Blankenau et al, 1990a, 1990b; Blankenau et al, 1992a, 1992b).

An examination of the physical and mechanical properties of a restorative material can be useful in predicting how that material will endure in the oral environment. Compressive strength is a measure of a material's resistance to fracture or failure when compressive loads, such as mastication, are applied. It, therefore, can provide an indication of how a restorative material will perform during function. Argon laser polymerization of microfilled and small particle resins resulted in slightly greater, but not statistically significant, compressive strength values when compared to those with visible light activation. At the very least, this demonstrates that argon laser activation of resin polymerization does not impair the attainment of current clinically acceptable compressive strength values. Interestingly enough, the attainment of these comparable compressive strength values was achieved with one fourth the polymerization time required by visible light activation.

Functional stresses in the oral cavity typically are not solely compressive in nature. Lateral forces that tend to elongate or stretch a restorative material are also present. Diametral tensile strength values should provide an indication of a material's resistance to these forces. Argon laser polymerization resulted in greater diametral tensile strength values for both microfilled and small particle resin-restorative materials, and these differences were statistically significant. It may be inferred that argon laser–polymerized restorations should be better able to resist these lateral, tensile forces generated during function. Functional stresses can also result in the distortion or deformation of a restoration.

Transverse flexural strength is a measure of a material's resistance to distortion. When results with argon laser polymerization were compared to those with visible light activation, the transverse flexural strength of a microfilled resin and a small particle resin were both improved with the difference being statistically significant for the microfilled material. Related to this concept of restoration deformation is the flexural modulus, which is a measure of a restorative material's stiffness or rigidity. This can be important clinically because if a large discrepancy exists between the flexural modulus of a resin restorative material and the surrounding tooth structure to which it is attached, shear forces could develop at that point of attachment (ie, the enamel or dentin bond). This would be most likely to occur when the less rigid resin restorative material bends as occlusal loads are applied and the more rigid or stiffer tooth structure does not. This could ultimately lead to margin failures of the restoration and the subsequent problems of interfacial staining, microleakage, and secondary caries. As observed with the transverse flexural strength, argon laser polymerization yielded flexural modulus values for both microfilled and small particle resins that indicated these materials would be more resistant to deformation than when conventional visible light activation was used, and these differences were statistically significant for the microfilled material.

It would appear that argon laser polymerization will at least meet, and quite possibly exceed, transverse flexural strength and flexural modulus values considered acceptable and achievable with current visible light polymerization technology. Once again, as with compressive strength, these results were accomplished with only 25% of the standard visible light exposure time (Kelsey et al, 1989). Application of currently available argon laser technology may result in the improvement of both the efficiency of dental health-care delivery and the physical properties of the restorative materials used during that process.

Although the exact mechanism of physical property improvement following argon lasing is not totally understood, it is probably the result of enhanced or more thorough resin polymerization. Studies have confirmed that a greater degree of resin polymerization is attainable with the argon laser than with conventional visible light. This was determined by measuring and comparing the amount of residual, unpolymerized resin monomer extracted from cured samples (Blankenau et al, 1991a). This would also partially explain some of the differences noted in physical property enhancement between microfilled and small particle resins.

Microfilled materials tend to have a greater resin content and a lower filler particle loading than their small particle counterparts. Since the microfilled materials have a greater resin content, it would appear that they have a greater relative component that is affected by the polymerization process. Since the argon laser represents a more effective means of polymerization, its results should be most apparent in those materials that have the greatest component in need of polymerization, in other words, the resin matrix. This could possibly explain the differences encountered between microfilled and small particle composite resin materials as well as account for the improvements noted with resin rich materials such as pit and fissure sealants (Blankenau et al, 1992b).

Interproximal Caries Detection

Scientific studies indicate that argon laser energy will offer diagnostic capabilities when used to illuminate teeth. Alfano et al (1981) used monochromatic light at 350, 410, and 530 nm and measured the visible emission spectra comparing carious to noncarious tissue. The result was a shift of the emission spectra to >540 nm, or the visible red range of the electromagnetic spectrum. Bjelkhagen et al (1982) used an argon laser for luminescence and studied the results through barrier filters. Again, a difference was detected, with the carious tissue appearing darker than the noncarious tissue. Kutsch (1992) reported clinical findings comparing carious and noncarious tissue illuminated with an argon laser with dark-field photography. The findings were compared with clinical appearance and radiographic analysis. The carious tissue was readily apparent with the laser illumination.

When illuminated with argon laser light, carious tissue has a clinical appearance of a dark, fiery, orange-red color and is easily differentiated from sound tooth structure. Decalcified areas appear as a dull, opaque, orange color. To examine a tooth, the power output should be set to the lowest available setting, normally 80 mW, continuous wave. Any size fiber can be selected, although we prefer the 300-μm fiber for almost all applications. This will create a 114 W/cm^2 power density at the tip of the fiber. The delivery fiber should be placed either lingually to the tooth and illuminated and observed from the buccal or facial aspects, or illuminated buccally or facially and observed from the lingual aspect with a mouth mirror. The fiber should be moved in and out of contact with the tooth and redirected to thoroughly expose and examine the entire clinical crown. Enamel fractures will also be readily apparent during this procedure. This procedure can be used in conjunction with radiographic examination of teeth; decay that does not appear radiographically will often be detected with the laser illumination. A hard copy of this examination can be captured with an intraoral photograph or videocamera.

Case 1. Transillumination

A 53-year-old white man with an unremarkable medical history presented for treatment. Oral examination revealed no incipient decay or decalcification on the maxillary right lateral incisor (Fig 15.1a). The periapical radiograph indicated no carious lesion (Fig 15.1b). Illuminated with the argon laser from the lingual side, the distal contact area had an incipient carious lesion, apparent as a distinct dark red area easily differentiated from the rest of the sound tooth structure (Fig 15.1c). When illuminated from the facial aspect, the lesion exhibited the characteristic fiery red coloration, and enamel fractures were readily discernable (Fig 15.1d). By moving the fiber over the surfaces, all areas of decay, decalcification, and fractures may be identified. Recurrent decay can even be diagnosed around metallic and resin restorations.

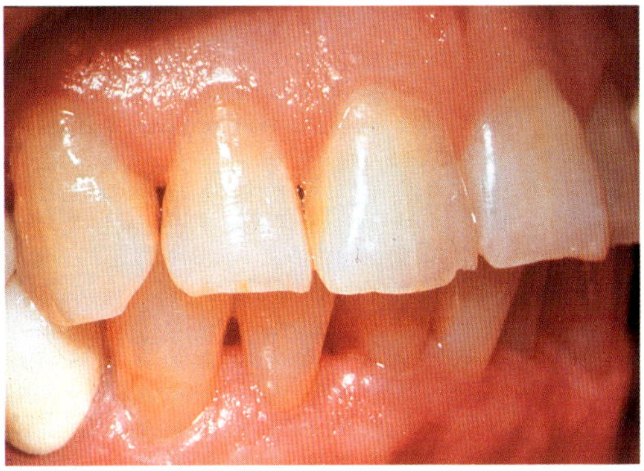

Fig 15.1a Maxillary right lateral incisor.

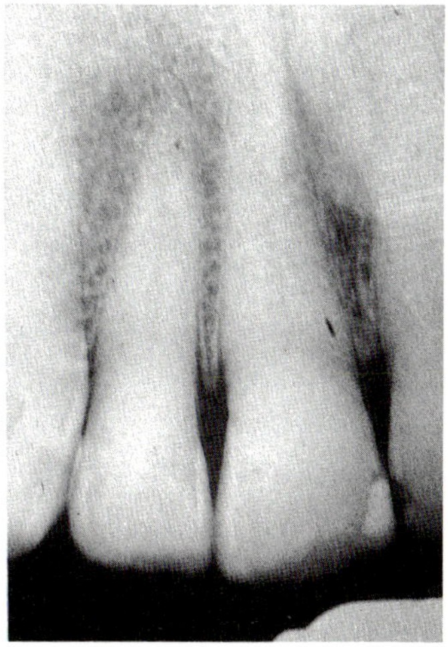

Fig 15.1b Periapical radiograph of the same lateral incisor.

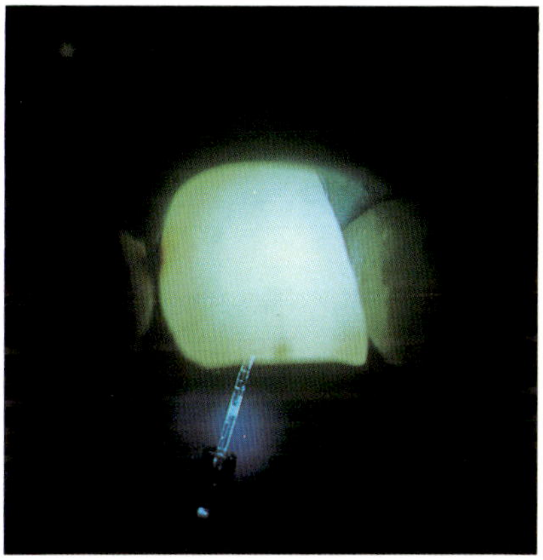

Fig 15.1c Argon laser illumination from the lingual surface.

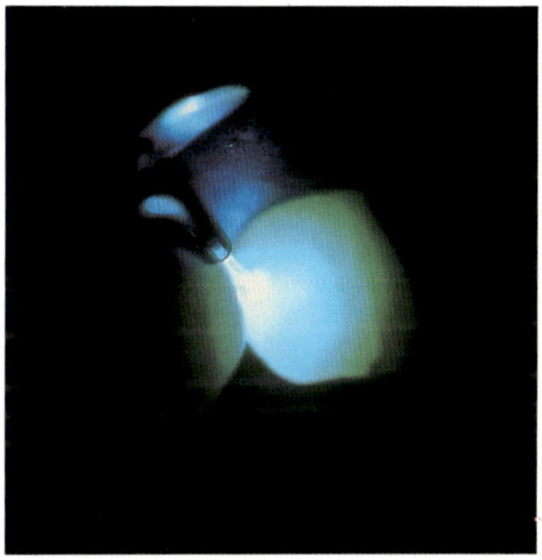

Fig 15.1d Continued argon laser illumination from the facial aspect.

Preventive Dentistry

Currently, the principal means of rendering teeth less susceptible to caries is to either chemically alter the surface characteristics of enamel through topical fluoride application or to bond a caries-resistant material, such as a sealant, to the tooth. The use of laser energy in dentistry may be able to be expanded to include preventive treatments and may have application in both changing enamel surface morphologic characteristics and in the placement of sealants. It has been demonstrated that a change in enamel morphologic characteristics that renders the tooth more resistant to acid attack can be effected by laser light exposure. Carbon dioxide and Nd:YAG lasers have been used for this purpose; however, care must be exercised due to concern about changing the pulp (Yamamoto and Sato, 1980; Yu et al, 1990; Nelson et al, 1986; Peters et al, 1990; Goodman and Kaufman, 1977; Boran et al, 1992). The argon laser has also been shown to alter the surface characteristics of enamel to make it more caries-resistant and to do so without as much danger to the pulp (Westerman et al, 1991, 1992). It has been shown that enamel displays a significant reduction in its acid solubility after argon lasing. When a topical fluoride treatment was performed after argon laser conditioning of enamel, an even more dramatic reduction in enamel acid demineralization was observed. Apparently, in addition to rendering the enamel less susceptible to caries attack, the argon laser also facilitates the tooth's uptake of fluoride to improve this desired result. Additionally, argon-lased enamel shows a high positive birefringence, suggesting the formation of microspaces within the enamel. These microspaces would impart an increased acid resistance to the enamel by trapping ions formed during acid demineralization rather than allowing them to escape into the surrounding solution.

The other method of reducing caries susceptibility involves the placement of an acid-resistant material on the teeth. Again, laser technology may prove helpful. A synthetic hydroxyapatite compound has been successfully attached to the enamel of extracted teeth with a CO_2 laser operating at energy levels that are less than those known to cause pulpal injury. As such, this technique has potential for use as a pit and fissure sealant. The argon laser would appear to have applications when considering conventional pit and fissure therapy with resin materials currently available.

When photopolymerizing unfilled resins, a 7- to 8-mm spot size for 5 sec at 300 mW is recommended. Opaque, filled pit and fissure sealant resins should be polymerized for 10 sec. Compared to a standard curing light, the small fiber size (300 to 600 µm) allows easy access for all difficult-to-reach places. When applied correctly, the argon laser is a valuable tool for photopolymerizing composite sealants, resulting in improved quality and significant time savings.

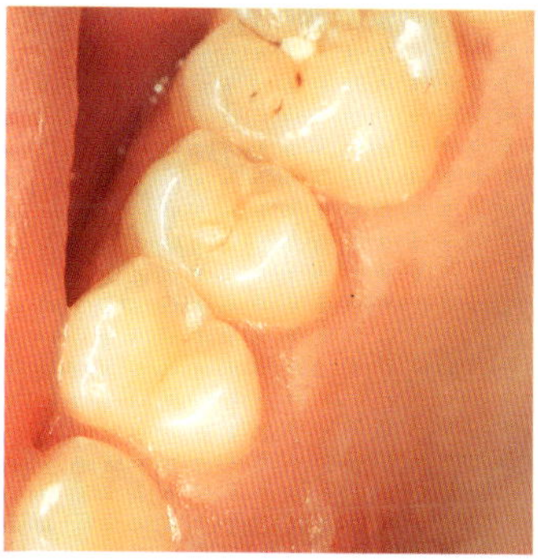

Fig 15.2a Occlusal view of typical case requiring sealant therapy before treatment.

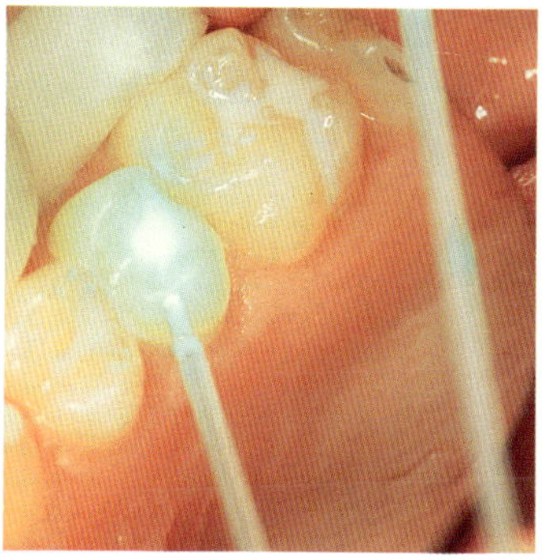

Fig 15.2b Photopolymerization of pit and fissure sealants with argon laser light.

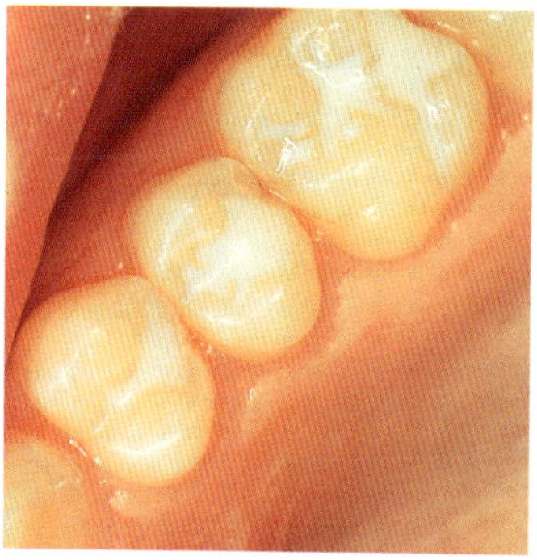

Fig 15.2c Appearance of sealed teeth after treatment.

Case 2. Argon Laser Use for Caries Prevention

This case demonstrates the use of argon lasers with conventional pit and fissure sealant therapy. Several teeth were in need of sealant therapy (Fig 15.2a). A common clinical problem associated with this type of treatment is sealant loss. The argon laser is used to polymerize a resin pit and fissure sealant (Fig 15.2b to 15.2c).

When compared to sealants polymerized by conventional visible light means, argon-lased sealants demonstrated less microleakage. Although sealants polymerized by these two methods provided a similar degree of caries prevention at the tooth-restoration interface, the argon laser–cured samples had a significant reduction in surface lesion depth. An improvement in sealant retention would be expected following argon laser polymerization as a result of improvement in the physical properties of diametral tensile strength and flexural modulus.

In addition to producing a better sealant, the use of the argon laser also seems to be well suited to improving the reliability of the procedure. Its reduced exposure time would tend to increase the probability of maintaining a dry field throughout the duration of the procedure (Blankenau et al, 1989b, 1990a, 1990b, 1992a, 1992b).

Argon Laser Photopolymerization of Composite Resins

During the 1980s, scientific studies demonstrated the ability of visible light to penetrate both composite material and tooth structure to photopolymerize camphorquinone-activated resins (Swartz et al, 1983; Forsten, 1984; Weaver et al, 1988). More recent studies have indicated that argon laser light is effective in photopolymerization of these systems and improves the physical properties of the restorations (Kelsey et al, 1989; Powell et al, 1989; Severin, 1989; Blankenau et al, 1991a, 1991b). When used to photopolymerize camphorquinone-activated composite resins, the argon laser increases the depth of cure, increases the diametral tensile strength, increases the adhesive bond strength, increases the degree of polymerization of the material, reduces the acid solubility of the surrounding enamel, and decreases the time of activation significantly. One weak link of light-activated composite resins, directional photopolymerization shrinkage, has not yet been reported with the argon laser in the scientific literature. With the growing demand for cosmetic dentistry and bonded restorations, the argon laser has a bright future in dentistry.

To cure composite resins, the power output of the argon laser should be set at 250 to 500 mW, depending on the type of composite selected. The pulse parameters should be set for a single pulse, with a duration of 10 sec. Any size fiber can be used; we prefer the 300-µm diameter bare fiber, but many clinicians use the 600-µm fiber. The key is to create approximately a 5-mm spot size on the target material. This will produce a power density of approximately 1.25 to 2.50 W/cm^2 throughout the 5-mm spot. The laser will adequately cure to a depth of 2 mm on most materials in 10 sec. Incrementally cure the restoration with maximum 2-mm increments 10 sec each. Do not exceed 600 mW for 40 sec on a given increment.

Case 3. Class III Composite Restoration of Lateral Incisor

A 53-year-old white man with an unremarkable medical history sought treatment. His maxillary right lateral incisor had a distal incipient carious lesion. After local anesthesia and isolation with a rubber dam, the lesion was exposed and debrided with a high-speed handpiece and carbide bur (Fig 15.3a). The composite restoration was then placed with standard procedures (Fig 15.3b). The argon laser was used to photopolymerize the material with 500 mW, 5-mm spot size, and 10-sec pulse (Fig 15.3c). The material may be cured from one position if the restoration does not exceed 2 mm in depth from the buccal to lingual aspects, or may be cured about 10 sec each from the buccal and lingual surfaces. This restoration was polymerized for a total of 10 sec (Fig 15.3d). When photopolymerizing anterior porcelain veneer restorations, expose the restoration incrementally with 5-mm spots at 500 mW, 10-sec duration, until the entire restoration has been covered.

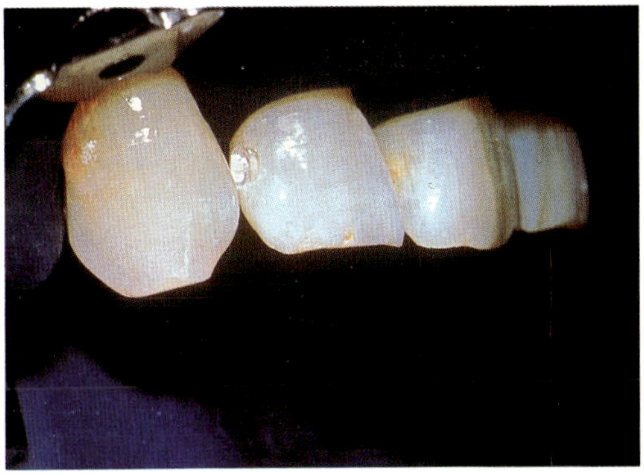

Fig 15.3a Exposure of the carious lesion with conventional instrumentation.

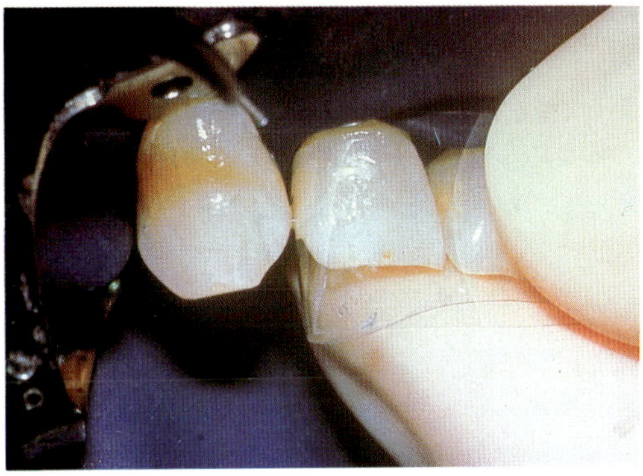

Fig 15.3b Placement of the composite material with a clear matrix retainer.

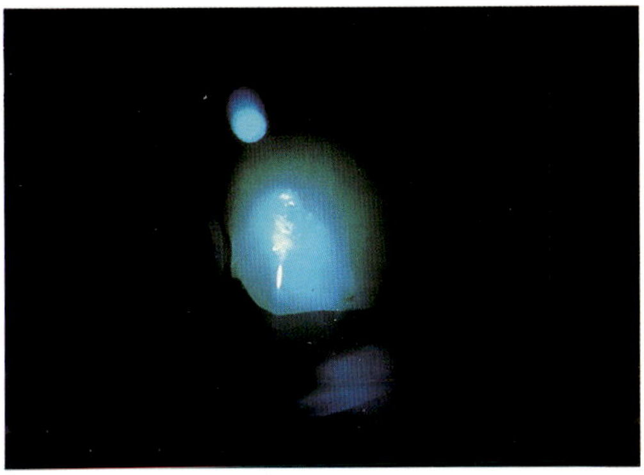

Fig 15.3c Photopolymerization of the restoration with the argon laser.

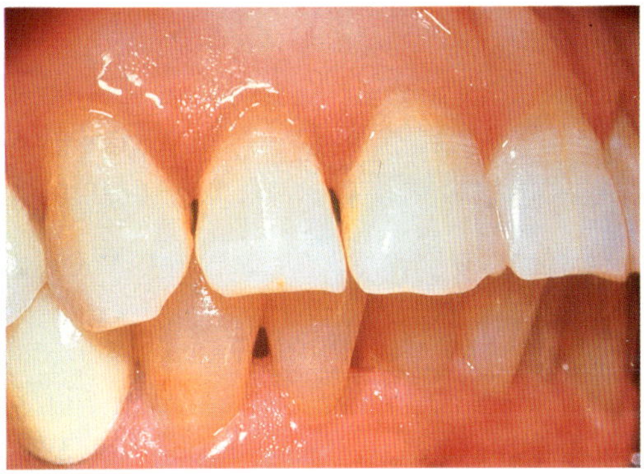

Fig 15.3d The finished restoration.

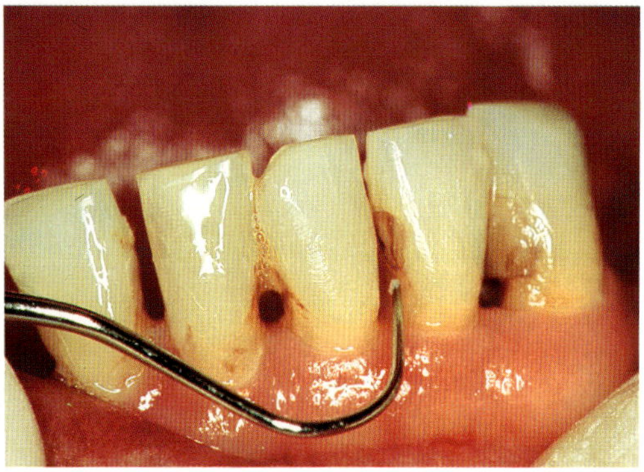

Fig 15.4a Interproximal cervical caries and gingival recession (typical).

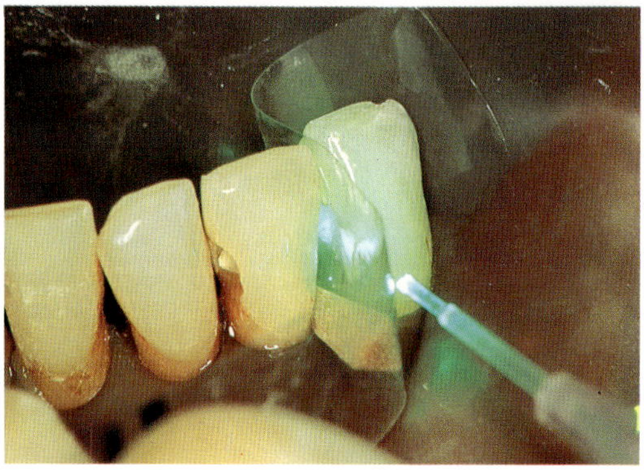

Fig 15.4b Matrix and wedge used for creating gingival contour of restoration.

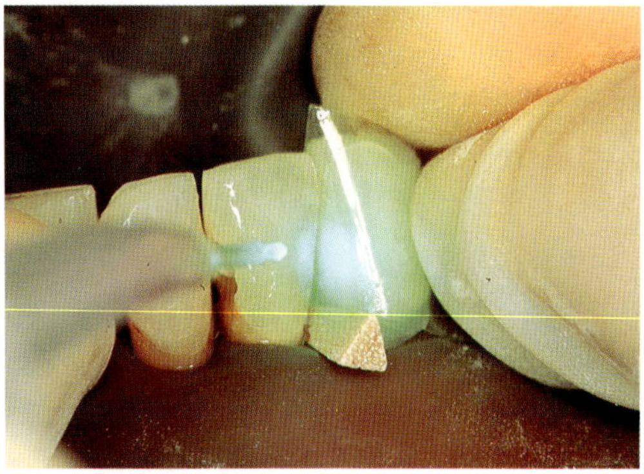

Fig 15.4c Photopolymerization of light-activated restorative material.

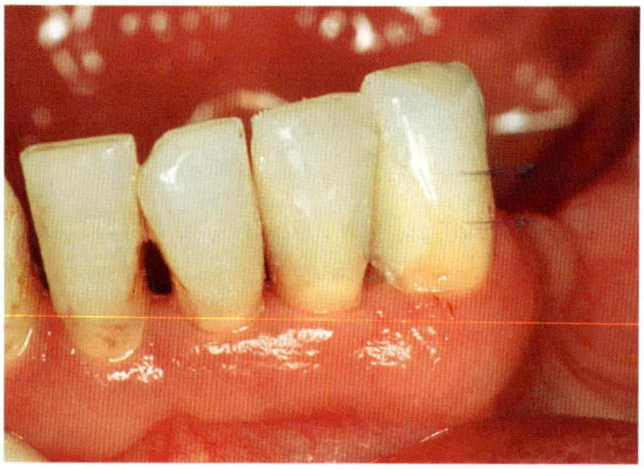

Fig 15.4d Completed class V restorations.

Case 4. Class V Composite Resin Restorations in a Geriatric Patient

Fig 15.4a shows a segment of the mandibular dentition of a geriatric patient who had serious cardiac problems, the complications of which contributed to a significant amount of recurrent decay. Most of the oral changes occurred within a 6-month period. An argon laser was used to polymerize conventional light-cured composite resin restorations (Figs 15.4b to 4d). In addition to improving the physical properties of the restorative material, this method of curing may be beneficial to the older patient because it has the potential to create a more acid-resistant surrounding tooth surface, which will enable the teeth to better resist the illness-related changes in the oral environment.

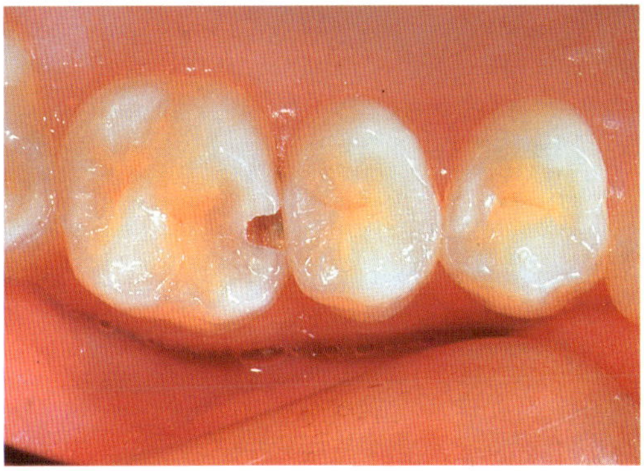

Fig 15.5a Preoperative appearance of the carious lesion.

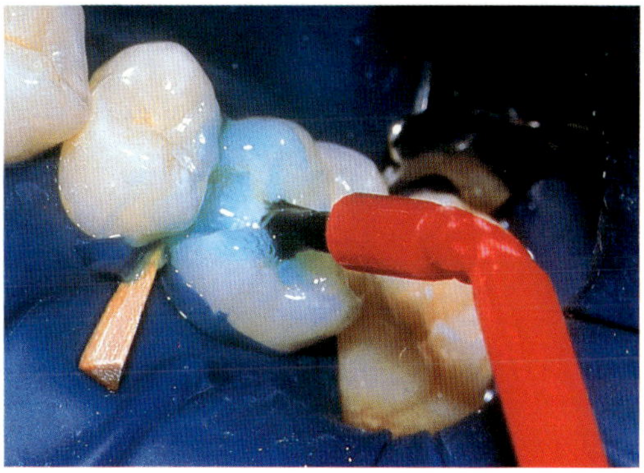

Fig 15.5b Acid-etching the dentin and enamel.

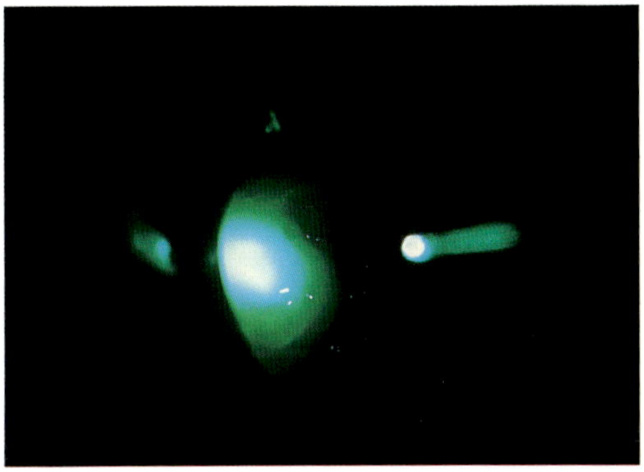

Fig 15.5c Photopolymerization of the restoration with the argon laser.

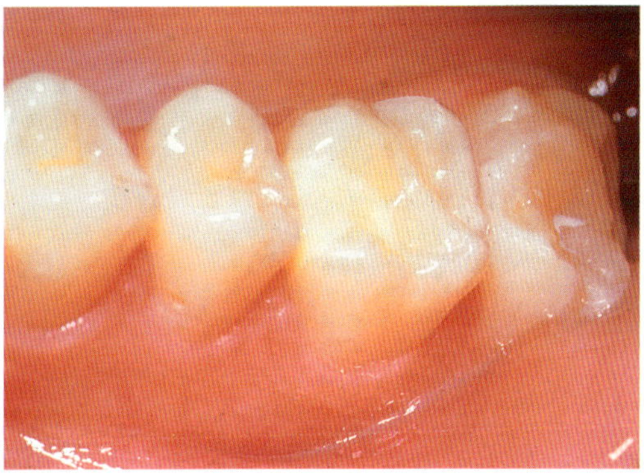

Fig 15.5d Twenty-eight-day postoperative appearance of the restoration.

Case 5. Conservative Class II Molar Restoration

A 16-year-old white male with an unremarkable medical history underwent an examination. The maxillary left first molar was diagnosed with a carious lesion on the mesial and occlusal surfaces (Fig 15.5a). After local anesthesia and isolation with a rubber dam, the lesion was exposed and debrided with a high-speed handpiece and carbide burs. The enamel and dentin were etched in preparation for the placement of a posterior composite restoration (Fig 15.5b). After the application of the adhesive, the unfilled resin was cured with the argon laser at 0.50 W for 5 sec. With a matrix retainer, the posterior composite filling material was placed according to the manufacturer's directions. The composite was then cured at 3-mm–deep increments at 0.50 W, 5-mm spot size, and single pulse of 10 sec for each increment (Fig 15.5c). At 28 days after placement of the composite, the posterior restoration demonstrated an excellent clinical appearance (Fig 15.5d). While the restoration may be cured with the fiber stationary, alternative techniques suggest moving the fiber continuously to assure even distribution of the laser energy within the restoration.

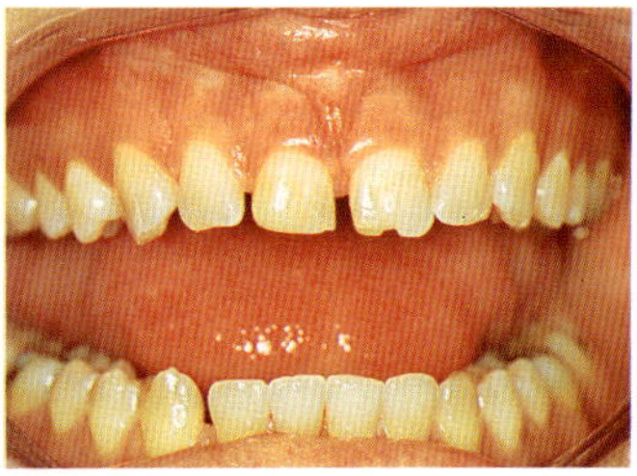

Fig 15.6a Pretreatment appearance of incisal fracture and diastema.

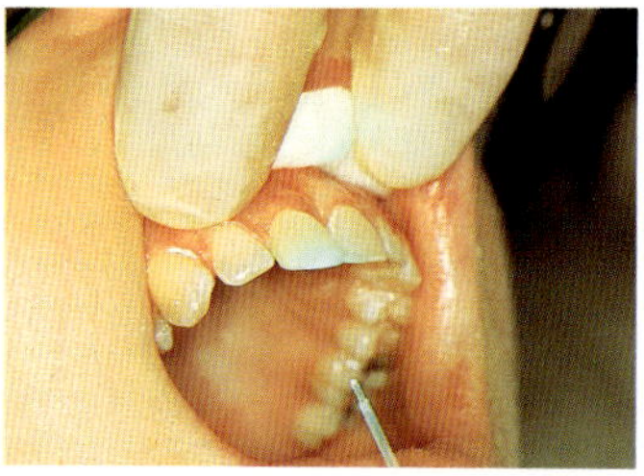

Fig 15.6b Curing of composite resin by argon laser.

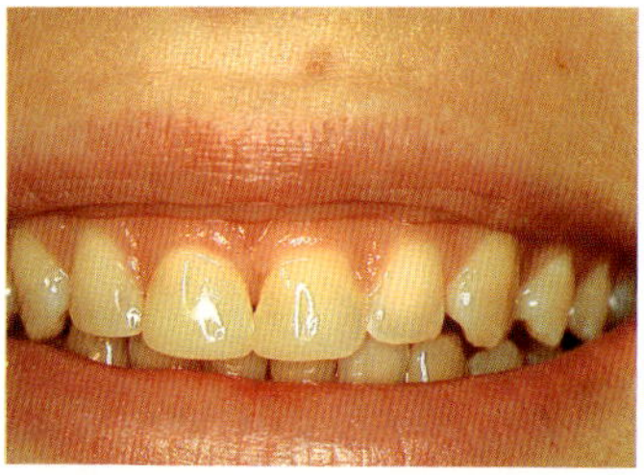

Fig 15.6c Incisal repair and diastema closure.

Case 6. Esthetic Dentistry

A patient sought treatment for the repair of an incisal edge defect on the central incisor and the diastema between the incisors (Fig 15.6a). The argon laser was used at 231 mW of power for a 10-sec cure cycle to polymerize each increment of composite resin (Fig 15.6b and c).

Composite resin was placed according to the manufacturer's directions. Normal placement, finishing, and polishing techniques were used. Because of the numerous increments required to properly restore this case, laser polymerization resulted in a considerable reduction of time to complete the treatment.

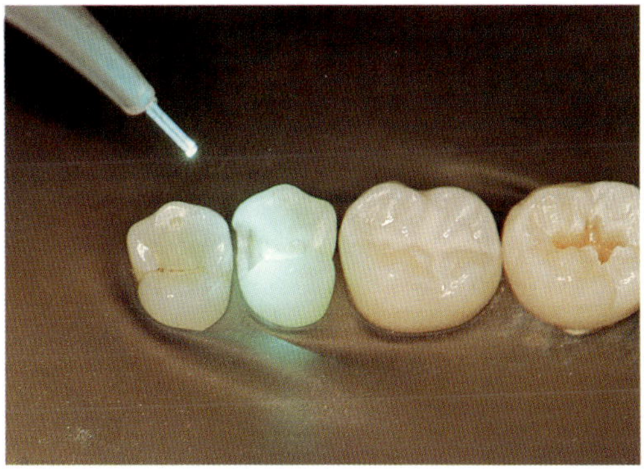

Fig 15.7a Light activation of glass ionomer restorative material being used as base/liner.

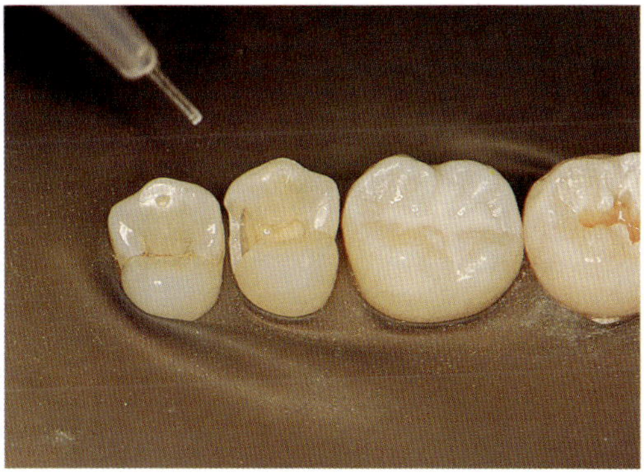

Fig 15.7b Cured base material in place. Final restoration by class II composite resin (not shown).

Case 7. Photopolymerization of Glass-Ionomer Base Material

The polymerization of light-activated bases and/or liners can also be accomplished with the argon laser. An argon laser was used at 231 mW of power for 10 sec to polymerize a typical light-activated base (Fig 15.7a), with an excellent result (Fig 15.7b).

Major problems associated with the use of light-activated bases and liners is the time required to polymerize them and gaining access in deep areas of preparations to bring the conventional light to these areas. The argon laser with a wide variety of fiber sizes provides access to all locations of a cavity preparation. The reduction in polymerization time is a benefit in each case.

The argon laser can be used to photopolymerize any light-activated restorative material with a camphoquinone-activated resin. This feature will most certainly make the argon laser a primary instrument for the general practitioner.

References

Alfano RR, Yao SS. Human teeth with and without dental caries studied by visible luminescence spectroscopy J Dent Res 1981;60:120–122.

American Dental Association, Council of Dental Materials, Instruments and Equipment. Visible light-cured composites and activating units. J Am Dent Assoc 1985; 100:100–103.

Benedicenti A, Daneo M, Verrando M, Guarneri L, Martino AR, Gherlone EF. Valutazione dell'usura di un composito, il durafill, polimerizzato in luce laser argon rispetto alla normal polimerizzazione. Paradontol Stomatol(Nuova) 1984;3:51–53.

Benedicenti A, Gherlone FE, Danoe M, et al. Tutto pui facile conil laser. Attual Dent 1986;2:52–61.

Bjelkhagen H, Sunderstrom F, Angmar-Mansson B, et al. Early detection of enamel caries by luminescence excited by visible laser light. Swed Dent J 1982;6:1–7.

Blankenau RJ, Barkmeier WW, Powell GL, Kelsey WP. Enhancement of physical properties of resin restorative by laser polymerization (abstract). J Dent Res 1989a; 68:742.

Blankenau RJ, Powell GL, Barkmeier WW, Kelsey WP. Argon laser effects on dentin adhesive systems (abstract). J Dent Res 1989b;68:1117.

Blankenau RJ, Taylor MH, Powell GL, Barkmeier WW. Microleakage of dental sealants cured with an argon laser (abstract). J Dent Res 1990a;228:959.

Blankenau RJ, Powell GL, Barkmeier WW, Kelsey WP. Power requirements for laser polymerization of dental resins. Presented at the Second World Congress ISLD, Paris, May 1990b.

Blankenau RJ, Kelsey WP, Powell GL, Shearer GO, Barkmeier WW, Cavel WT. Degree of composite resin polymerization with visible light and argon laser. Am J Dent 1991a;4:40–42.

Blankenau RJ, Powell GL, Kelsey WP, Barkmeier WW. Postpolymerization strength values of an argon laser cured resin. Lasers Surg Med 1991b;11:471–474.

Blankenau RJ, Powell GL, Cavel WT, Kelsey WP, Anderson D. Argon laser polymerized pit and fissure sealants. ISLD Third International Congress on Lasers in Dentistry; 1992a:21.

Blankenau RJ, Powell GL, Cavel WT, Barkmeier WW, Anderson D. The comparison of diametral tensile strength values of pit and fissure sealants polymerized with an argon laser and a conventional light source. Lasers Surg Med 1992b;21:75.

Boran TL, Peters JFM, Zakariasen KL. Effects of fluoride and CO_2 laser radiation on enamel demineralization. J Dent Res 1992;71:201.

Cook WD. Spectral distribution of dental photopolymerization sources. J Dent Res 1982;61:1436–1438.

Craig RG. Photopolymerization of dental resins. In Taylor DE (ed): Posterior Composites: Proceedings of the International Symposium on Posterior Composite Resins. Chapel Hill: North Carolina University Press; 1984:243–254.

DeMichelis B, Fagnoni V, Piccoli S. Il laser per la polymerization dei compositi. Attual Dent 1986;2:15,22–23, 27.

Forsten L. Curing depth of light activated composites. Acta Odontol Scand 1984;42:23–28.

Goodman BD, Kaufman HW. Effects of an argon laser on the crystalline properties and rate of dissolution in acid of tooth enamel in the presence of sodium fluoride. J Dent Res 1977;56:1201–1207.

Kelsey WP, Blankenau RJ, Powell LG, Barkmeier WW, Cavel WT, Whisenant BK. Enhancement of physical properties of resin restorative materials by laser polymerization. Lasers Surg Med 1989;9:623–627.

Kutsch VK. Caries illumination with the argon laser: a clinical trial. ISLD Third International Congress on Lasers in Dentistry; 1992:22.

Nelson DGA, Shariati M, Golena R, Shields CP, Featherstone JDB. Effects of pulsed low energy infrared laser irradiation on artificial caries like lesion formation. Caries Res 1986;20:289–299.

Peters JFM, Zakariasen KL, Boran TL, Borron JR. Effects of pulsed/nonpulsed CO_2 laser energy on enamel demineralization (abstract). J. Dent Res 1990;69:302.

Potts TV, Petrou A. Argon laser initiated resin photopolymerization for the filling of root canals in human teeth. Lasers Surg Med 1991;11:257–262.

Powell LG, Kelsey WP, Blankenau RJ, Barkmeier WW. The use of an argon laser for polymerization of composite resin. Aesthetic Dent 1989;1:34–37.

Severin C, Maquin M. Argon laser beam as composite resin light curing agent. Lasers Dent 1989;1:241–246.

Swartz ML, Phillips RW, Rhodes BF. Visible light activated resins—depth of cure. J Am Dent Assoc 1983;106: 198–202.

Weaver WS, Blank LW, Pelleu GB. A visible light-activated resin cured through tooth structure. Gen Dent 1988;36:236–237.

Westerman G, Hicks MJ, Flaitz CM, Blankenau RJ, Powell GL. Argon laser-cured sealants and reduced caries formation. J Dent Res 1991;70:493.

Westerman G, Hicks MJ, Fliatz CM, Blankenau RJ, Berg J, Powell GL. Argon laser irradiation in root surface caries (abstract). J Dent Res 1992;71:201.

Yamamoto S, Sato K. Prevention of dental caries by Nd:YAG laser irradiation. J Dent Res 1980;59:2171–2177.

Yu D, Wong J, Otsuka M, Powell GL, Fok JL, Higuachi WI. Laser irradiated human enamel dissolution: influence of inhibitors (abstract). J Dent Res 1990;69:302.

Chapter Sixteen

Laser Processing of Dental Materials

Heidemarie Dobberstein, Herbert Dobberstein, Annegret Schwarz, Rainer Zuhrt, and Yoshiaki Tani

Lasers have been investigated for potential use in working with dental materials since the mid-1960s. The results of industrial applications of lasers for machining and processing materials have had stimulating effects on dentistry. Previous investigations into the laser treatment of dental materials addressed attempts to fuse dental materials on or into the tooth's surface (Beyer et al, 1986) and attempts to fuse or repair dental alloys (Beyer et al, 1984). These investigations sought to examine the possibility of treating dental ceramics with lasers and to test the laser's ability to weld dental precious and nonprecious metal alloys.

Welding of Ceramic Materials

Processes for laser-induced modification of ceramic materials are currently being investigated under laboratory conditions (Zscherpe et al, 1984). There is little in the existing literature about laser treatment of dental ceramic masses. The strength of ceramic materials in the presence of temperature changes is low. This is evidenced by high elasticity, low tensile strength, and low plastic workability, which normally are displayed only with high temperatures. During laser treatment, steep local temperature changes in the heating and cooling phases create internal tensions that can damage the materials. It is necessary therefore to use appropriate laser operating parameters (Reisse et al, 1984).

The CO_2 laser is well suited for the treatment of ceramic materials because its emission wavelength is almost totally absorbed by ceramic. During the process of heat induction of ceramic surfaces with a focused CO_2 laser, conchoidal tears appear, which are typical effects of surface warming (Fig 16.1).

The use of a defocused CO_2 laser beam produces a local gloss firing on the surface of the dental ceramic, which when compared to the main vacuum firing (Fig 16.2, left) and the furnace gloss firing (Fig 16.2, center) makes an impression due to its macroscopic homogeneous surface. After the main vacuum gloss firing, irregular wavelike structures with dendritic crystal features are found on dental ceramics. After the furnace gloss firing, these structures are leveled off, but the crystal features are not removed. However, with the

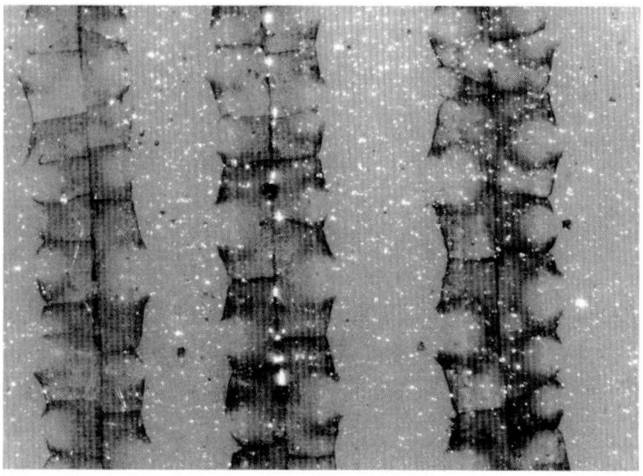

Fig 16.1 Surface of a sample of dental ceramics after exposure to laser (CO_2 laser, pulse energy).

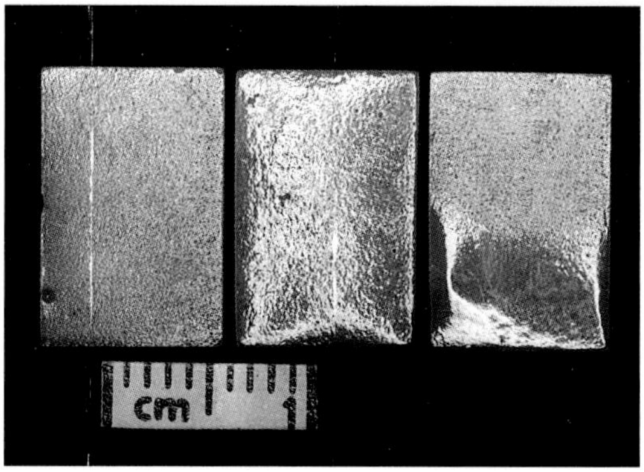

Fig 16.2 Surface of samples from dental ceramics: *left,* after main vacuum firing; *middle,* after furnace gloss firing; *right,* after laser gloss firing (original magnification × 6).

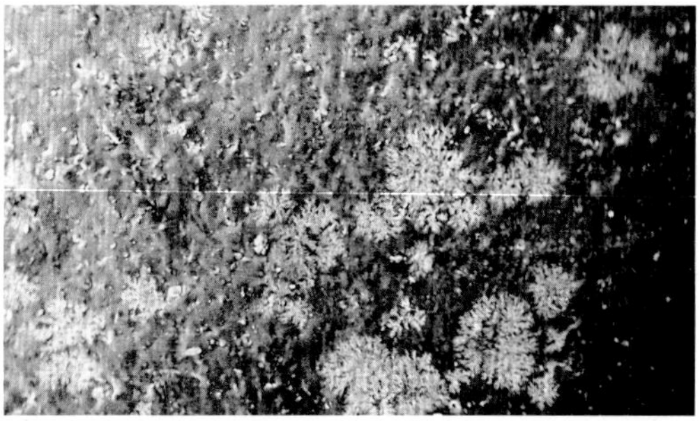

3a

Fig 16.3 Surface of samples from dental ceramics: **(a)**, after main vacuum firing; **(b)**, after furnace gloss firing; **(c)**, after laser gloss firing (raster electron microscropy; magnification, × 96).

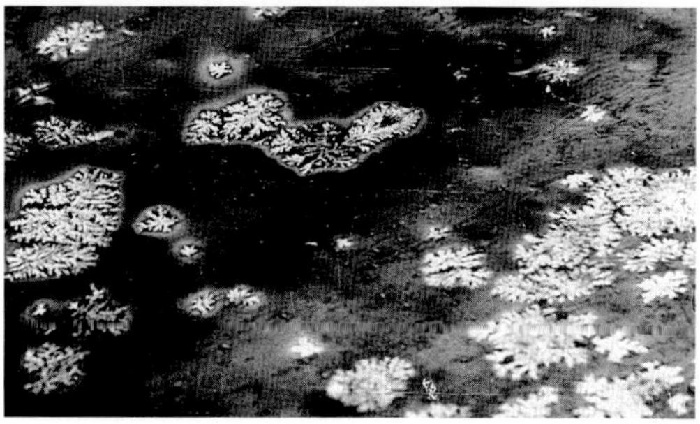

3b

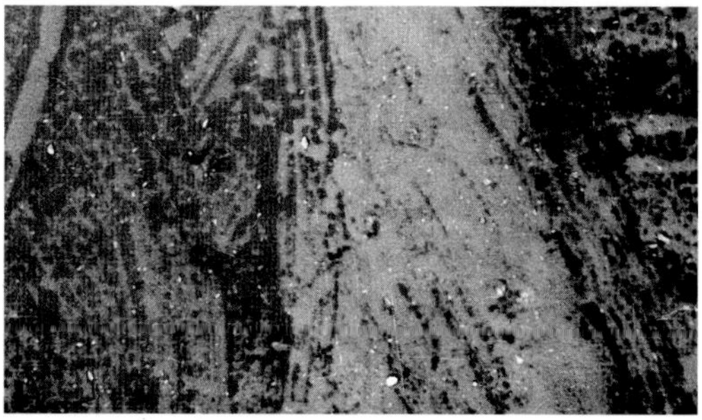

3c

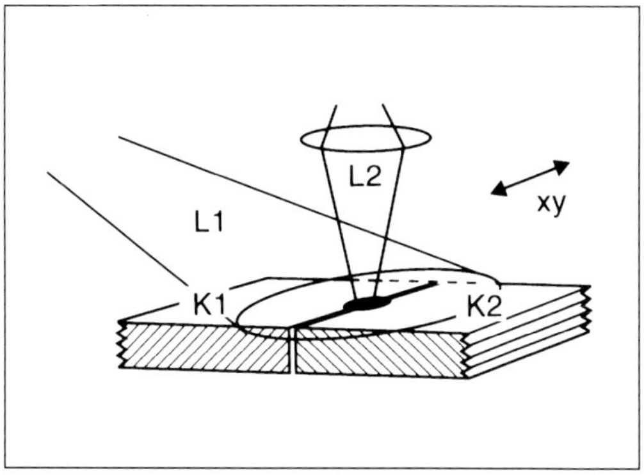

Fig 16.4 Diagrammatic representation of the laser double-beam process for the welding of dental ceramics. L1 = first laser beam, L2 = second laser beam, K1 = first ceramic sample, K2 = second ceramic sample, xy = movement of the x-y table.

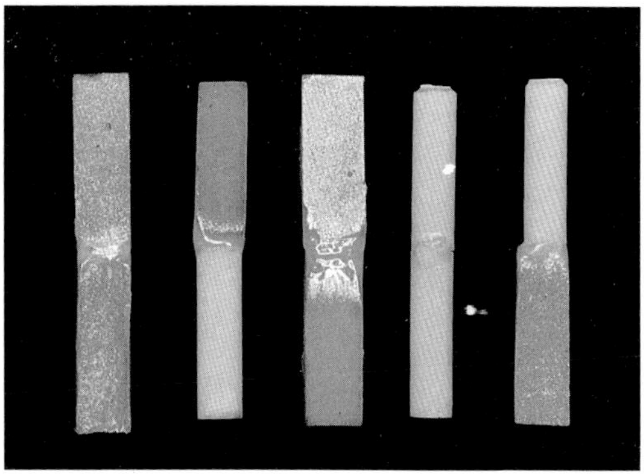

Fig 16.5 Laser-welded samples of different dental ceramic masses (from left to right). 1 = nucleus mass, 2 = two aluminum oxide cross sections, 3 = two sample bodies of dentin mass, 4 = dentin mass with aluminium oxide cross section, 5 = two sample bodies of nucleus mass (magnification, × 3).

laser gloss firing (Fig 16.2, right), a full leveling of the surface is achieved, and even with scanning electron-microscopic examination, any remaining structures are hardly noticeable (Fig 16.3 a to c).

Double-Beam Laser Modification

One possible solution for problem-free laser treatment of dental ceramics, in contrast to the prevailing laser treatment methods, is the preheating of relatively large areas of the ceramic surface prior to high temperature treatment. After laser-induced modification of ceramic surfaces (patent no. WP DD 231 522 A1), a laser double-beam process has been developed for the laser-induced joining of dental ceramic materials. In this process (Fig 16.4), a pulsating, 200-W, defocused CO_2 laser beam (L1) with a gaussian-shaped beam profile distribution, is used for preheating, which when used at an angle of 45 degrees warms a fundamentally larger area than the weld site. The other continuous-wave, 100-W CO_2 laser beam (L2), which falls vertically onto the target, actually performs the laser welding. The first laser maintains a temperature below the fusion temperature, and the second produces a higher temperature, which softens the dental ceramic. The area of influence of the second laser beam lies temporally and locally within the sphere of influence of the first laser beam. The maximum intensity of the second laser beam is found within the range of the first laser beam, so that the necessary depth in the material for the laser welding is reached. For the preheating of the lateral surface area needed for laser welding, a ratio of 10:1 is chosen for the cross-sectional surface of the first and second beams on the ceramic surface. Through the coordination of the reaction length and intensity distribution of both laser beams on each other and on the dental ceramic material, it is possible to produce the required heating and cooling temperature-place-time profiles. These profiles are necessary for the area of influence of the second laser beam to the ceramic materials.

With this process, samples of dentin mass and nucleus mass, as well as one of them in combination with aluminum-oxide particles, were fused together (Fig 16.5).

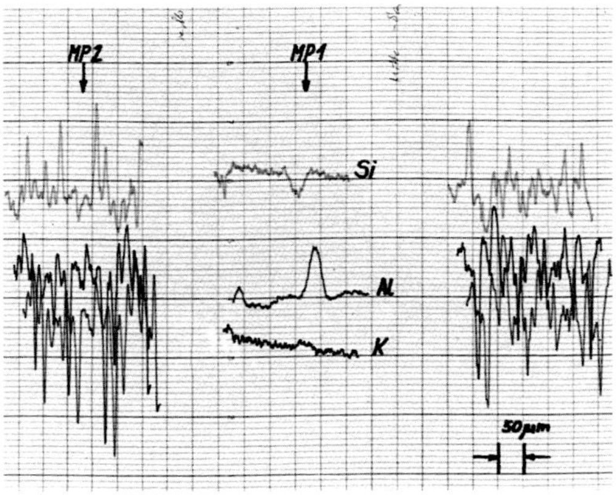

Fig 16.6 Electron-beam microprobe element analysis of Si, Al, and K in the raw material and in the welded area of a laser-welded sample of dentin.

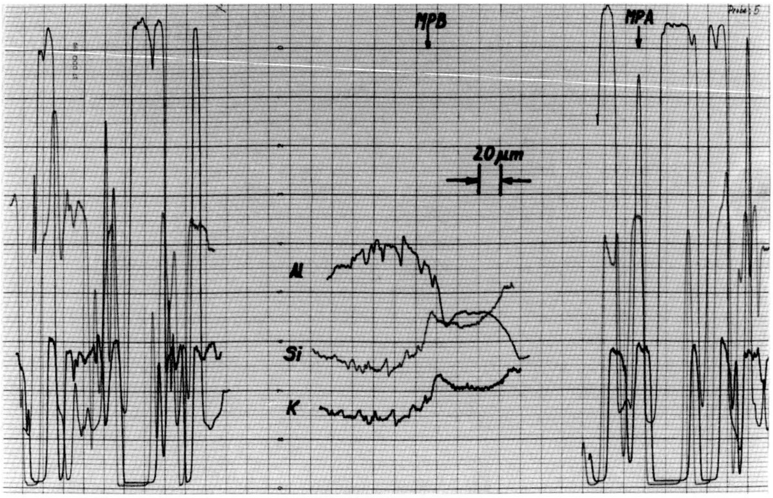

Fig 16.7 Electron-beam microprobe element analysis of Si, Al, and K in the raw material and in the welded area of laser-welded samples of nucleus mass

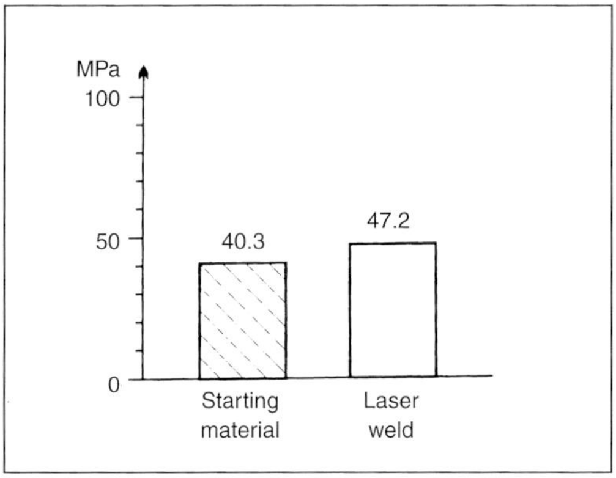

Fig 16.8 Bending strength of dentin mass: raw material compared to the laser-welded material.

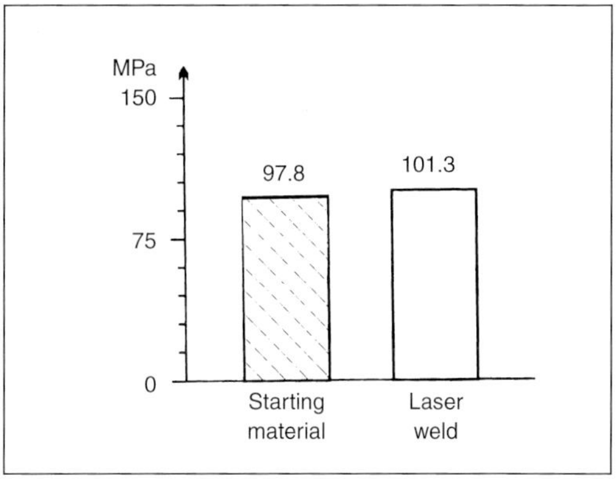

Fig 16.9 Bending strength of nucleus mass: raw material compared to the laser-welded material.

Different laser operating parameters were used for the different combinations. With use of electron-beam microprobe analysis, compression and homogenization of the raw material were verified with the dentin mass and the nucleus mass, which indicates a profound joining of both samples (Figs 16.6 and 16.7).

Investigations into the bending strength of the laser welds, as compared to the raw materials yielded by the dentin mass and nucleus mass, showed a slight rise in the bending strength after double-beam laser welding (Figs 16.8 and 16.9). This improved weld strength over that of the raw material can be attributed to the higher density and condensation of the ceramic substratum after laser treatment.

Because of these promising results, it is possible to consider a number of applications for laser treatment of ceramics in dentistry. With laser surface homogenization of the dental ceramics, it is possible to remove local surface defects and polishing marks without the need to reconstruct a complete correction firing. It is also possible that by using the laser double-beam process, one could expand the use of ceramics to a number of intraoral applications. As a further point of interest, it would be possible to test the laser treatment of new ceramic systems, such as In-ceram and glass ceramics. Up to now however, experiments have indicated that the laser treatment of ceramics in the oral cavity is not possible because of the need for high-energy densities and long exposure times.

Welding of Dental Alloys

Laser welding can help solve the technical problems encountered in the repair of various dental alloys. Laser welding belongs to the field of melt-weld processing.

The efficiency of laser beam treatment is determined by the absorbed optical energy of the material in use and is proportional to the degree of absorption of the material. Metals with a high reflection have a small degree of absorption in the visible and infrared spectral areas. These metals include the dental alloys, as indicated by the reflection curves of some of the main constituents of these alloys (Landoldt-Björnstein, 1982).

With the Nd:YAG laser, the degree of absorption of nonprecious metal alloys and titanium is slightly better than that of the precious metal alloys. If, however, a laser beam with a performance concentration of 10^6 W/cm^2 is used, an increase in absorption can usually be seen (Beyer et al, 1984; Dorn et al, 1980).

Nd:YAG Laser Welding

We investigated the use of the Nd:YAG laser on dental alloys. The tests were carried out with a pulsed Nd:YAG laser (wavelength, 1.06 µm; pulse duration, 2.0 to 5.0 msec; focal length, 50 and 100 mm; pulse repetition frequency, 0.1 to 10.0 Hz) on three dental cast alloys and titanium.

Initially, attempts were made at surface fusing with the laser beam to determine the influence of energy on the configuration of the structure after the re-fusing. This was examined to deduce the characteristics of the points of joining by this method. From the wide range of alloys used in dentistry, a silver-palladium cast alloy (Sipal) was chosen from the group of precious metals. From the group of nonprecious metal alloys, a cobalt-chrome-molybdenum cast alloy with added nitrogen (KCM) and a nickel-chrome-aluminium cast alloy (NCA) were chosen. Test samples were made for the experiment with standard dental laboratory fabrication methods (production of the molds by wax-melting process, warming of the mold, casting of the melt, and a cooling to room temperature). The sizes of the samples were 5 × 20 × a mm (a = 0.5/0.8/1.0 mm).

The interaction between the laser and material is determined by the characteristics of the material being used, ie, degree of absorption, thermal conductivity and capacity, and the composition of the surface. The choice of laser parameters and thus the energy density of the beam greatly influence the quality of the weld (Beyer et al, 1986; Dorn et al, 1980; Herziger, 1983).

To define the optimum laser parameters for each of the alloys that were examined, the parameters for the pulsed operation were varied while the other parameters remained constant. The parameters in question were pulse energy, pulse duration, focus diameter (spot size), speed, and pulse repetition frequency. The selection of the optimum parameters was made by means of metallographic microsection and was judged on the following criteria: (1) homogenous, tear-free and pore-free weld; and (2) maximum depth and breadth of weld.

During these experiments, it was determined that the geometry and the quality of the welded area vary in relation to the dependence on the laser parameters and are subject to material-specific, laser-technological irregularities. The development of the geometry of the melting bath is mostly influenced by the variation of the pulse energy. With increasing pulse energy, while the other parameters remain constant, the width and depth of the laser trace showed an increase that was directly proportional to the pulse energy (Figs 16.10 and 16.11). With nonprecious metal alloys, one can observe tear-free weld zones with a focused laser beam at a pulse energy of 5 J; and with Ag-Pd alloys, at a pulse energy of 4 J; whereas pure titanium shows flawless weld zones at a pulse energy of 8 J. The efficiency of the laser beam on pure titanium is more favorable because of the good absorption characteristics and low heat conductivity of titanium compared to those of other dental alloys.

The inner fused areas show a finer consistency of structure than the raw materials. A shallow inner fusion is made with a pulse energy of 5 J in a Co-Cr alloy (Fig 16.12). With a pulse energy of 7 J on pure titanium, a deeper inner fusing is achieved (Fig 16.13). A lower heat-influenced area at higher pulse energy is clearly seen with

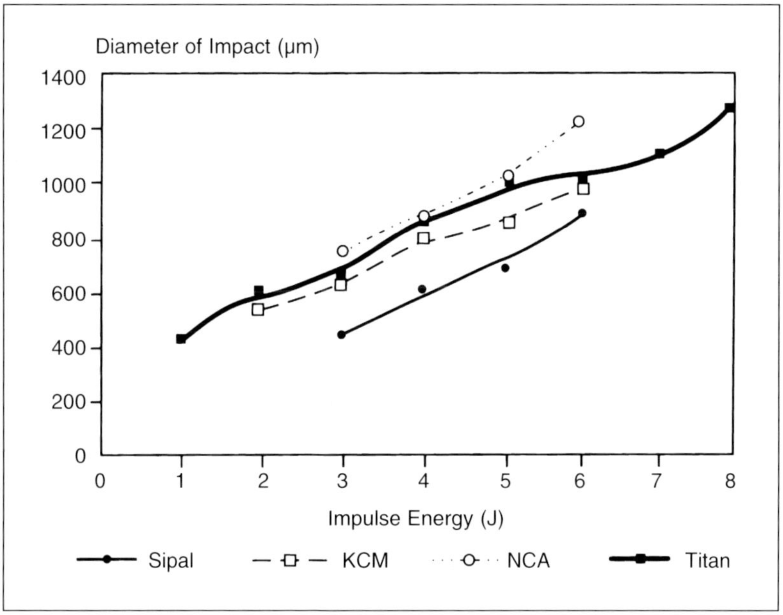

Fig 16.10 Change in the laser trace width is dependent on the change in the impulse energy.

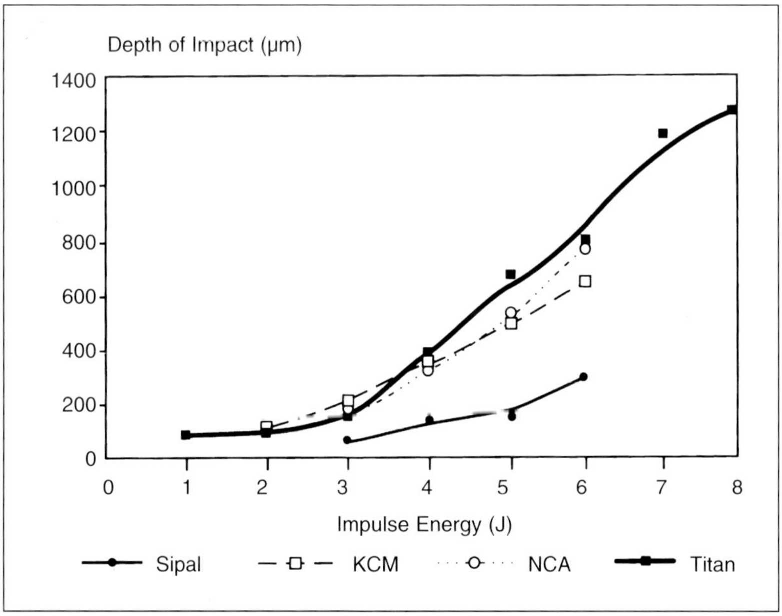

Fig 16.11 Change in the laser trace depth is dependent on the change in the impulse energy.

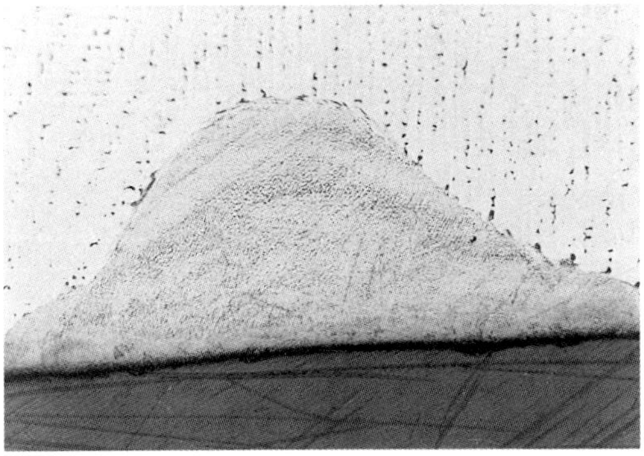

Fig 16.12 Laser welding with refined cobalt-chrome-molybdenum alloy with an impulse energy of 5 J.

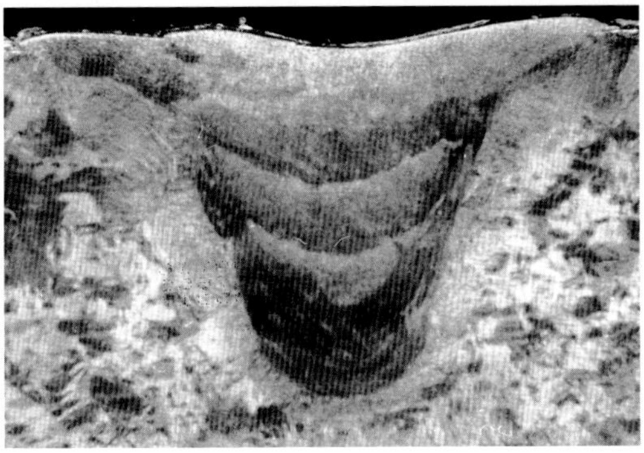

Fig 16.13 Laser welding with pure titanium and an impulse energy of 7 J.

pure titanium, whereas with a light microscope hardly any heat-influenced areas can be seen on Co-Cr alloys. The finer consistency of structure that is created by all dental alloys in laser welding is mainly responsible for the better tensile and bending strengths of the welds in comparison to those attained with the conventional soldering (Dobberstein, 1990). The optimum laser parameters for the welding of the researched dental alloys were selected on the basis of metallographic microsections (Table 16.1).

Identical samples 0.8-mm long and 5-mm thick of the same alloys, and combined samples of different alloys, were welded bluntly and double-sided. The tensile and bending strengths of the laser welds exceeded the values that were achieved with conventional soldering methods (Figs 16.14 and 16.15).

Evaluation of Corrosion Resistance

By coordinating the type of laser and its parameters with the material that is to be used, a high efficiency can be achieved. Pure titanium is a very good material for use with laser treatment. Apart from the strength factors, the corrosion reaction of a point of joining is another important criterion for its quality and use. Soldered points of joining (solder joints) in partial dentures have been weak with regard to strength and corrosion resistance. The fol-

Table 16.1. Optimum Laser Parameters for the Welding of Researched Dental Alloys

Parameters	Cobalt-chrome-molybdenum	Silver-palladium	Nickel-chrome-aluminum
Pulse energy	5 J	4 J	4.5 J
Pulse repetition frequency	5 Hz	5 Hz	5 Hz
Pulse duration	5 ms	5 ms	5 ms
Focal length	100 mm	100 mm	100 mm
Speed	1 mm/s	1 mm/s	1 mm/s
Defocusing	0	0	0

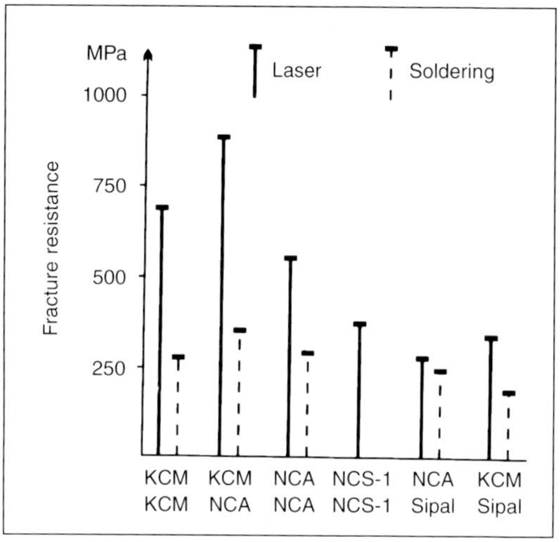

Fig 16.14 Tensile strength of laser combination welding compared to that of soldering.

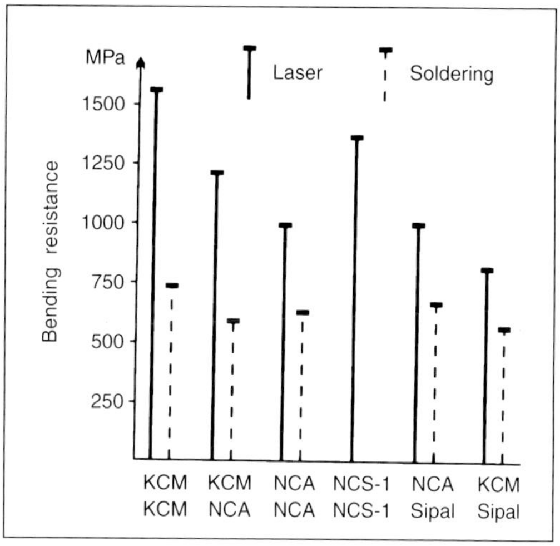

Fig 16.15 Bending strength of laser combination welding compared to that of soldering.

lowing effects could be expected due to insufficient oral durability: galvanic currents, toxicity, allergic reactions, and risk of cancer.

With regard to biocompatibility, laser welding could also be an interesting alternative to the conventional fusing processes in laboratory technology. Research was carried out on the aforementioned laser-welded alloys and solders. According to the current literature, electrochemical analysis is the preferred method for evaluating corrosion resistance. We were unable to fully determine the effects of laser welding on the samples tested because the points of joining that were researched were too small in comparison to the general electrode. The verdict on corrosion on the points of joining was not possible or was only partially predictable with electrochemical analysis. The anodic polarization curve could be measured only as a total curve of all areas; thus, no statements about singular structural areas could be made.

For this reason, the immersion procedure was used as a method of quality comparison to define the continuance of corrosion (electrolyte solution: 0.1 M lactic acid and 0.1 M sodium chloride at ph = 2.4 and 37°C). The electron-beam microprobe analysis and the immersion test were used for quantification of the results.

The points at which the electron-beam microprobe analysis was to be carried out were marked with hard micro-impressions before the immersion tests. During the immersion tests, analyses for corrosion were performed with light microscopy every 2 days. Laser welds were shown to be superior to the soldered welds, since the corrosion attacks took place much later on all laser-welded samples than on soldered samples (Figs 16.16 and 16.17).

With the Co-Cr and Ni-Cr alloys, a selective corrosion at the edges of the grain of the raw material was observed. In the weld zone, the areas where the lenses overlap are especially affected. A selective corrosion due to the fine consistent structure is not apparent. The different corrosion reaction of the thermally influenced areas (transition zone between the weld and raw material) shows that not only the

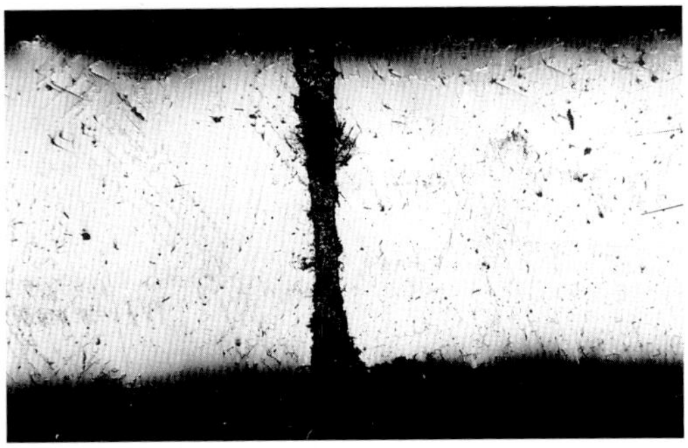

Fig 16.16 Corrosion on a KCM solder after soaking 15 days in electrolyte solution (Auflicht and Hellfeld; magnification, × 58).

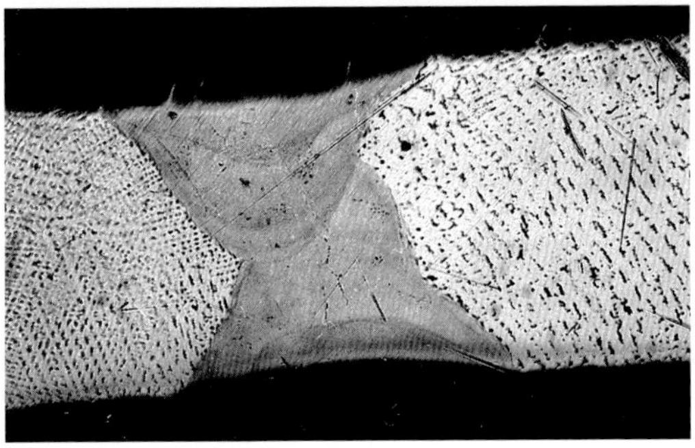

Fig 16.17 Corrosion on a KCM laser weld after soaking 20 days in electrolyte solution (Auflicht and Hellfeld; magnification, × 50).

type of structural composition but also the thermal toning of the sample during the welding is important for the corrosive reaction.

Electron-beam microprobe analysis was carried out for each sample before and after the immersion tests. In the evaluation of the point analysis and element distribution graph, the composition of the laser weld before the immersion test is equivalent to the raw material in quantity and quality—this requirement was not achieved with solder.

The concentration of oxygen as a measurement of corrosive activity represents an important factor in the characterization of electrochemical processes. Before the immersion tests, an increased oxygen content was generally found in all soldered joints compared to that in the raw material and in the laser weld. On the contrary, an unconditional low oxygen concentration was found in the laser welds before the immersion tests. After the immersion test, the change in oxygen concentration in the weld was negligible. The oxygen concentration of the soldered joint rose further after the immersion test, which suggests intensive electrochemical occurrences (Table 16.2).

Table 16.2 Oxygen Concentrations Before and After Immersion Test

	Oxygen Concentrations Before/After Immersion Test (mass %)	
Sample	Laser-welded sample	Soldered sample
Silver-palladium		
Raw material	2.25 / 5.74	3.42 / 5.09
Transition zone	3.03 / 2.72	—
Weld	0.64 / 2.46	6.02 / 9.51
Cobalt-chrome-molybdenum		
Raw material	1.05 / 1.99	2.15 / 3.27
Weld	1.20 / 3.12	3.26 / 5.74
Nickel-chrome-molybdenum		
Raw material	3.78 / 6.03	2.97 / 5.97
Transition zone	5.73 / 8.97	—
Weld	1.18 / 2.08	4.09 / 8.12

These corrosive processes influence not only the strength factors but also the biologic compatibility of dentures. With further microprobe analysis, concentration changes of individual elements during the immersion test were observed in the points of joining. This suggests a release of metal ions. After the immersion test, concentration changes in palladium, gold, and copper take place in the soldered joint of the sample silver-palladium—whereas only negligible concentration changes were registered in the welded joints of similar samples (Table 16.3).

In the sample combinations of the nonprecious metal alloys, changes in the concentration of chrome, nickel, cobalt, and aluminum occurred. In the cobalt-chrome-molybdenum weld, the concentration of cobalt changes. In the nickel-chrome-aluminum weld, no concentration changes were registered, while in the area of transition a change in the concentration of chrome and nickel was registered. With an intensive corrosive process in the point of joining of the dentures, one must expect an interaction of the organism and the aforementioned elements.

The corrosion features, typical for all alloys, were also registered in the different combination welds, whereby the different corrosion features of the welded joints point to a mixing of the alloys during welding and no standardized structuring takes place. This was seen above all in the combination welds of nonprecious metal alloys and precious metal alloys and was confirmed with element dispersion graphs.

Welding of Titanium with the Nd:YAG Laser

Laser beam welding of titanium for prosthodontics has begun to be investigated by a number of researchers. Titanium is a metal that displays minimal corrosion and therefore is highly safe in vivo. Because of its excellent biocompatibility, the use of titanium as an implant material has become widespread in dentistry.

Following recent advances in high-temperature, vacuum casting technology, it is now possible to use titanium as a prosthetic material (eg, partial dentures, crowns, and bridges). Clinical applications

Table 16.3 Elemental Changes in Alloys

	Elemental Changes Before/After Immersion Test (mass %)	
Sample Element	Laser-welded alloy	Solder-welded alloy
Silver-palladium		
Pd	24.64 / 26.10	17.58 / 21.38
Au	2.47 / 2.75	6.24 / 2.15
Cu	8.79 / 9.80	13.70 / 10.09
Cobalt-chrome-molybdenum		
Co	54.81 / 50.34	11.22 / 7.25
Cr	22.92 / 20.76	17.49 / 13.79
Mo	3.39 / 3.46	1.91 / 2.92
Al	0.87 / 0.74	0.53 / 1.16
Nickel-chrome-aluminum		
Co	0.43 / 0.53	6.97 / 5.10
Cr	19.89 / 22.00	27.06 / 14.96
Ni	68.67 / 65.63	71.60 / 33.75
Al	4.20 / 5.20	0.79 / 14.03

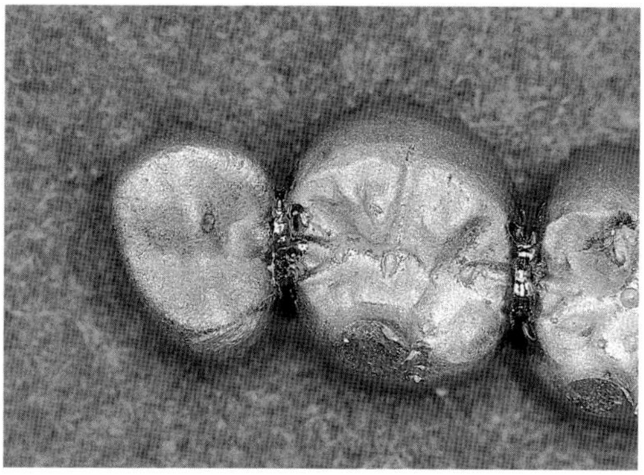

16.18

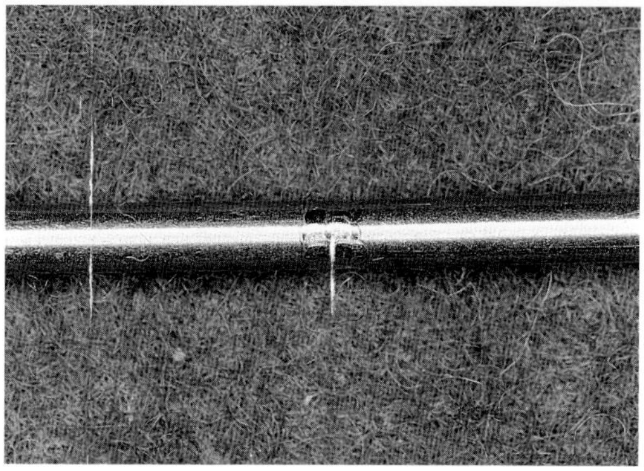

16.19

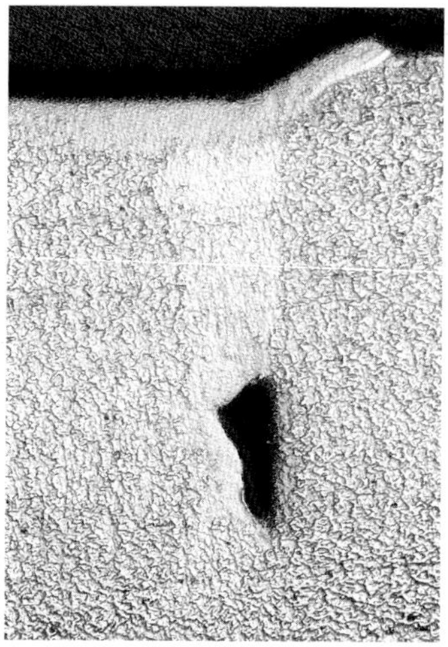

16.20

Fig 16.18 Titanium crowns welded with normal pulsed Nd:YAG (ML-2310A, Miyachi Technos Co). Pulse width = 6 msec.

Fig 16.19 Weld of titanium rods. Pulse width = 5 msec.

Fig 16.20 High magnification of weld joint of titanium rods showing fine grain structure of the solidified material.

Fig 16.21 Seam weld of titanium plates.

Fig 16.22 Spot weld of titanium plates.

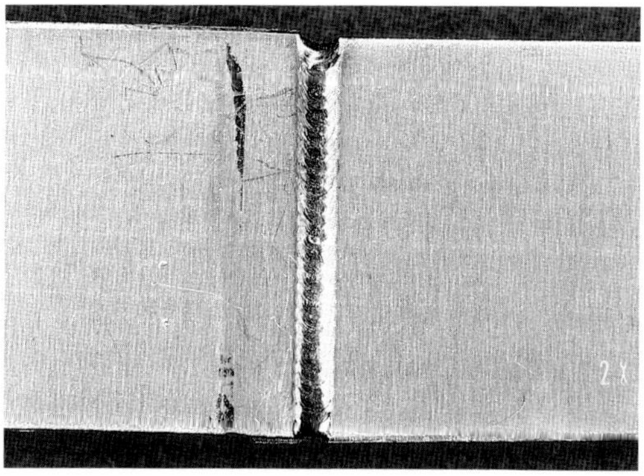

16.21

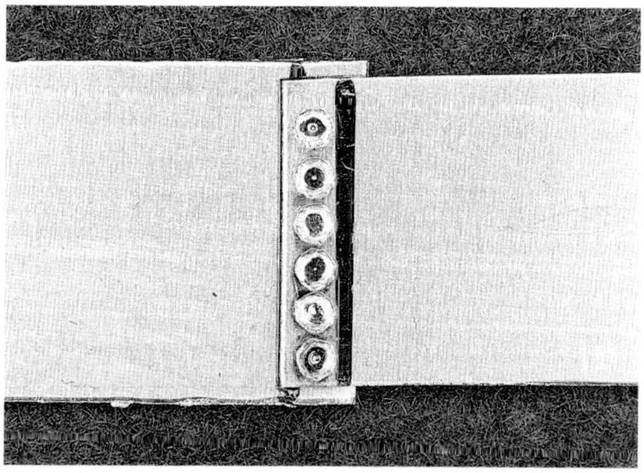

16.22

of titanium are expanding. Although titanium has a high relative strength and excellent corrosion resistance, the use of titanium for prostheses has been hampered by difficulties in processing because of its high melting point (about 1,700°C) and susceptibility to oxidation. Within the dental field, soldering has generally been used to join metallic materials. Titanium, however, is very difficult to solder because of its high melting point. As an alternative method, laser welding of titanium is more practical and may offer some distinct advantages.

Laser welding can be characterized by: (1) high bond strength and corrosion resistance, since laser welding is a form of sweating that does not use solders of different metals; (2) reduced oxidation when argon gas is applied during welding; and (3) decreased thermal influence and greater precision in processing than with soldering or other techniques.

Industrially, titanium is usually welded by tig or mig welding. When precision welding is required or when alteration of the metal's properties from heat must be avoided, high-energy-density welding techniques are used. These include electron beam welding, plasma arc welding, and laser beam welding.

In preliminary experiments, we attempted to weld cast crowns and prefabricated rods of 2-mm diameter pure titanium with a pulsed Nd:YAG laser. Test specimens were composed of JIS type II titanium. Pulse widths were 6 msec for crowns and 5 msec for the rods at 300 V. During welding, the rods were rotated around their center at a rate of one rotation per 2.7 seconds. The total energy output for crowns was 7 J and 6 J for rods. Argon gas was applied to the region during welding to suppress oxidation during welding.

Glossy, strong unions with pure titanium crowns were achieved by moving the laser spot from one point to another along the contact areas (Fig 16.18). The results of welding pure titanium rods with the same method were equally good (Fig 16.19). Since no solder was added, there was a slight loss of material in the welded area (Fig 16.20).

At high magnification, the appearance of the solidified structure of the welded region can be evaluated. The crystallization of the welded region has a finer grain structure than the nonwelded portion of the same metal (see Fig 16.20). Unlike soldering, laser welding does not involve contamination with different metals; therefore, the joint is more uniform and resistant to corrosion.

Other experiments were performed to evaluate the bond strength of laser-welded titanium. Two methods of welding were tested: seam welding and spot welding. During seam welding (Fig 16.21), the overlapped ends of two test pieces were welded by moving the laser beam along the line of contact. With spot welding (Fig 16.22), the laser beam was applied to the two overlapped plates of titanium to penetrate deeply into the plate thickness. A series of nine specimens for each test condition was performed. The parameters used for each method are listed in Table 16.4.

The results of the shear tensile strength test are summarized in Table 16.5. In general, it may be concluded that because seam welding results in a continuous union of the two materials, the application of tensile force results in failure of the nonwelded portion of the material in most cases. The mean shear bond strength of the seam-welded titanium was high (>106 kgf). Apparently the finer grain structure of the welded material contributes to higher shear strengths as compared to the raw metal. In most of the spot-welded

Table 16.4 Laser Welding of Titanium

Type of Weld*	Output	Pulse Width (msec)	Spot Diameter (mm)	Pulse Rate (pps)
Seam	75 W	3	0.8	15
Spot	13.5 J	4	0.8	single pulse

*Specimen size = 40 × 10 × 0.3 mm; width of lap joint = 2 mm.

Table 16.5. Results of Shear Tensile Test of Titanium Plates Welded by Normal Pulse Nd:YAG Laser*

Type of Welding	Region of Failure	Number of Specimens	Shear Bond Strength (Actual)
Seam welding	Welding part	2	72 (32)
	Parent metal	7	>106 (5)
Spot welding	Welding part	9	56 (4)
			Units: kg

*From Tani Y, Nambu T, Watanabe C. Welding of titanium using normal pulse Nd:YAG laser. J Jpn Soc Laser Dent 1992;3:45–49.

samples, failure under tension occurred in the region of the welded area. Thus, the bond strengths were lower with spot welding than with seam welding based on these experiments.

Conclusions

The available research results lead to the conclusion that lasers are suitable for the processing of dental materials. Their uses will, for the time being, be in dental laboratories, because a beam with a very high performance concentration is used and intraoral use entails high risk to the patient.

By coordination of the type of laser and its parameters with respect to the material being used, it is possible to achieve a high efficiency result with the laser beam. Apart from the dental alloys, pure titanium is a material that can be manipulated very well with a laser; the advantages of this technology are: (1) the laser treatment is contact-free; (2) the good focusing ability makes an extremely high-performance concentration possible, which assures low thermal stress on the material; (3) many varieties of dental materials can be treated with the laser; (4) the ability to reproduce the laser beam assures a consistent quality in the results of the treatment; (5) the laser is an excellent tool for treating micromaterials because of the small focus diameter; (6) and lasers save time. Further technical advancements and the objective use of knowledge about laser-material interaction will lead to the use of lasers in technologic processes in dentistry.

References

Beyer E, Behter K, Petschke U. Schweissen mit CO_2-Lasern. Laser u. Optoelektronik 1986;18:35–46.

Beyer E, Wissenbach K, Herziger G. Werkstoffbearbeitung mit Laserstrahlung, Teil 4. Absorption von CO_2-Laserstrahlung während der Bearbeitung. Feinwerktechnik/Messtechnik 1984;92:141–143.

Dobberstein H. Laserbearbeitung von Dentallegierungen mit einem Festkörperlaser—ein Beitrag zu den Grundlagen der Laseranwendung in der Zahnmedizin. Med Diss B 1990, Berlin (HUB).

Dorn L, Jäkle G, Ohlschläger E, Smernos S. Einfluss der Strahlparameter beim Laserstrahlimpulsschweissen auf das Aufschmelzverhalten und die Eigenschaften von Schweissverbindungen. DSV Berichte Strahltechnik 1980;63:158–163.

Herziger G. Werkstoffbearbeitung mit Laserstrahlung, Teil 1: Grundlagen und Probleme. Feinwerktechnik/Messtechnik 1983;91:156–162.

Landoldt-Björnstein. Optische Konstanten. In: Zahlenwerte und Funktionen aus Physik, Chemie, Astronomie, Geophysik, Technik. 6 Auflage. Berlin: Springer-Verlag; 1962;Band II:8 Teil.

Reisse G, Seifert U, Zscherpe G. Laserinduzierte Modifizierung von Keramikwerkstoffen. IHM Wiss Arb 1984;4:113–122.

Reisse G, Seifert U, Zscherpe G. Verfahren zur laserinduzierten Modifizierung von Keramikwerkstoffen. Patentschrift, WP DD 231 522 Al.

Schwarz A. Vergleichende Korrosionsuntersuchungen zwischen lasergeschweissten und geloteten Nahten. Med Diss, 1992, Berlin (HUB).

Zscherpe G, Reisse G. Stand und Entwicklungstendenzen der Lasermaterialbearbeitung. IHM Wiss Arb 1984;4:1–18.

Chapter Seventeen

Biostimulation and Photodynamic Therapy

Elliot Abt

Photodynamic therapy (PDT) is an experimental cancer treatment that is based on a cytotoxic photochemical reaction. This reaction requires molecular oxygen, the photoactive drug dihematoporphyrin ether (DHE), a hematoporphyrin derivative, and intense light, which is typically delivered by a laser. DHE, which is selectively retained in malignant tissue after several days, is given intravenously to a patient. Laser light at a wavelength corresponding to the absorption peak of the drug (red light at 630 nm) is used to activate the drug to an excited state. The drug then reacts with molecular oxygen to produce singlet oxygen, a highly reactive free radical, which ultimately leads to tissue necrosis. The drug is thought to localize in macrophages (Bugelski et al, 1981; Chan et al, 1988) and endothelial cells (Weintraub et al, 1988), and PDT is thought to destroy tumor vasculature, which leads to tumor necrosis.

Tissues containing high amounts of porphyrins fluoresce under blue light, and this phenomenon is exploited as a diagnostic aid in the detection of small satellite lesions typically found with carcinomas (Figs 17.1 and 17.2). Fluorescence microscopy has shown drug localization in the stroma and a lack of activity in tumor parenchyma. Conceptually, because the drug localizes in malignant tissue, PDT is selective for tumor necrosis. In actuality, both drug and laser light dose must be carefully controlled to achieve this selectivity, and, in fact, both clinically and experimentally, damage to normal tissue has occurred (Harris, 1991). Patients undergoing cancer treatment with PDT are extremely sensitive to sunlight (see Fig 17.3). Photodynamic therapy has been used clinically for malignant disease that has not responded to conventional therapy and for palliation in end-stage disease. Current applications include PDT for carcinomas of the skin, mucous membranes, bladder, lung, brain, and upper respiratory tract.

Basis of Photodynamic Therapy

The interaction of light and plant cells containing chlorophyll, a type of porphyrin, is responsible for the photosynthetic process, which allows aerobic life to exist. However, light can cause the formation of

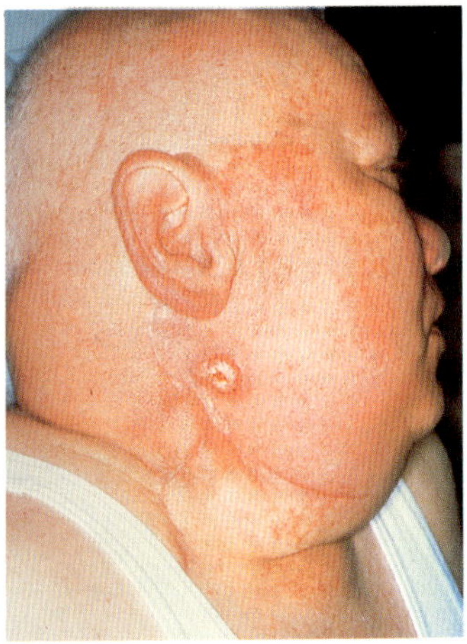

17.1

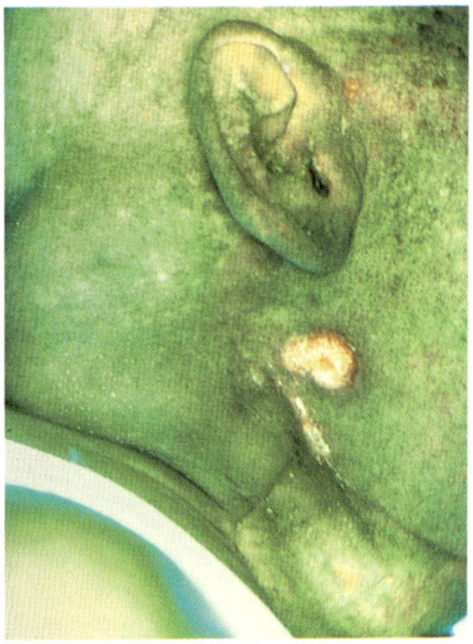

17.2

Fig 17.1 Metastatic squamous cell carcinoma of the neck. (Courtesy of Wenske Laser Center; Chicago, Illinois.)

Fig 17.2 Fluorescent detection of the lesion following HpD injection. (Courtesy of Wenske Laser Center; Chicago, Illinois.)

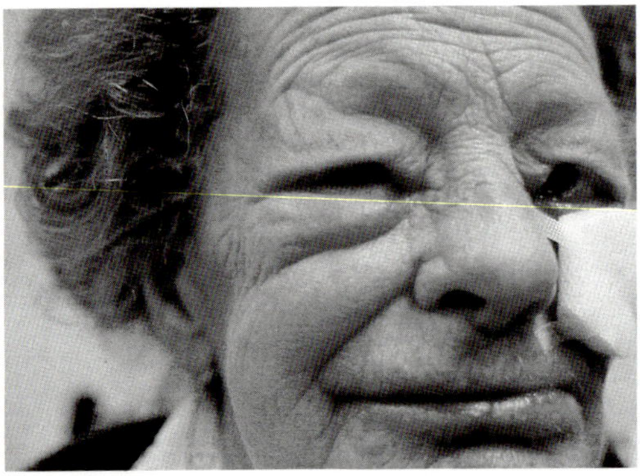

Fig 17.3 Skin photosensitivity following HpD administration: edema of the face.

singlet oxygen in plants, which would rapidly lead to cell death if not for the presence of carotene pigments. Porphyrins are also found in many animal species and include hemoglobin, myoglobin, and the cytochromes. In diseases of porphyrin metabolism, referred to as porphyrias, excess production of porphyrins can lead to central nervous system disorders and skin sensitivity to sunlight. This photosensitization is characterized by singlet oxygen production and cell death via the same mechanism proposed in PDT.

After the systemic administration of DHE, patients undergoing PDT are instructed to completely avoid sunlight and high-intensity lamps since severe burning of the skin may result (Fig 17.3). This type of phototoxic reaction has been exploited to treat vitiligo and psoriasis in addition to cancer.

Photochemotherapy

The emergence of photochemotherapy took place in the early 1900s. Von Tappeiner and Raab studied the effects of quinine and acridine on malaria (Daniell and Hill, 1991). Quinine was quite effective in vivo whereas acridine showed efficacy only in vitro. Thus, serial dilution of acridine was performed to test its potency on the paramecia in vitro. The investigators came upon a great paradox simply by chance. Two sets of studies yielded very different results. In one, the paramecia lived for 1 hour after a 1:20,000 dilution of acridine was added to the specimen. In the other experiment, the paramecia lived for almost 18 hours. The only difference between the two studies was in the amount of light exposure on the specimens because of a thunderstorm. This phenomenon was exploited to yield experiments in which light was added as a variable. Subsequent investigations showed that when light was added to acridine exposed paramecium, a much greater toxicity was observed than with either the light or acridine alone, or acridine exposed to light and then added to the paramecium samples. This allowed von Tappeiner and Raab to postulate that some product of the fluorescence, and not the light itself, was responsible for the observed toxicity (Pope and Bown, 1991).

In 1903, von Tappeiner and Jesionek treated skin cancer and lupus with topical eosin followed by exposure to white light. They reported that oxygen was required for the photosensitization to occur. The dye was either applied topically or injected directly into the lesion, and the area was then exposed to sunlight or an arc lamp. These were some of the first experiments with PDT.

In 1907, von Tappeiner's series of experiments was published as a textbook, and the term *photodynamic therapy* was used to describe the process of oxygen-dependent photosensitization. These investigations certainly established the groundwork for the current body of research and clinical study in photodynamic therapy.

Photosensitizers

The experimental uses of porphyrins date back to the mid-1800s when Scherer discovered that by washing dried blood with concentrated sulfuric acid, the precipitate was iron-free. This residue could then be washed with alcohol to render a red-colored liquid, demonstrating that iron was not responsible for the color of blood. This substance was referred to as iron-free hematin, or hematoporphyrin.

Subsequently, it was discovered that when protozoa and rodents were injected with hematoporphyrin and exposed to intense light, they became extremely photosensitive. This did not occur with all types of porphyrins. The earliest documentation of human photosensitivity was in 1913 when Meyer-Betz, a German scientist, injected himself with hematoporphyrin and noticed swelling in light-exposed areas. He remained photosensitive for several months. In 1924, Policard was the first to discover the spontaneous fluorescence of experimental tumors under a Wood's lamp and postulated that this phenomenon was due to the presence of porphyrins. This finding is significant in that tumor fluorescence under blue light is a diagnostic tool used today. The ability of tumors to selectively retain porphyrins and fluoresce has been recognized since 1942. Auler and Banzer showed that tumors retain a greater amount of hematoporphyrin than the surrounding normal tissue. They also performed histologic studies on experimentally induced carcinomas and sarcomas injected with hematoporphyrin and illuminated with intense light and found large areas of tumor necrosis. This was the earliest work in PDT with porphyrins.

In the 1950s, the high toxicity of hematoporphyrins in humans became apparent. Schwartz et al (1955) were the first to investigate the composition of hematoporphyrin and found it to be a complex mixture of porphyrins with different chemical properties. After fractionation, other porphyrins were shown to have a much higher affinity for tumor localization than hematoporphyrin. This non-hematoporphyrin fraction was called hematoporphyrin derivative (HpD), an acetic and sulfuric acid porphyrin with enhanced tumor localizing properties. In 1961, Lipson and others, working at the Mayo Clinic, examined tumor fluorescence in several ex-

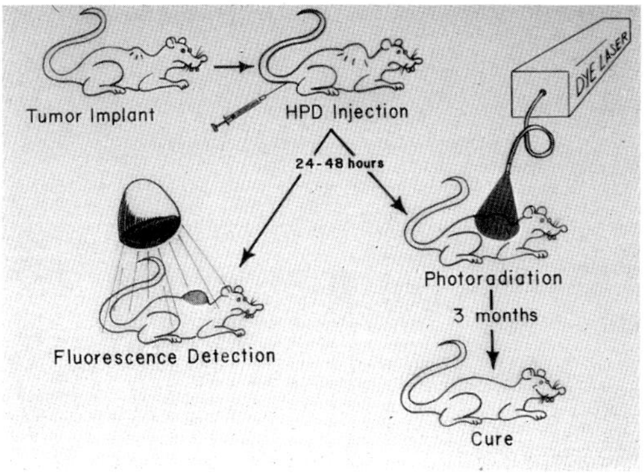

Fig 17.4 Mechanism of action of PDT in animal model. (Courtesy of David Harris.)

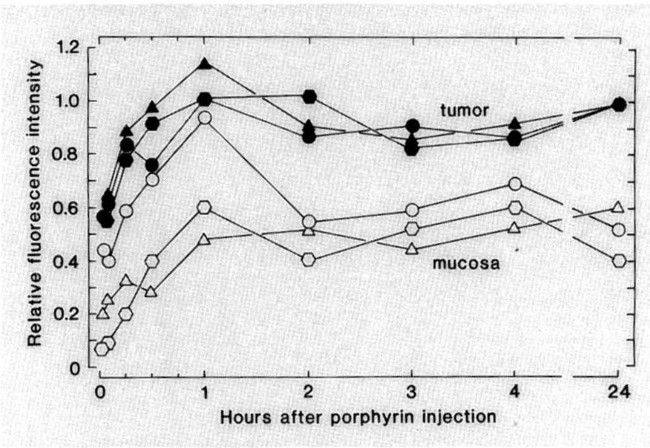

Fig 17.5 Relative uptake of porphyrin by tumor cells and normal mucosa by fluorescent detection. (Courtesy of David Harris.)

perimental models after injection of HpD (Fig 17.4). Early clinical trials then followed in 1966 with HpD administered with a xenon arc lamp for recurrent breast carcinoma. These tumors exhibited a partial response to therapy (greater than 50% reduction in tumor size without complete eradication). Clinical trials then lapsed until 1975 when Kelly and Snell investigated the effects of HpD in malignant and premalignant lesions of the bladder with a mercury vapor lamp. The results were favorable, and in 1978 Dougherty et al began a series of clinical trials on cutaneous malignant tumors in patients using HpD and red light. More than 100 carcinomas of the breast, colon, and prostate were treated and no lesions were shown to be unresponsive to therapy.

Modification of the original HpD composition prepared by Lipson and Schwartz was achieved by Dougherty in 1978. Hematoporphyrin derivative contains a mixture of porphyrin monomers and oligomers linked by some ester or more commonly by ether bonds. Only the oligomeric porphyrins are retained long enough in malignant tissue to render a therapeutic effect. Hematoporphyrin derivative contains approximately 45% of the oligomeric porphyrins, whereas a purified type of HpD called Photofrin II contains 80% to 90% of the oligomeric material. Experimental and clinical studies have confirmed that only oligomeric porphyrins are retained in malignant tissue and monomeric porphyrins are rapidly excreted. Photofrin II is the photosensitizer that is used in clinical and experimental PDT today.

Research continues in an effort to find new photosensitizers. The purpose is to find new drugs that will render patients less photosensitive and will absorb light at longer wavelengths than Photofrin II to allow deeper penetration of light into body cavities. Among the new drugs being studied are the naphthalocyanines, purpurins, benzoporphyrins, and the phthalocyanines. As yet, none of these drugs have been tested in patients, and their ability to fluoresce is unclear.

Distribution. After intraperitoneal injection of HpD, only 1% of the dye is found in the circulation (Fig 17.5). Drug clearance from the circulation is also rapid after intravenous administration. Fluorescence microscopy and fractionation studies have shown that the liver, spleen, kidney, and

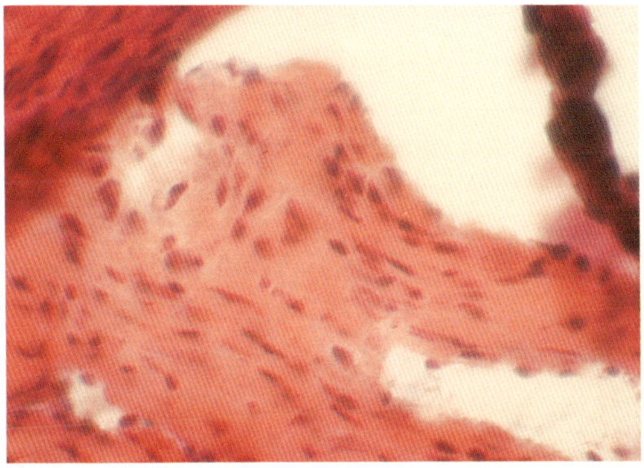

Fig 17.6a Histologic section (hematoxylin and eosin) of mouse squamous cell carcinoma transplant from human.

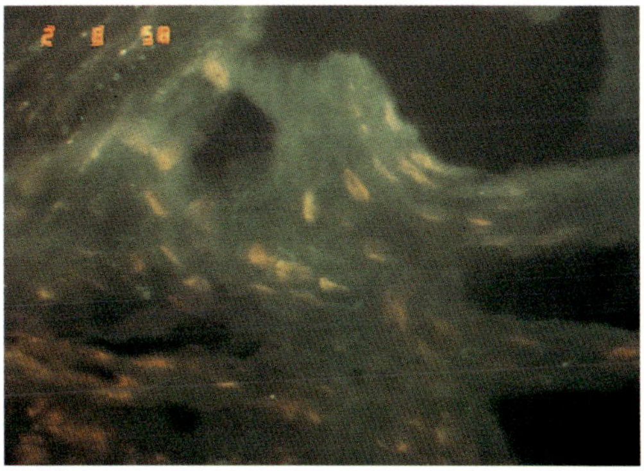

Fig 17.6b Serial section from 17.6a (fluorescent microscopy).

small intestine retain the greatest amount of drug 12 days after injection. Fluorescence microscopy has also shown HpD localization in stromal tissue elements (Bugelski et al, 1981).

Specific areas of dye localization have been controversial. Musser observed localization in connective tissue fibers, while Harris has suggested fibroblasts as the active site (Figs 17.6). Intravascular and extravascular reticuloendothelial cells such as mast cells (Kerdel et al, 1987), macrophages, and scavenger cells of the liver and spleen have also been suggested (Moan et al, 1989; Bugelski et al, 1981). Another commonly mentioned site of HpD localization is endothelial cells (Fig 17.7). Histologic observation of pyknotic endothelial cells after PDT is commonly observed (Abt et al, 1992), and Weintraub noted the localization of phthalocyanine in the endothelial cells of the spleen and lymph nodes of mice. Erythrocytes and leukocytes have not shown demonstrable drug accumulation (Henderson and Bellnier, 1989; Chan et al, 1988). Henderson and Bellnier suggest that with low doses of photosensitizer, singlet oxygen formation and subsequent destruction of the vascular bed are responsible for tumor

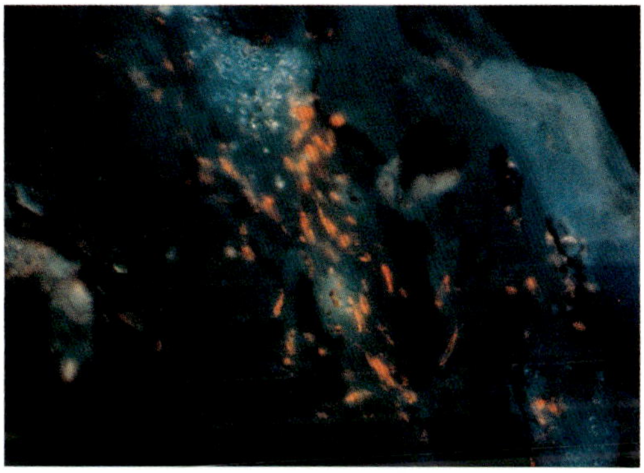

Fig 17.7 Fluorescent section of hamster oral mucosa (x 400) illustrating localization of photosensitizer within fibroblasts of tumor parenchyma. (Courtesy of Dr David Harris.)

necrosis. With drug doses high enough to cause direct tumor necrosis, tumor hypoxia from the damaged vascular supply would again be the mechanism of PDT since this would occur prior to irreversible changes in the tumor parenchyma.

The intracellular localization of photosensitizer has also been investigated. Subcellular fractionation studies have shown a general trend of lipophilic dyes (protoporphyrin) to localize in mitochondria and hydrophilic dyes (uroporphyrin) to accumulate in lysosomes. Ultrastructurally, drug

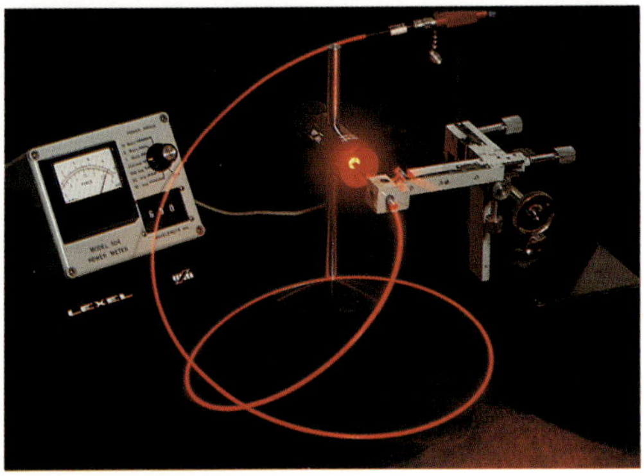

Fig 17.8 Typical fiber delivery apparatus used with tunable dye laser.

localization has been observed in the plasma membrane and mitochondria (Moan et al, 1989). Fluorescence microscopy has confirmed the presence of lipophilic porphyrins in the plasma, mitochondrial, and nuclear membranes (Berns et al, 1982).

Light Delivery Systems and Dosimetry

Lasers have replaced conventional incandescent and arc lamps as the standard light source for PDT. The advantage of using lasers over conventional lamps is the ability to deliver high energy densities (J/cm^2) through small optical fibers at a specific wavelength (Fig 17.8). With optical fibers, light can be delivered endoscopically or interstitially. The laser that is most commonly used for PDT is the argon-pumped dye laser. This is a tunable laser that is normally set at 630 nm to match the absorption spectrum for Photofrin II, but can be set at different wavelengths depending on which photosensitizer is used. The disadvantages of the argon-pumped dye laser are the high cost, poor reliability, and lack of mobility of the unit.

New photosensitizers are being developed that absorb at longer wavelengths (650 to 850 nm), which allows deeper light penetration into body cavities, are more selective for malignant tissue, and allows greater photoactivation efficiency. Along with these developments arises the need for improved laser technology. Technical advances are being accomplished with the diode and the solid-state lasers. As the wavelength of light is increased, the depth of penetration increases. Also, less hemoglobin absorption would occur by increasing the wavelength from 630 nm, which would facilitate further light penetration. Light penetration depth increases from 1 to 2 mm at 630 nm to about 2 to 4 mm at ranges of 700 to 850 nm (Wilson, 1989). Bown (1986) has shown a well-defined zone of necrosis subjacent to the treated area as opposed to a gradual change in tissue vitality. The production of singlet oxygen is proportional to the product of the light fluence (energy density) and the absorption coefficient of the photosensitizer. At 1 to 5 mg/kg of administered HpD, adequate laser light at 630 nm would give a therapeutic depth of penetration of 5 to 10 mm in solid tumors. Presently, dosage for PDT is described in light fluence (J/cm^2) and concentration of photosensitizer (mg/kg). In the future, dosage will be expanded to include the depth distribution of the light, the concentration of drug in the tumor, and tumor oxygenation.

Clinical Applications

Because of the limitations on depth of light penetration, PDT is currently most effective with skin and mucosal tumors, or small lesions accessible through procedures such as endoscopy and cystoscopy. All clinical applications are based on two thresholds that must be exceeded if a therapeutic result is to be achieved. The

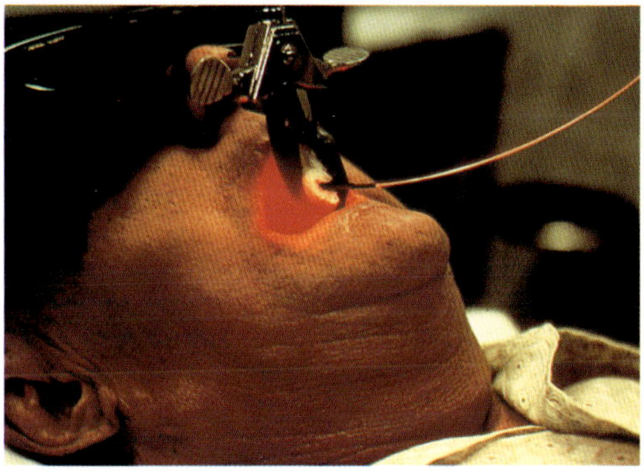

17.9a

Fig 17.9 Intraoral treatment of squamous cell carcinoma of the palate. **(a)**, Fiber delivery system for PDT. **(b)**, 24 hours after treatment. **(c)**, Remission observed 3 months after treatment. (Courtesy of Dr James Hill.)

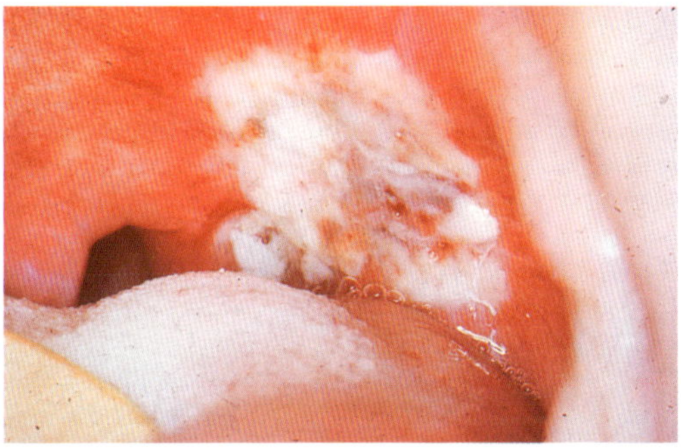

17.9b

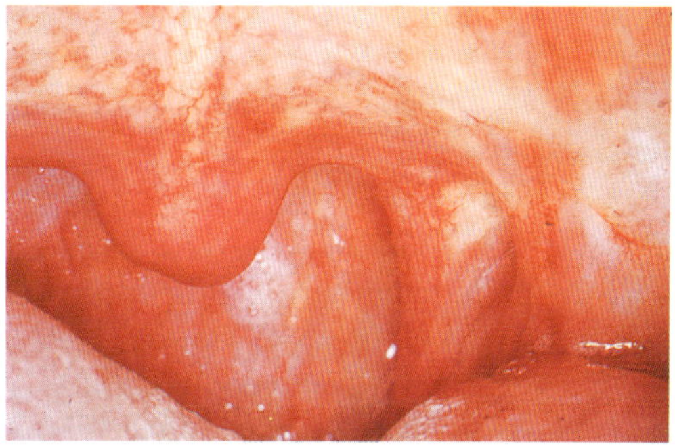

17.9c

first threshold is a minimum concentration of photosensitizer, which must be present in the target tissue. The second threshold is the product of the concentration of photosensitizer and the total light energy absorbed by each point in the tissue (Pope and Bown, 1991). With future advances in laser technology and photosensitizer chemistry, applications for PDT should continue to expand.

Head and Neck Cancer. Otolaryngology is another field where clinical PDT has been reported extensively. Overall success rates for head and neck cancer, generally reported in the 20% to 40% range, are less than those for bladder cancer, primarily due to the limited depth of light penetration into larger tumors. Originally, PDT had been used only in end-stage disease for palliation when patients had undergone surgery and/or radiation therapy. Where PDT has been successful is in early carcinomas (T1), especially in the oral cavity. The oral cavity is quite accessible with current technology, and postoperative edema does not cause airway problems as it does in the pharynx. Tumors further down the respiratory tract are typically much larger, and this decreases the effectiveness of PDT as laser light penetration is decreased. Implantable diffusion tips have been used in these larger tumors with inconsistent results.

Mucosal tumors of the oral cavity are more responsive to PDT than skin lesions, as the mucosa is thinner and does not usually contain adnexa such as sebaceous and sudoriparous glands, hair follicles, or great amounts of melanin (Fig 17.9).

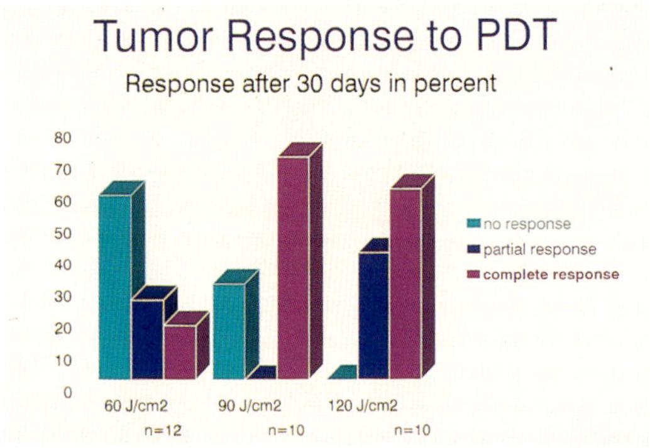

Fig 17.10 Tumor response to PDT. (Courtesy of David Harris and Elliot Abt.)

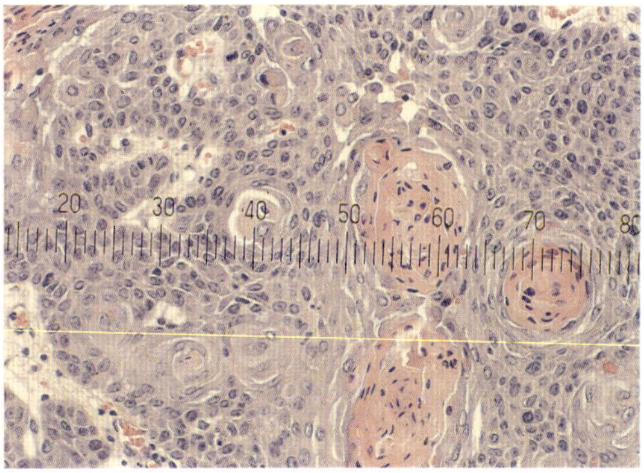

17.11a

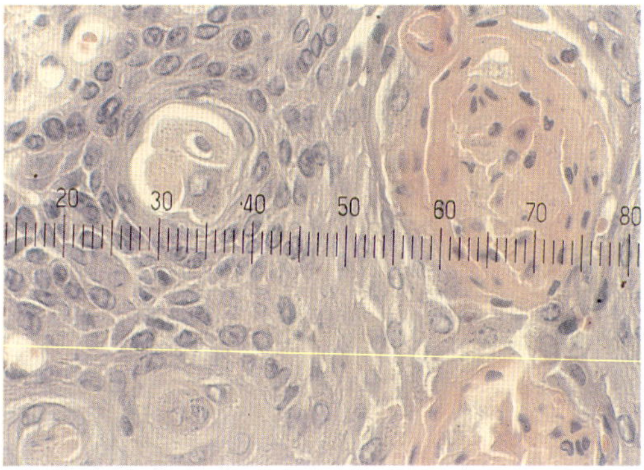

17.11b

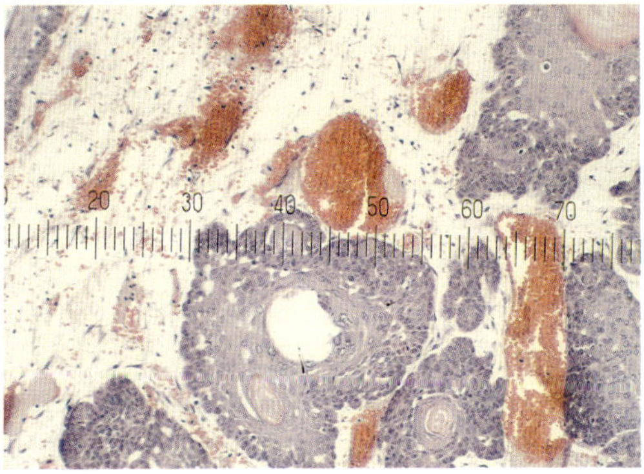

17.11c

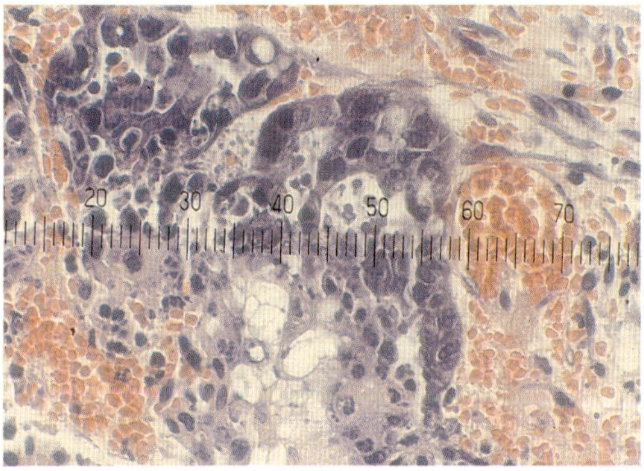

17.11d

Fig 17.11 Histologic appearance of squamous cell carcinoma of buccal cheek pouch in hamster. **(a)**, Untreated tumor: keratin pearls (K) and islands of epithelium (E) within the tumor parenchyma display good differentiation. **(b)**, Higher power magnification of keratin pearls (K) and pyknotic nuclei (P) of tumor parenchyma (untreated specimen). **(c)**, Vasodilatation and engorgement of blood vessels appear within 1 hour after PDT. **(d)**, At 12 hours after PDT, tumor parenchyma displays a loss of architecture and disruption of intercellular contacts. Note the absence of inflammatory cell infiltrate. (Courtesy of David Harris and Elliot Abt.)

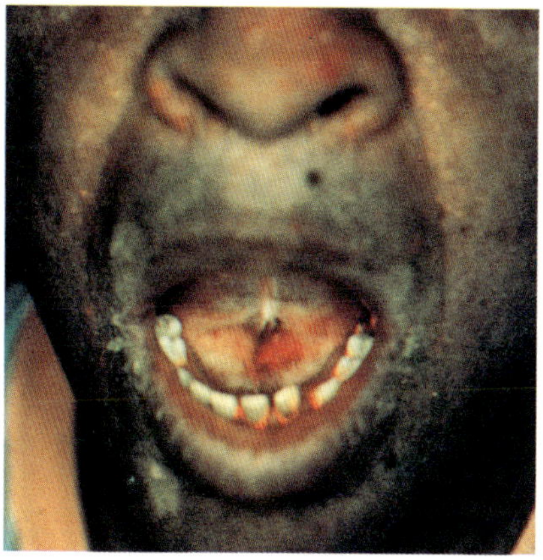

Fig 17.12 Autofluorescence of plaque (marginal gingiva) in a patient undergoing PDT for squamous cell carcinoma of the tongue.

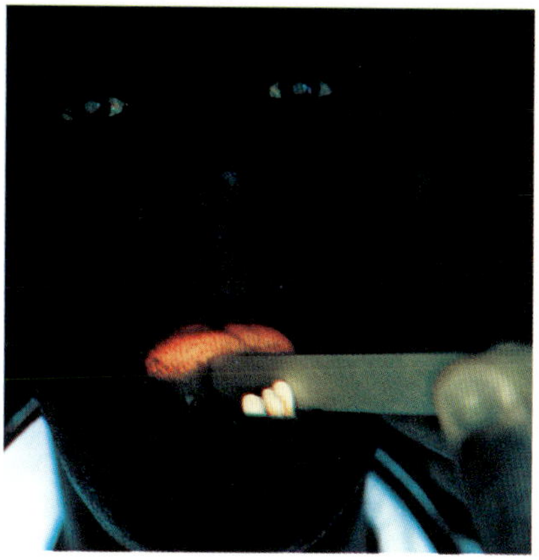

Fig 17.13 Autofluorescence of bacteria on the surface of the tongue.

Where PDT shows great promise in the treatment of oral tumors is in its detection of small satellite lesions that typically accompany the primary tumor. If the photosensitizer is administered 24 hours preoperatively, areas of malignancy or dysplasia are easily seen with a Wood's lamp or similar light source.

Investigations have also examined the differential response of tumors and normal mucosa (Fig 17.10). Abt et al found insignificant changes in surrounding normal tissues when a partial or complete response was observed in hamster squamous cell carcinomas (Fig 17.11). This is clinically significant in that pharyngeal edemas may become more predictable. Future applications of PDT in otolaryngology will study effects on benign tumors and viral infections.

Future Applications

Photodynamic therapy has been used with promising results in the treatment of malignancies of the cervix, brain, and lung. As with other types of cancers, PDT was originally used for palliation of end-stage disease. However, both experimental and clinical investigations have shown that PDT is effective either alone or in combination with surgery, radiation therapy, or chemotherapy. This is especially true with cerebral gliomas, where the lesions spread quickly and diffusely, making conventional treatment very difficult. With new photosensitizers and newer laser technologies being developed, applications for PDT should continue well into the future. Fluorescent detection of specific autofluorescent bacteria found in the oral cavity may also prove to be of benefit as a diagnostic modality for dentistry (Figs 17.12 and 17.13).

Biostimulation

Biostimulation, which also includes bioinhibition, is the use of low-energy laser light on tissues to achieve a clinical effect. Biostimulation has been used clinically for pain reduction and wound healing.

Low energy or soft lasers transmit at energy levels and frequencies that do not cause visible damage to mammalian tissues. Examples include the helium-neon laser, which has a red beam at 632.8 nm, and the gallium arsenide laser at 820-nm wavelength. Many claims of therapeutic potential for a wide variety of conditions were initially made for these laser systems. Many of these claims appear to have had no scientific basis, and the use of low energy fell into disrepute.

Nevertheless, in vitro studies have shown that these lasers do have effects on tissues in culture and can stimulate fibroblast proliferation (Abergel et al, 1987). This has stimulated some renewed interest in the clinical uses of low energy lasers and the results of controlled studies are awaited with interest. Recent reports have included its use in extraction sockets, where it may reduce postoperative pain and trismus (Carrillo et al, 1990), accelerate dental extraction socket healing (Takeda, 1988), and aid in physical therapy for temporomandibular joint disorders (Hansson, 1989; Bezuur et al, 1988). The helium-neon laser has not been shown to have any advantages in the treatment of hypersensitive dentin, gingivitis, pulp-capped teeth, herpes labialis, and aphthous ulcers, although patients have reported a very positive attitude toward the techniques (Wilder-Smith, 1988; Howell et al, 1988). A study on hamsters showed that helium-neon laser may inhibit plaque formation (Iwase et al, 1989). Strang et al (1988) offers a good review of the soft laser debate in dentistry.

The basic mechanism for biostimulation occurs at the molecular level. Laser light penetrates through tissue and strikes a chromophore, or photosensitive molecule, which in this case is the cytochrome contained within mitochondria. There are other photosensitive molecules, such as rhodopsin needed for vision, chlorophyll for photosynthesis, and HpD used in PDT. Mitochondrial cytochromes are responsible for converting adenosine diphosphate (ADP) to adenosine triphosphate (ATP), thus supplying energy to the cell and driving cellular metabolism. The ability of laser light to affect target molecules is dependent on the absorption spectra of biomolecules and tissue optics. There are no major absorbers between 500 and 1,200 nm. It appears that wavelengths near 1 µm penetrate best into tissue, but shorter wavelengths are better chromophore absorbers.

Biostimulation occurs with power densities below 300 to 400 mW/cm^2. At these energies, there is a photochemical effect as in PDT, rather than a thermal effect as with a CO_2 laser. Because low-energy laser light can increase cellular metabolism by increasing ATP production, several phenomena have been observed. With low-level laser irradiation, cell culture studies have shown an activation of suppressor T cells, which inhibit B lymphocytes from antibody production. Fewer antibodies translates into decreased production of histamines and kinins and a decreased inflammatory response in cases where B lymphocytes are relevant. Studies have also shown the restoration of the sodium pump necessary to maintain the negative resting potential of neuronal membranes. With inflammation, the normal resting potential of nerve fibers is decreased, leading to hypersensitivity. Returning the resting potential to normal could decrease pain transmission. This area of biostimulation is clinically important in pain reduction.

Biostimulation is also effective in increasing metabolism and cell replication in fibroblasts and endothelial cells. This is clinically important in wound healing, especially in diabetic patients' leg ulcers that are resistant to traditional therapy.

References

Abergel RP, Lyons RF, Castel JC, Dwyer RM, Uitto J. Biostimulation of wound healing by lasers: experimental approaches in animal models and in fibroblast cultures. J Dermatol Surg Oncol 1987;13:127–133.

Abt E, Harris DM, Palit M, Kotlarz J, Nelson-Bacos B. Gross and histologic effects of photodynamic therapy on hamster cheek pouch carcinoma. Proc Third Int Congress Lasers Dent 1992;73–74.

Berns MV, Dahlman A, Johnson FM. In vitro cellular effects of hematoporphyrin derivative. Cancer Res 1982; 42:2325–2329.

Bezuur NJ, Habets LLMH, Hansson TL. The effects of therapeutic laser treatment in patients with craniomandibular disorders. J Craniomandibular Disorders 1988;2:83–86.

Bown SG, Tralan CJ, Coleridge-Smith PD, Akdemir DTJ, Weiman TJ. Photodynamic therapy with porphyrin and phthalocyanine sensitization: quantitative studies in normal rat liver. Br J Cancer 1986;54:43–52.

Bugelski PJ, Porter CW, Dougherty TJ. Autoradiographic distribution of hematoporphyrin derivative in normal and tumor tissue of the mouse. Cancer Res 1981;41:4606–4612.

Carrillo JS, Calatayud J, Manso FJ, Martinez JM, Donado, M. A randomized double blind trial on the effectiveness of helium neon laser in the prevention of pain, swelling, and trismus after removal of impacted third molars. Int Dent J 1990;40:31–36.

Chan WS, Marshall JF, Lam GYF. Tissue uptake, distribution, and potency of the photoactivatable dye chloroaluminium sulfonated phthalocyanine in mice bearing transplantable tumors. Cancer Res 1988;48: 3040–3044.

Daniell MD, Hill JS. A history of photodynamic therapy. Aust NZ J Surg 1991;61:340–348.

Dougherty TJ, Kaufman JE, Goldfarb A, et al. Photoradiation therapy for the treatment of malignant tumours. Cancer Res 1978;38:2628–2635.

Hansson TC. Infrared laser in the treatment of craniomandibular disorders, arthrogenous pain. J Prosthet Dent 1989;61:614–617.

Harris DM. Biomolecular mechanisms of laser biostimulation. J Clin Laser Med Surg 1991;8:277–280.

Henderson BW, Bellnier DA. Tissue localization of photosensitizers and the mechanism of photodynamic tissue destruction. Photosensitizing compounds: their chemistry, biology, and clinical use. Ciba Found Symp 1989,146:112–130.

Howell RM, Cohen DM, Powell GL, Green JG. The use of low energy laser therapy to treat aphthous ulcers. J Am Dent Assoc 1988;47:16–18.

Iwase T, Saita T, Wara Y, Morioka T. Inhibitory effect of He Ne laser on dental plaque deposition in hamsters. J Periodont Res 1989;24:282–283.

Kelly JF, Snell ME, Berenbaum MC. Photodynamic destruction of human bladder carcinoma. Br J Cancer 1975;31:237–244.

Kerdel FA, Soter NA, Lim HW. In vivo mediator release and degranulation of mast cells in hematoporphyrin derivative-induced phototoxicity in mice. J Invest Dermatol 1987;88:277–280.

Lipson RL, Baldes EJ, Olsen AM. The use of a derivative of hematoporphyrin in tumour detection. J Natl Cancer Inst 1961;26:1–11.

Mester E, Spiry T, Szende B, Tota JG. Effects of laser rays on wound healing. Am J Surg 1971;122:532–535.

Moan J, Berg K, Kvam E, et al. Intracellular localization of photosensitizers. Photosensitizing compounds: their chemistry, biology, and clinical use. Ciba Found Symp 1989;146:95–111.

Pope AJ, Bown SG. Photodynamic therapy. Br J Urol 1991;68:1–9.

Schwartz SK, Absolon K, Vermund H. Some relationships of porphyrins, x-rays, and tumours. Univ Minn Med Bull 1955;27:7–8.

Strang R, Moseley H, Carmichael A. Soft lasers: have they a place in dentistry? Br Dent J 1988;165:221–225.

Takeda Y. Irradiation effects of low energy laser on alveolar bone after tooth extraction. Int J Oral Maxillofac Surg 1988;17:388–391.

Weintraub H, Abramovici A, Altman A. Toxicity, tissue distribution and excretion studies of aluminium phthalocyanine tetrasulfonate in normal mice. Lasers Life Sci 1988;2:185–196.

Wilder-Smith P. The soft laser: therapeutic tool or popular placebo. Oral Surg Oral Med Oral Pathol 1988; 66:654–658.

Wilson BC. Photodynamic therapy: light delivery and dosage for second-generation photosensitizers. Photosensitizing compounds: their chemistry, biology, and clinical use. Ciba Found Symp 1989;146:60–77.

Part IV

Current Technology and Future Directions

Chapter Eighteen

Analysis of Excimer Laser Interactions with Hard Tissue

Joseph Neev

New possibilities for the application of lasers in dentistry have recently been proposed based on the use of excimer lasers. Excimer (for "excited dimers") lasers are a class of gas lasers, which are formed by the excitation of rare earth gases and their subsequent reaction with halide atoms such as chlorine or fluorine. Since these molecules exist only in their excited state and dissociate instantly upon emission of radiation, they constitute an ideal system for population inversion, which is the precondition for lasing action. Because their relaxation mechanism involves transition between electronic states with a relatively large energy gap, excimer laser radiation is always in the ultraviolet (UV) range of the electromagnetic spectrum.

Excimer lasers define a different regime of laser-tissue interaction, because ultraviolet photons are energetic enough to result in direct bond breaking in organic molecules. This mechanism of energy absorption, combined with the very short pulse duration, virtually eliminates thermal damage. Additional benefits arise from the fact that organic tissue absorbs UV radiation well and the tissue ablation rates can, thus, be controlled with extreme precision.

The application of excimer lasers for the ablation of organic material was first suggested in the pioneering work of Srinivasan (Srinivasan and Mayne-Banton, 1982; Srinivasan and Leigh, 1982) in the early 1980s. Srinivasan called the process "ablative photodecomposition" (APD), which was soon afterward applied to the etching of a variety of materials from polymers to human corneas to atherosclerotic plaque (Srinivasan, 1986). Despite the considerable volume of research on excimer laser ablation, the precise mechanism of the interaction remains unclear and the physical process of tissue removal is only partly understood.

Although short pulse excimer lasers were found to have a relatively low removal rate of hard dental tissue (Tasev et al, 1990; Neev et al, 1991), they were useful because of several characteristics: (1) they leave an extremely smooth surface essentially free of thermal damage; (2) the heat production is apparently highly confined to the ablation region, resulting in thermal fusion of the ablated surface, but only minor temperature changes in the rest of the tissue; (3) at least in the far ultraviolet (UV) region, they appear to show high variation in the ablation efficiency from tissue to tissue (ie, the ablation of dentin is much higher than ablation of enamel, which in turn is lower then that of calculus and soft tissues). These variations are large enough to make this type of laser attractive for selective tissue removal; (4) excimer laser radiation induces strong plume luminescence with an emission spectrum that can be used to detect and monitor removal of diseased tissue.

Research into Applications of Excimer Laser

Dentists and scientists began considering uses of excimer lasers in dentistry in the late 1980s, and initial investigations were reported as early as 1989. In one of the first studies (Frentzen et al, 1989a), the possible use of photoablation with excimer laser to create retentive surfaces was investigated as an alternative to conventional enamel conditioning methods using acids. Surfaces of untreated enamel and of prepared cavities were irradiated with an ArF laser at 193 nm and evaluated with scanning electron microscopy (SEM). The bond strength of composites to these surfaces was measured in tear tests. The laser treatment left the surfaces almost as rough as those treated by chemical etching. The tear tests with human tooth enamel showed bond strength values corresponding to approximately 75% of those obtained by acid etching techniques.

In another study by Frentzen et al (1989b), the researchers attempted to show that caries removal and conditioning of tooth surfaces by an ArF excimer laser can be an alternative to conventional preparation methods without thermal and mechanical irritations. They discovered that the photoablative process leads to retentive surfaces of the treated cavities, which showed promise for good results in adhesive techniques. They indicated that in vitro studies demonstrated that photoablation of dental tissue is effective enough to make clinical use possible.

Vernole et al (1989) used 28 samples of human enamel to measure fluoride absorption after treatment with UV radiation. Samples treated with topical application presented only limited fluoride absorption in enamel surface (up to 0.5 μm deep). The absorption rate was higher with a UV lamp. In the samples treated with the excimer laser, fluoride absorption was much higher in the surface layer and was deeper (3 μm).

Liesenhoff et al (1989a) assessed the usefulness of an excimer laser (wavelength, 308 nm) to remove enamel and dentin by examining micromorphologic changes in the irradiated surfaces. Their results demonstrated that it is possible to remove dentin and enamel with the excimer laser in a controlled fashion. The temperature in the pulp cavity rose as a function of the distance to the site of irradiation (corresponding to distance between temperature measuring probe and irradiated tooth surface) and the duration of exposure and amounted to 3.5°C to 18.3°C. Differences in the micromorphologic appearances of the surface structures were observed as a function of the material (enamel or dentin) and the duration of irradiation. The same authors also demonstrated with 308-nm excimer lasers and SEM investigations that a good retention of filling materials could be achieved. Transmission electron microscopic (TEM) investigations of irradiated dental hard tissues demonstrated that there were no structural changes in the ultrastructure below the irradiated surface.

In 1989, Pini and coworkers reported the first study of the application of excimer lasers in dentistry for the treatment of dental root canals. High-energy UV radiation emitted by an XeCl excimer laser (308 nm) and delivered through suitable optical fibers was used to remove residual organic tissue from the canals. Ultraviolet ablation thresholds of dental tissues have been measured, showing a preferential etching of infiltrated dentin with respect to healthy dentin, at laser fluences of 0.5 to 1.5 J/cm^2. This technique has been tested on extracted tooth samples, simulating a clinical procedure. Fibers of decreasing core diameters have been used to treat different sections of the root canal down to its apical portion, resulting in an effective, easy, and fast cleaning action.

In 1990, Liesenhoff et al (1990) conducted SEM studies that showed that irradiation in the energy density range of 4 to 6 J/cm^2 resulted in the removal of hard tooth structure without causing thermal alterations of the tissues. In the process of photoablation, they showed, the natural structures of the tissues are exposed. The surface structure, which is produced in dentin, depends on whether the dentin tubules are hit transversally or longitudinally and varies accordingly. The surface structure of enamel is also determined by the alignment of the prisms. When the laser beam was adjusted to energy densities of 4 to 6 J/cm^2 and peripheral fading of the beam was achieved, no structural changes could be demonstrated in the depth of the tissue.

Ochiai (1990) investigated the possibilities of bone and soft tissue ablation without thermal damage with the 248-nm KrF excimer laser. The KrF laser was also investigated as an alternative for acid etching (Ruppenthal et al, 1991). Morphologic effects of enamel conditioning with a pulsed KrF excimer laser and SEM examinations revealed a surface similar to that produced by peripheral etching and no signs of thermal damage were seen. It should be noted, however, that while the KrF laser possesses many of the same laser-tissue characteristics as others in the excimer family, it is generally avoided in clinical applications because of the proximity of its wavelength to the 260-nm DNA absorption peak.

Frentzen et al (1990) studied the temperature increases occurring in the dental pulp during laser irradiation. They found that infrared laser radiation (CO_2 and Nd:YAG) had great thermal effects on the pulp tissues. At an average power output level of 5 W, temperature rises of approximately 40°C occurred within 100 sec, and they found the effect of a cooling system to be negligible. On the other hand, radiation from an ArF excimer laser (193 nm) at an average output of 5 W caused only slight thermal changes when an airstream was used to remove the fragments of photoablative decomposition of the dental tissues. The temperature in the pulp chamber increased by approximately 5°C after 6 min. They thus concluded that only ArF excimer lasers may be effective in the mouth without producing unacceptable thermal effects in the dental pulp. The same study revealed that during preparation of hard tooth structures with a 193-nm ArF excimer laser, the laser beam produces a specific fluorescent light, the spectrum of which is governed by the structure of the specimen. These fluorescence spectra allow an analysis of the removed tissues, and the data may be used to control the laser system so that only specific structures, such as carious tissue, are removed. Reproducible fluorescence spectra were established with standardized samples (pure synthetic hydroxyapatite ceramics, enamel, dentin, and carious dentin), and the characteristic absorption bands (peaks) for the different substances were measured. With the aid of data processing, these reference spectra could be compared with the fluorescence spectra obtained during preparation. When a spectrum differed from the predefined limits of relative intensities, preparation was stopped. Since ablation per pulse is only to a small depth (0.04 to 4 μm) with the 193-nm ArF excimer laser, this feedback system of ablation and fluorescence spectroscopy allows decisions about continuing or stopping the preparation process to be taken within the range of a few micrometers.

Frentzen et al (1991) studied XeCl as an alternative method to mechanical methods for root canal treatment. In a light microscopic investigation, undecalcified sections of laser-treated extracted human teeth showed that it was not possible to remove dentin in the root canal. Pulpal tissues remained in all wall areas. The available energy densities of this laser type seem not to be sufficient to ablate pulpal tissues or wall dentin. These observations appear to contradict those of Pini et al (1989).

Arcoria et al (1992) showed that the reaction of enamel, dentin, and pulpal tissues to exposure from a laser beam depends on the type of laser medium used. The objective of their study was to examine the pulpal response in rat molars after external enamel surface treatment with either an ArF excimer laser or acid-gel application. Maxillary right molar occlusal surfaces in 22 animals were irradiated (energy density, 45.0 J/cm^2). Maxillary left molar occlusal surfaces were treated with 37% phosphoric acid for 30 sec. Untreated mandibular right molars served as control sites. At two postoperative times (1 and 6 weeks), molars were removed, sectioned, stained, and scored. Data analysis indicated no significant difference between molars with ArF irradiation and control sites at 1 week. Treatment with laser or acid-etching left a similar degree of pathosis at 1 and 6 weeks. Although the ArF excimer laser produced a more exaggerated pulp response than that in control sites at 6 weeks, tissue vitality was maintained. They thus concluded that the ArF excimer laser may be useful for ablating vital tooth structure since pulpal tissue in rat molars exhibited no damage in response to low-power irradiation.

Feuerstein et al (1992) exposed human enamel surfaces to ArF excimer laser and examined the results with light microscopy and SEM. The enamel surface was irradiated at three different areas with different energy fluences. It was demonstrated that the ArF excimer laser causes ablation of the calcified hard enamel tissue. Ablation curves were measured. There was no significant difference found in the etch depth between the three different areas of enamel surface. The morphologic characteristics of the irradiated areas seen with SEM were found to be dependent on energy fluence. With an increase in energy fluence, the appearance changed from that of being etched to that of a smooth, fused, glazelike surface. At very high energy fluences, a rough surface was produced. The influence of the laser irradiation was confined to the irradiated area only, with no visible heat damage to surrounding tissues. These results suggest that the excimer laser could be applied in a controlled and defined manner for the treatment of enamel in dentistry.

Arima and Matsumoto (1993) exposed round enamel and dentin surfaces of sound and carious extracted human teeth to an ArF excimer laser for up to 180 sec. Thermographic measurements indicated that the temperature increase due to heat accumulation caused by laser irradiation on these enamel and dentin surfaces was up to 19°C (10 Hz with 540 J/cm^2), and the temperature returned to the pre-irradiation value within 10 sec after the irradiation was stopped. With light microscopy, no carbonization was evident on these surfaces, and a simple recess was formed by abrasion or vaporization in the irradiated regions. In the secondary SEM, uniformly distributed fine pores and prism structures appeared on the enamel surfaces. Between the peritubular and the intertubular dentin, distinct differences in the dissolved area appeared. The laser almost completely removed carious regions on the enamel and the dentin, and penetration extended beyond the carious regions. In the backscattered electron SEM, highly mineralized layers were observed on the enamel and dentin surfaces treated by the laser.

Arcoria et al (1993) conducted a study on laser-induced roughened enamel surfaces and showed that they provided a greater acid-resistance and enhanced restorative material/enamel bond strength. Extracted tooth enamel was irradiated with several lasers: CO_2/Nd:YAG (continuous wave), CO_2 (superpulse), Nd:YAG (continuous wave), Nd:YAG (Q-switched), argon (continuous wave), and ArF excimer. Additional teeth were acid-etched. Energy densities were standardized at 25.47 J/cm^2 for all mediums. Surface profile analyses were conducted with a profilometer to determine the amount of enamel surface roughness. They found that acid-etched samples exhibited both a greater amount of surface roughness and a qualitatively different type of enamel surface morphology than the laser-treated specimens. They found that coaxial CO_2/Nd:YAG beam displayed surface roughness approaching that of the acid-etch samples. Different lasers produce enamel surface morphologic characteristics that are characteristic of a variety of inherent lasing parameters.

Finally, a recent study (Stabholz et al, 1993) has shown that XeCl lasers are effective as a sterilizing agents. A short pulse (15 nsec) excimer with radiation at 308 nm was used and *Streptococcus mutans* was killed effectively. The bactericidal effect of the laser was shown to be directly proportional to irradiation time, as well as to the laser fluence level. Additional excimer laser studies have been conducted (Neev et al, 1991; 1992), as discussed on the following pages.

Current Status of Excimer Laser Research

The number of studies on the use of excimer lasers in dentistry is still relatively small with conflicting results. Part of the reason for these conflicting results is the lack of a systematic approach in the field and the great variety of research disciplines involved. Additionally, the work that has been conducted is often limited with respect to the range of the laser parameters involved and poorly represents the huge number of possible parameter combinations. Selection of laser parameters is often done either on a trial-and-error basis or is simply dictated by the random availability of a particular system.

The situation resembles the general status of research on the interaction of excimer lasers with matter, where a complete understanding of the underlying mechanisms continues to elude researchers. Indeed, despite the large volume of work in this field (Dingus et al, 1990; Dingus and Scamon, 1991; Zyung et al, 1989; Izat et al, 1991; Jackjin et al, 1988; Vogel et al, 1986; Vogel and Lauterborn, 1988; Walsh, 1990), controversies about the dominating mechanisms and their relative importance prevail. Here, too, the processes appear complicated primarily because of the large range of parameters (both in terms of the number and range of variables). Thermal, mechanical, and photochemical reactions take place often simultaneously. Many nonlinear processes come into play as laser variables are changed. Absorption, scattering, and re-radiation all attenuate and redirect laser energy into new directions, thereby changing the laser output characteristics and making correct analysis difficult.

If, however, the parameter range is systematically divided into segments that can be explored individually, a predictable pattern can often be uncovered. Thus, the rationale for the use of lasers for applications on hard dental tissue is that they can interact efficiently, selectively, and in a minimally invasive manner with the various structures of the tooth. While it is quite certain that almost all the time all three ablation mechanisms (photothermal, photochemical, and photomechanical) contribute to the interaction of laser light with hard dental tissue and will determine the safety and efficacy of the treatment, a new understanding of the relationship between a dominant mechanism and the laser setting will allow clinicians to predict the treatment outcome with a high degree of confidence and reliability. Maximum efficiency and minimal injury to adjacent dental tissue or pulp will then be achieved.

This chapter reviews several investigations that have been conducted in the past 4 years, comparing some of the most important characteristics of the interaction of several short pulse excimer lasers with hard dental tissue. Most of the investigations described are basic research in nature, and no clinical studies are included. A 15-nsec pulse from two sources was used: 193-nm wavelength radiation from an ArF excimer laser, and 308-nm radiation from a XeCl excimer laser. Additionally, a XeCl laser with comparable energy and laser pulse repetition rates (PRR), but with much longer pulses of 120 nsec was also used. Ablation rates, tissue thermal responses, surface quality, plume emission spectra, and plume trajectory dynamics following the ablation pulse were compared. These interaction characteristics were studied as a function of PRR, fluence levels (pulse energy per unit area), pulse duration, and spot size.

Hard Tissue Ablation and Antibacterial Investigations

The specific laser systems used in the experiments were: (1) a Lambda-Physik model EMG 103 MSC with ArF fill, emitting pulses of a rectangular beam profile at 193 nm; (2) a Lumonics HyperEX-400 with XeCl fill, also with rectangular pulses of 308-nm radiation; and (3) a long pulse (120 nsec) excimer with a XeCl gas fill. Generally, laser radiation is attenuated to achieve the desired energy and then focused on the treated surface. Laser pulse duration (FWHM) was 15 nsec in systems 1 and 2, and maximum laser energy at the laser output was 200 mJ for the ArF laser, and 150 mJ for the Lumonics XeCl. Fluence levels used in our experiments ranged from 0.5 J/cm^2 to over 25 J/cm^2 in the case of the ArF, and from 1.0 J/cm^2 to 15.0 J/cm^2 in the case of the XeCl laser. Excimer laser repetition rates used in most of our measurements were 1, 5, and 10 Hz, as well as single pulses on demand. Pulse repetition rates as high as 100 Hz were used to assess thermal effects on the tissues. The spot size of the excimer laser and actual profile were measured with a linear photodiode array to within 25 μm (Reticon K-Series with 25 μm center-to-center spacing) and was usually kept at 0.9 mm.

Ultrafast photography of the ablation plume at various stages of its evolution was obtained by using a secondary probe laser to illuminate the plume at the desired time. An Nd:YAG pulsed laser with a KTP nonlinear crystal (Quantel model YG 48 1A) generated 532-nm pulses of 15 nsec (FWHM) duration at repetition rates of 1, 5, and 10 Hz, as well as single pulses on demand. The Nd:YAG beam was used as a probe after its intensity was attenuated to minimize interference with the ablation process, and its shape modified to allow an optimal cross-sectional illumination of the plume. The Nd:YAG beam was perpendicular to the ablating beam (and tangential to the surface), allowing for illumination of the excimer-generated plume. By electronically delaying the Nd:YAG pulse with respect to the excimer laser emission, the Nd:YAG laser was made to function as a stroboscopic light, allowing fast photography of the plume at different stages of its evolution. By simply redirecting the probe beam so it forms an image on a screen, the formation and propagation of shock waves (which appear as dark bands on the bright laser background) were observed and monitored in the air above the ablated dental section.

Laser ablation efficiency was studied by slicing dentin to a prescribed thickness and measuring the duration necessary (at a given repetition rate) for the excimer beam to ablate the material. A weak continuous wave (cw) He:Ne laser beam (< 5 mW), co-linear with the excimer beam, detected the precise moment of drilling completion as it appeared on a screen on the other side of the ablated section. Thermal camera measurements (Inframetrics Model 600 scanning at 60 Hz) allowed studying the effects of the ablating pulse repetition rate and fluence on the surface temperature. Although our thermal camera time response could not resolve temperature distribution on the time scale of the ablation pulse, it did show the material's steady-state thermal response for different pulse repetition rates and fluence levels.

The He:Ne laser was used to ensure that the tooth was positioned at the proper height and that the ablation spot was aligned with the collection optics for each experiment. The control circuit was built with digital electronics and designed to synchronize all the equipment within tens of nanoseconds. The control circuit triggered the excimer lasers, triggered the optical multichannel analyzer OMA (Tracor Northern, Middleton, WI), gated the intensified photodiode array PA (NI-TEC, Niles, IL), and triggered the storage oscilloscope (Tektronix 7834, Irvine, CA). The photodiode was used to detect the onset of emission so that time zero could be ascertained. The intrinsic time delay of the electronics was measured by transferring the gate to the oscilloscope as indicated by a dotted line. The adjustable time delay (t) was then corrected for tint by electronically adjusting the control circuit to t + tint. Also, the gate width could be measured and adjusted electronically to the desired time window. For spectra at different time delays, fresh positions on the target were chosen with an XYZ-precision translation stage.

Spectroscopic information was obtained by focusing the plume emission region onto the input slit of a monochromator. The focusing was achieved with a spherical quartz lens with a focal length of 15 cm, and an f-number that matched the internal optics of the monochromator. The lasers in this case were fired at a PRR of 0.75 Hz so that thermal effects were minimized. The ArF and XeCl laser energies were, respectively, 58.2 ± 2.1 mJ and 57.4 ± 1.0 mJ with a spot size of 1.2 mm^2. The spectra were obtained by adding successive measurements and then subtracting the background with the laser beam blocked. The spectra were then processed by a Macintosh SE/30, where the wavelength calibration was assigned to the data. The wavelength calibration was determined by using He:Ne lasers in the red and the green spectra. All spectra were not corrected for the spectral response of the detector.

The effect of the XeCl excimer laser on the growth of *Streptococcus mutans* in liquid media and on agar plates was studied by placing a bacterial suspension in 96 wells of a culture plate. The contents of 72 wells (three experimental groups of 24 wells each) were exposed to the laser beam for different durations (2, 4, and 8 sec). The remaining 24 wells were not exposed to the laser and served as control samples. Samples were withdrawn from all wells and examined for surviving bacteria. In addition, blood agar plates were inoculated with *S. mutans* and lased with different fluences. Zones of bacterial inhibition were measured. An analysis of variance test was used to determine statistical differences.

Dentin and enamel sections were used for ablation rate studies, while whole teeth, bisected teeth, and sections were used for infrared (IR) thermography and spectroscopic and SEM studies. Freshly extracted third molars were used. Dentin sections 0.5- to 1.0-mm thick were cut from the middle section in a plane perpendicular to the occlusal-cervical direction. Teeth were treated with 0.5 M ethylenediamine tetraacetic acid (EDTA) for 2 minutes to remove the smear layer, then stored in 10% thymol solution until treatment. Enamel samples were sliced parallel to the crown and washed with demineralized water.

Ablation Efficiency Measurements

The ablation rates in dentin obtained with the ArF and XeCl lasers were determined (Fig 18.1). The etch depth per pulse (in µm) was plotted as a function of fluence for PRR of 1 Hz, 5 Hz, and 10 Hz. Each data point was obtained by dividing the total depth ablated by the number of pulses required to achieve this depth. Thus the data typically represent an average over several hundred pulses.

The curve for the ArF ablation at 5 Hz (see Fig 18.1a) shows an etch depth per pulse that increases exponentially from 0.3511 µm/pulse at 0.8 J/cm^2 to 1.13 µm/pulse at 10.0 J/cm^2. A similar exponential increase of etch depth/pulse is observed at the ablation rate of 10 Hz. Here, the etch depth/pulse ranges from 0.36 µm/pulse at 0.8 J/cm^2 to 1.18 µm/pulse at 10.0 J/cm^2. Thus, variations in repetition rate in this regime do not significantly affect dentin ablation efficiency. Lower repetition rates, however, do seem to have a more significant effect on ablation efficiency. At 1 Hz, etch depth per pulse is about 0.4 µm for dentin ablation, even at a fluence level as high as 10.0 J/cm^2. (This is about half the etch rate of the laser at 5 Hz and 10 Hz). Measurements at 1 Hz and low fluence levels are slow and tedious as ablation efficiency is considerably lower, and ablation times become very long. Thus, accurate ablation efficiencies were not obtained in the case of ablation with 193-nm radiation in the low fluence regime and 1-Hz PRR. In this regime, the fast photography technique was helpful in recognizing that active ablation (including ejection of debris, plasma formation, and shock wave generation) was occurring.

The ablation of dentin by the XeCl 308-nm radiation at the higher fluence regime is considerably more efficient than that of the ArF (see Fig 18.1b). The etch depth at 1.0 J/cm^2 is about 0.68 µm/pulse both 5 Hz and 10 Hz, and only slightly lower, 0.4911 µm/pulse, at 1 Hz. Note that these values are not much different than the values obtained with the ArF system. This is no longer true when the laser fluence is in-

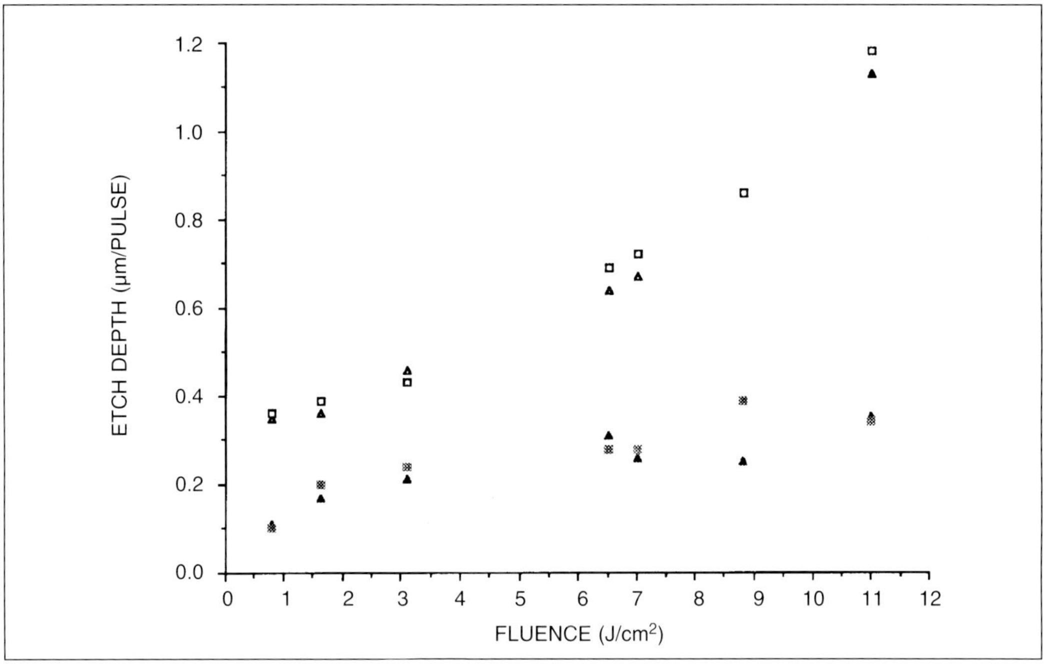

Fig 18.1a Etch depth per pulse vs fluence in dentin (hollow symbols) and enamel (solid symbols) ablation, at 5 Hz (triangles) and 10 Hz (squares) with ArF laser.

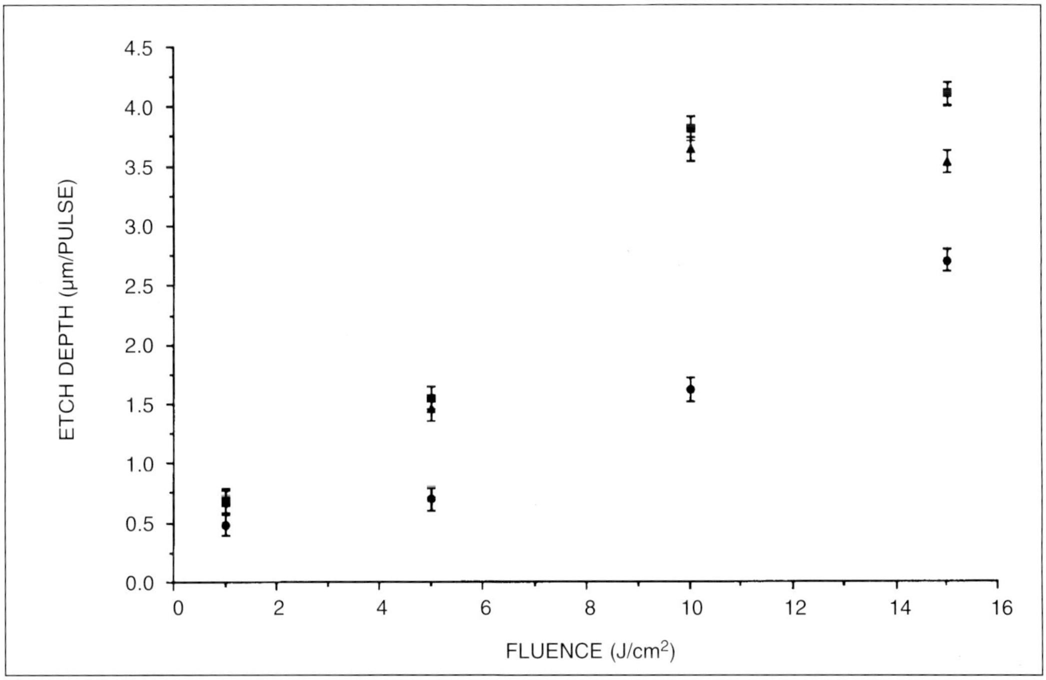

Fig 18.1b Dentin ablation rates with the XeCl laser at 1 Hz (circles), 5 Hz (triangles), and 10 Hz (squares).

creased. At 10.0 J/cm^2 we find the etch rate to be 1.621 μm/pulse at 1 Hz, 3.64 μm/pulse at 5 Hz, and 3.82 μm/pulse at 10 Hz. These values are about three times larger than the corresponding ablation rates of the ArF laser. Interestingly, the ablation rate curves at 5 and 10 Hz level off with further increase in fluence. The entire curve has two inflection points and forms an S shape: initially, the curves show a weak exponential increase, then, with a further increase in fluence level, they saturate at about 3.7 μm/pulse. Thus, at 15.0 J/cm^2, there is a 3.53 μm/pulse at 5 Hz and a 4.1 μm/pulse at 10 Hz. The 1-Hz curve at this fluence shows, as expected, a lower ablation efficiency of 2.7, 11 μm/pulse, although the second inflection point and saturation are not yet observed. We believe that this curve has the same characteristics as those of the 5-Hz and 10-Hz curves, but the S shape is not observed because the entire curve is stretched in the direction of increasing fluence. Also, note that at low fluence levels, ablation efficiencies at all PRR converge to the same value, as the importance of the thermal component diminishes and the ablation threshold is approached. Finally, observe that similar to the behavior of the ArF laser, ablation efficiencies of the XeCl system at 5 Hz are very close to the efficiencies at 10 Hz. The main effect of increased PRR is that the heat generated by one pulse is affecting the interaction of the tissue with the following pulse. The similar response to increasing PRR, therefore, suggests that the thermal component of the ablation plays a similar role in both lasers, despite the significant difference in wavelength.

Light Microscopy Observations

Light microscopy observations of treated enamel and dentin surfaces after irradiation by 5.0 J/cm^2 of 193-nm light at 10 Hz for 5 minutes showed that there was practically no thermal damage to the exposed surfaces and they were extremely smooth and free of cracks and fractures. This was always the case at all fluences up to PRR less than 20 Hz. Only at higher PRR (over 50 Hz) do we begin to observe thermal damage such as charring and cracking. At very low fluence levels (such as 0.3 mJ/cm^2 and 10 Hz), we find an incomplete ablation with a rough surface and pillar-like structures.

Surfaces ablated with the XeCl system also showed no evidence of thermal damage or charring at the lower PRR (below 50 Hz). The ablation by the 308-nm laser is more efficient than that of the 193-nm laser. This is a consequence of the larger penetration depth of light at this longer wavelength. The longer penetration depth means that a larger volume of material is affected and ejected from the crater. This larger volume of ablation debris and gases is confined to a crater of the same lateral dimension as in the 193-nm radiation and will, therefore, result in stronger lateral stresses on the crater's wall and in a higher likelihood of mechanical fracturing of the surface. Indeed, this could be observed in light microscopy photographs of the XeCl laser–treated dentin: very small cracks and microfractures are observed at almost all fluence levels and all PRR, even though no thermal damage or charring is detected. The surface damage is likely due to mechanical stresses as previously explained. Note, however, that similar to the ArF system, very high PRR (> 50 Hz) do result in thermal damage and charring.

Thermal Camera Measurements

An IR thermal camera (Inframetrics Model 600 Imaging Radiometer, Bedford, MA) with a scan speed of 30 frames per second was used for temperature measurements. The center temperature adjustment ranges from 20°C to 1,500°C. The camera field of view (FOV) could be adjusted from 1:1 to 8:1 and was maintained at 2:1 or 4:1. The camera detector was a liquid nitrogen–cooled Hg:Cd:Te with spectral sensitivity from 8 to 12 µm. The thermal camera was placed so that the surface temperature (ST) could be viewed directly. The camera was operated in the point mode so that center temperature could be read with the camera-specified accuracy of ±0.5 degrees. For thermal penetration depth (TPD), the camera was placed at a ninety-degree angle to the treatment site and operated in the isotherm mode, which yielded contour areas of equal temperature within ±5.0°C. Dentin and enamel sample preparation was performed as previously described, except when TPD was studied, where teeth were simply bisected longitudinally along the sagittal plane.

ArF Laser (193 nm, 15 nsec). Initial experiments showed linear dependence of ST on PRR in both enamel and dentin. Fluence levels ranged from 50 mJ/cm^2 to 25 J/cm^2. Pulse repetition rate was tested from 1 to 100 Hz. Temperature increased linearly with PRR for both enamel and dentin (Fig 18.2a) and, for the same parameters at higher fluences, enamel surface temperatures reached higher values than those of dentin. If PRR of 20 Hz or lower were used, temperatures of dentin and enamel remained below 50°C and below 60°C, respectively. If higher PRR were used (50 and 100 Hz), surface temperatures reached 150°C or even 200°C in dentin and 200°C and 300°C in enamel. Because ST (which are the highest temperatures on a target) remained relatively low (below the level of coagulation) during treatment with the ArF laser, we did not investigate TPD and thermal diffusion into the root canal.

XeCl Laser (308 nm, 15 nsec). Thermal camera studies monitored the effect of PRR, fluence, beam spot size on ST, and TPD into the treated tooth and the root canal. Pulse repetition rates ranged from 10 to 35 Hz and fluences from 0.5 to 5.0 J/cm^2. Spot size ranged from 0.4 to 10 mm^2. The studies showed (as for ArF) a linear dependence on PRR with surface temperatures below 80°C at all PRR for fluences of 1 J/cm^2 or smaller. At 5 J/cm^2 and PRR of 25 Hz or higher, temperatures reached a range of 100 to 140°C, even for this small spot size of 0.4 mm^2. Temperature depended linearly on spot size, and for 1 J/cm^2 and 25 Hz temperatures ranged from 70°C at 0.4 mm^2 to about 600°C at 10 mm^2. For a relatively small spot size of 2 mm^2 and a fluence of 0.5 J/cm^2, TPD did not reach the root canal at any of the PRR used (Fig 18.2b). However, at the higher fluence of 5 J/cm^2 and PRR of 35 or 25 Hz, the studies showed that TPD extended 3 to 4 mm from the surface and thus reached into the vicinity of the root canal (temperature increase at this depth is about 5°C greater than ambient temperature). One must keep in mind that since the tooth was cut in half, this temperature rise is about twice what one would expect for a whole tooth.

Scanning Electron Microscopy

Scanning electron microscopy investigations in our laboratories were performed on dentin sections or bisected teeth prepared as previously described. Following irradiation, each dentin section was washed briefly with 100% ETOH and mounted on a stub with colloidal silver liquid (Ted Pella Inc, Redding, CA) with the

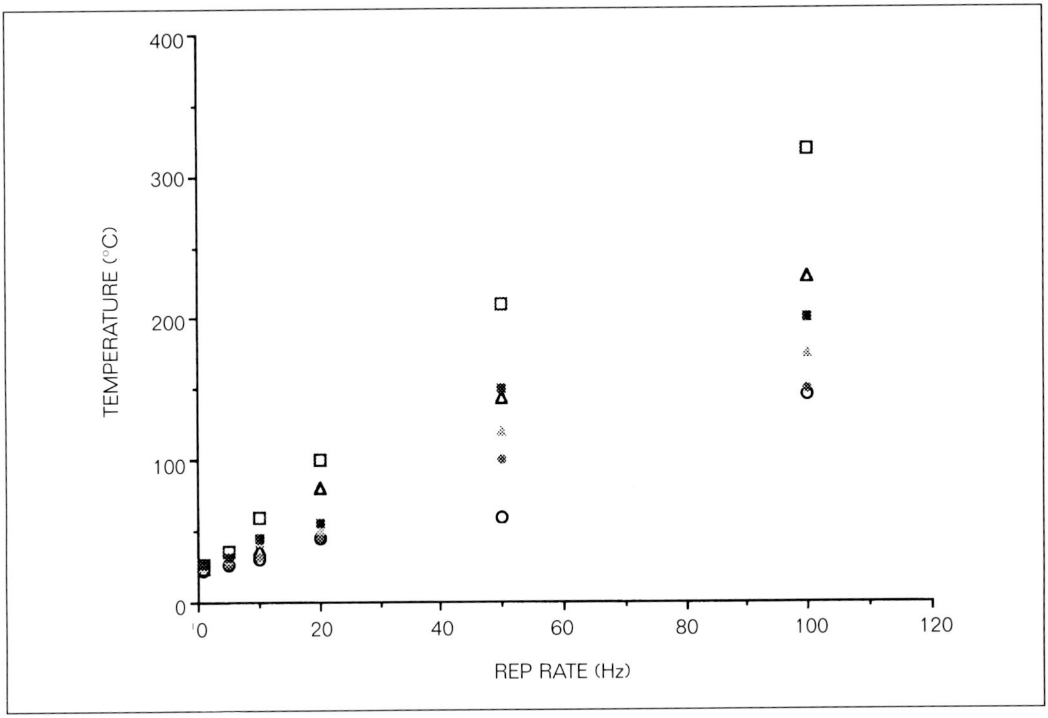

Fig 18.2a ArF ablation of dentin (solid symbols) and enamel (hollow symbols). Surface temperature vs PRR for 4 J/cm^2 (circles), 10 J/cm^2 (triangles), 20 J/cm^2 (hollow squares), and 25 J/cm^2 (solid squares).

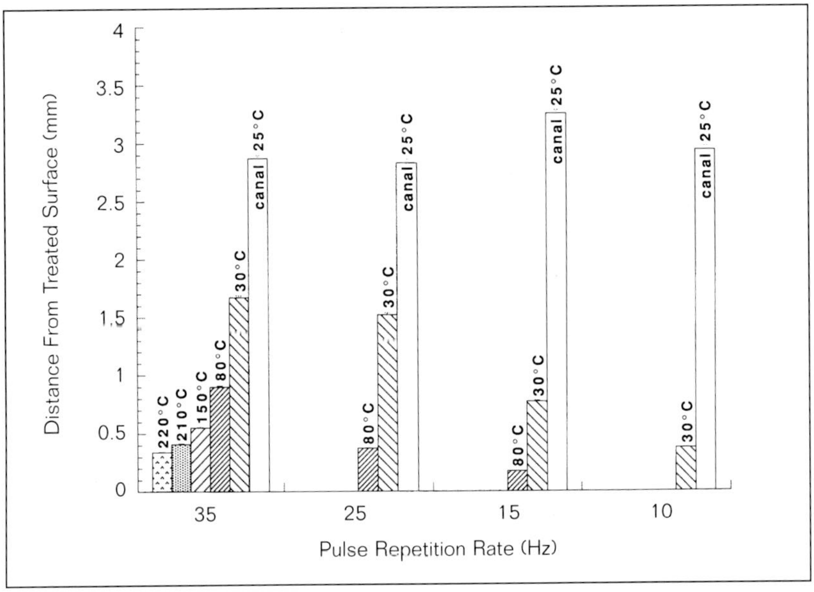

Fig 18.2b Heat penetration profiles as a function of pulse repetition rate in XeCl ablation of dentin. The position of the root canal is indicated in each case. Respective temperatures (°C) at each depth are shown on top of the bars.

and 4 takes account of the light field compression effect.

In the calculation results of the intensity attenuation of collimated and diffuse fluxes in enamel and dentin calculated according to equations 3, 4, 5, the rate of attenuation in dentin is substantially lower than that in enamel and the intensities of both fluxes in dentin are very close (Fig 19.6).

Nonlinear Optical Characteristics of Tooth Hard Tissues

There are no experimental data on nonlinear characteristics of tooth hard tissues in the literature. Meanwhile, the studies in this field could serve as a good basis for new diagnostic methods. The main substance of hard biotissues (hydroxyapatite) is not highly nonlinear. Therefore, one may hardly expect strong nonlinear effects in tooth hard tissues. Generally speaking, they must be observed in the field of short powerful light pulses (shorter than 10 to 7 sec) when the intensity is close to the damage threshold. Nevertheless, the level of this intensity can vary by several orders of magnitude less for enamel and dentin organic components.

Electron Nonlinearity

First of all, this is the generation of optical harmonics, or the doubling and tripling of the incident light frequency. Since hydroxyapatite crystals are not centrally symmetric, frequency doubling can exist in a tooth. A certain order of these crystals as well as the existence of waveguiding structures could enhance this effect. These factors could substantially enhance transformation into the third harmonic. Harmonic generation could be expected when there is reflection from the enamel surface and at the enamel-dentin junction. These effects are probably observed in the field of extremely short light pulses.

Effects connected with the electron nonlinearity of the refractive index would hardly be of significance because of the high microheterogeneity of hard tissues. The nonlinearity of electron absorption, however, could be substantial in the blue and near ultraviolet (UV) range. Effects of local field enhancement on microparticles forming dental hard tissues and the electron nonlinearity of surface conditions could be displayed in the same spectrum range.

Electron-Oscillation Nonlinearity

Electron oscillation of non-linearity causes effects of stimulated Raman scattering (SRS). High light attenuation due to elastic scattering substantially decreases the probability of observing this effect in a tooth. Nevertheless, waveguide effects, especially in dentin, hopefully will allow achievement of the threshold of SRS.

Lattice Nonlinearity

This kind of nonlinearity is displayed in the range of photon absorption in hydroxyapatite crystals. The lattice nonlinearity of the refractive index would hardly be of significance; nevertheless, the lattice absorption nonlinearity will have a substantial effect on the interaction of powerful infrared (IR) radiation with enamel and dentin.

Heat Nonlinearity

The heating of teeth by laser radiation must first of all cause changes in the absorption index in the near IR range. The mechanism of this effect is displayed in the temperature shift of absorption bands observed with H_2O molecules situated in hard tissues. It could be important for the development of the prethreshold condition for laser induced tooth destruction.

Laser-Induced Destruction of Dental Hard Tissues

Laser destruction of hard media is one of the most important aspect of laser physics. Until recently, basic works in this field dealt with the studies of mechanisms of laser destruction of metals, semiconductors, polymers, optical crystals, and glasses. Detailed studies of laser destruction laws were carried out, and theoretical models were developed for the previously mentioned media. Nevertheless, despite the enormous number of published studies, one can hardly imagine that all of the problems have been solved in this area of laser physics.

Many specialists dealing with lasers for hard tissue processing (enamel, dentin, bone tissues) still think that it is possible to operate without first performing the fundamental studies necessary to determine the basic mechanisms and principles of laser destruction. For example, the practice of laser surgery was developed, strictly speaking, on an exceptionally empirical basis. As our experience shows, such an approach is hardly applicable to hard tissues. High-quality processing of hard tissues (for instance, tooth hard tissues) can be carried out only when the characteristics (parameters) of laser radiation are controlled within a very narrow range. The operating mode selected must provide for the following conditions to be effective:

1. The rate of tissue removal must provide a permissible duration of laser operation.
2. The level of tooth overheating must not cause thermal damage of the pulp and the tissues adjacent to enamel and dentin.
3. Thermal stresses must not be above the threshold to cause macrocracks and microcracks on the laser cavity surface.
4. The recoil moment (mechanical and/or acoustic pressure) must not cause contusion of the pulp or patient discomfort during laser treatment.
5. The laser cavity created on the enamel or dentin surface must provide the appropriate conditions for the stable adhesion and adaptation of dental filling materials.

What is this range? This question can be answered only by the proposed theory of laser destruction and through detailed investigations. At present little is known about the mechanisms of hard tissue destruction. It is clear that the basic knowledge of laser destruction developed for homogeneous media (such as crystals, glasses, optical polymers) could be inapplicable to hard tissues because enamel, dentin, and bone tissues have a complicated heterogeneous structure. New, specific mechanisms of laser destruction, however, could be developed. For example, consider a case in which the laser radiation wavelength coincides with the absorption peak of one of the components of the medium. Then, with powerful laser irradiation, the actively absorbing component will expand on heating, which will result in the generation of nonbalanced mechanical stresses. This will cause disruption of the irradiated volume without melting and evaporation. Such a mechanism of "cold" destruction requires minimal energy and is accomplished with minimal heat.

To develop a proper model of hard tissue laser destruction, it is necessary to know the destruction mechanisms. This chapter considers only the model of laser heating (temperature propagation within a tooth during exposure to laser radiation) that takes into account the geometry of teeth and their thermophysical characteristics. In most cases, laser destruction of teeth is accompanied by heating, which will be a part of the complete model of laser destruction. Furthermore, this model allows conditions to be defined when there is no thermal damage to human dental tissues (for instance, to define a moment when the limiting permissible overheating of tooth pulp is achieved).

Thermophysical Model

When analyzing the destruction of dental hard tissue, it is necessary to first work out the most adequate descriptions that allow a real tooth to be substituted with a certain model. It is necessary to take into account its complicated geometric shape and the fact that a real tooth is a complex nonhomogeneous object in terms of optics as well as thermophysics. Additionally, the magnitudes of the observed optical and thermophysical characteristics can vary substantially during destruction.

When considering material destruction and removal with laser pulses, the process of laser action on a tooth within a pulse can be divided into three sequential stages: (1) pre-threshold heating; (2) destruction; and (3) post-destruction heating. The first stage begins simultaneously with the beginning of a pulse and terminates when the laser destruction threshold is achieved. In this stage, there is a quasi-adiabatic heating of a certain tissue volume up to the following temperature:

$$T(r,z)= \frac{\beta(r,z)}{C_p(r,z)g(r,z)}\int_0^{\tau_p} I(r,\tau)\exp[-\aleph(r,z)]d\tau \quad (6)$$

Where Tr, z = temperature, the spatial coordinates, $\aleph$ = the light attenuation, β = the absorption index, Cp, g = the specific heat capacity and density of tissue, respectively, β = the absorption coefficient of the medium, I = the function describing the spatially temporal distribution of a laser pulse incident on the surface, τ = the time, τp = pre-threshold heating duration.

Within the next stage (destruction), the process of tissue removal takes place, accompanied by travel of the destruction boundary in the direction $Z > 0$. This stage is described with the following equation:

$$C_p(r,z)g(r,z)V(z)\frac{\partial T}{\partial z}+\frac{\partial}{\partial z}\left[\lambda(r,z)\frac{\partial T}{\partial z}\right] + \frac{1}{r}\frac{\partial}{\partial r}\left[\lambda(r,z)r\frac{\partial T}{\partial r}\right] = \beta(r,z)I(r,\tau)\exp[-\aleph(r,z)] \quad (7)$$

with corresponding boundary conditions. Here $\lambda(r,z)$ = the thermal conductivity of tissue, and V = the velocity of destruction boundary travel in the direction $Z > 0$.

An adequate definition of V is a complicated task when there is no clear understanding of destruction mechanisms. On the other hand, this function can be specified phenomenologically, based on the experimental findings of destruction processes.

The next stage begins at the trailed edge of a pulse (when due to a power decrease, the destruction process terminates) and ends when a pulse ceases. Within this stage, the remaining pulse power is absorbed and the thermal disturbance is then relaxed within the geometry of the object that was changed by the pro-

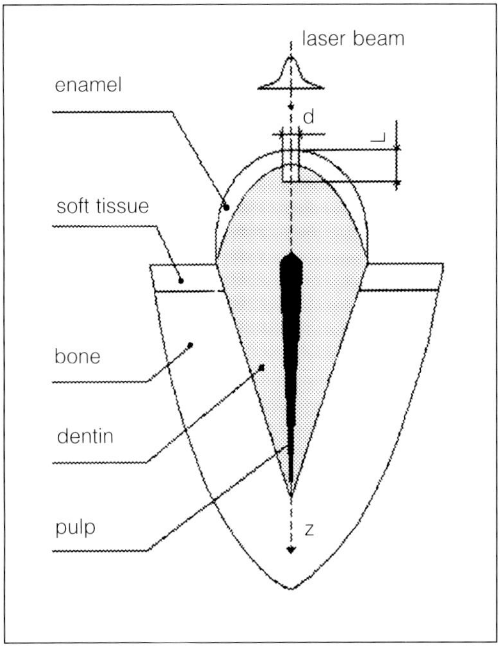

Fig 19.7 Geometric model of a tooth used in mathematical simulations.

cessing. The following equation corresponds to this case:

$$C_p(r,z)g(r,z)\frac{\partial T}{\partial \tau}+\frac{\partial}{\partial z}[\lambda(r,z)\frac{\partial T}{\partial z}] + \frac{1}{r}\frac{\partial}{\partial r}[\lambda(r,z)r\frac{\partial T}{\partial r}] = \beta(r,z)I(r,\tau)\exp[-\aleph(r,z)] \quad (8)$$

It is clear from this equation that the calculation results of every preceding stage determine the initial and boundary conditions for a subsequent stage. The same can be said about the simulation of a pulse train action. The description of thermal relaxation within a pulse interval is similar to the description of a subsequent stage of laser action at I $(r,\tau) = 0$. In the tooth geometric model, which is used in our thermophysical model, the apex (cusp tip) of an anatomic crown is considered a hemisphere, with its sides being cylindrical (Fig 19.7). The root's apex is visualized as a cone. The anatomic crown exchanges heat with the surroundings and coolant (in the case of forced cooling). This is taken into account by means of the boundary conditions of type III. The tooth root is in thermal contact with the gingival periodontal ligament and bone, which is taken into account by means of the boundary conditions of type IV. Geometric dimensions of the model are quite close to the real ones.

The described model is nearly universal and allows different patterns of laser interactions to be simulated. For example, compare the results of Nd, Ho, and Er laser radiation effects on human tooth enamel. Laser energy densities, focusing conditions, and repetition rates are chosen from the point of view of achieving maximum ablation efficiency. Heat exchange conditions in this example are also maximized by forced water cooling. At the chosen conditions for this experiment, the Nd laser provides for a very shallow processing depth of approximately 60 µm (Fig 19.8). If the processing is continued, laser radiation will cause pulp overheating. The Ho:YAG laser can penetrate enamel to a depth of 1.6 mm before its radiation starts causing trauma. The Er:YAG laser is most efficient, with a maximum cut depth up to 13 mm.

The same model can be used to work out the relationship between the temporal structure of repetitively pulsed radiation and pulp chamber overheating. In our example, erbium laser radiation has the following parameters: pulse energy = 0.2 J, number of pulses = 25, and the gaussian beam radius on the enamel surface = 200 µm, with forced surface cooling. In the first case, the total duration of the pulse train is set at 25 sec which corresponds to the pulse repetition rate of 1 Hz; in the second and third cases, it is fixed at 2.5 (10 Hz)

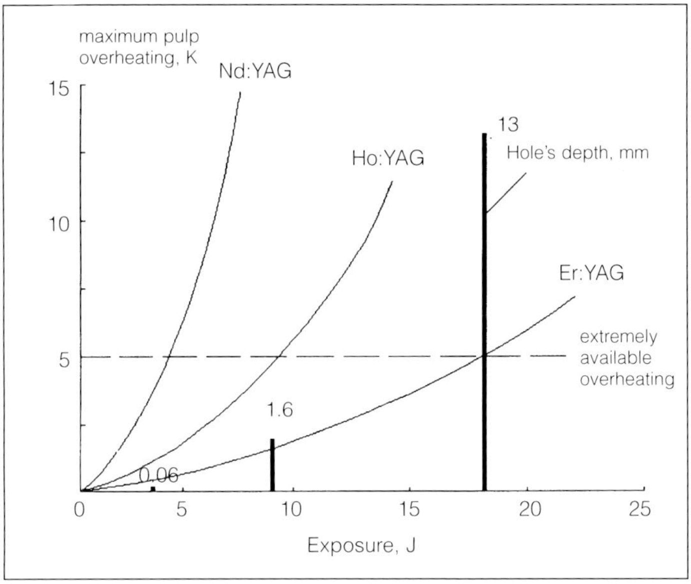

Fig 19.8 The relationship between pulp chamber overheating and laser radiation exposure, where the parameters are as follows: Ho:YAG laser = 0.2-mm spot diameter, energy 0.2 J, pulse rate 10 Hz; Er:YAG laser = 0.4-mm spot diameter, energy 0.2 J , pulse rate 10 Hz; Nd:YAG laser = 0.1-mm spot diameter, energy 0.2 J, pulse rate 10 Hz.

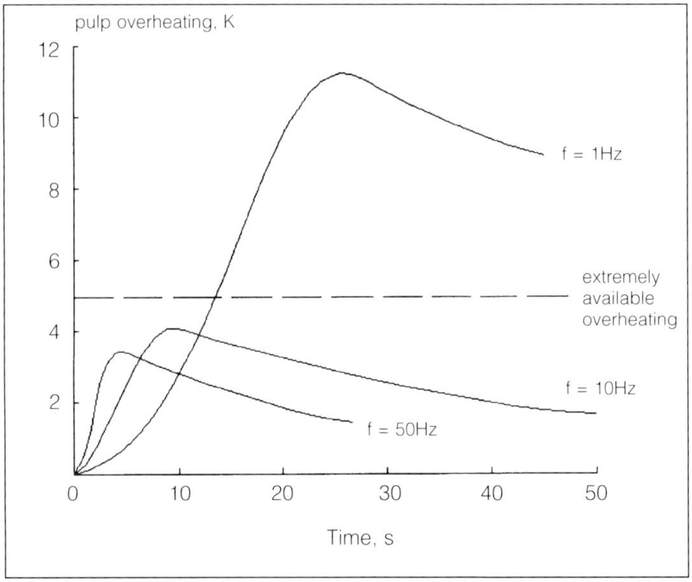

Fig 19.9 The relationship between pulp chamber overheating and Er:YAG laser pulse repetition rate (radiation exposure was equal in all cases).

and 0.5 sec (50 Hz), respectively. In all three cases, the laser cavity depth is equal (Fig 19.9). Based on the results of these calculations, heating dynamics is highly dependent on the pulse repetition rate. As seen here, there should be a maximum repetition rate that once exceeded, will inevitably result in pulp chamber overheating. As we see, the computer simulation model is a powerful instrument enabling scientists to make reasonable predictions of probable laser-tissue interactions and to optimize irradiation modes. It is also clear that when there is no reliable information on the mechanisms of laser destruction, the mathematical model is substantially

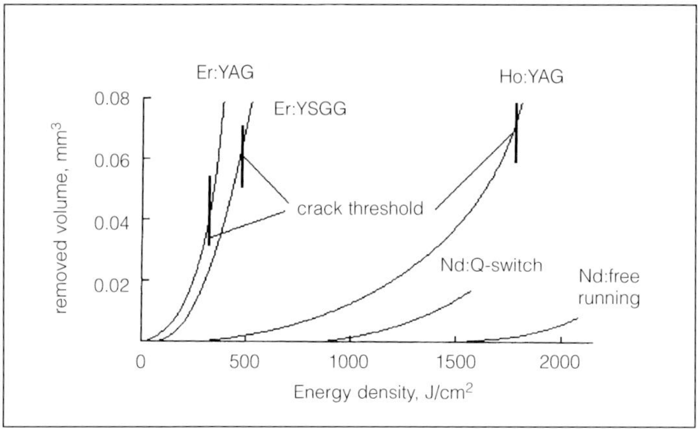

Fig 19.10 The relationship between enamel ablation efficiency per pulse for various laser types and energy density.

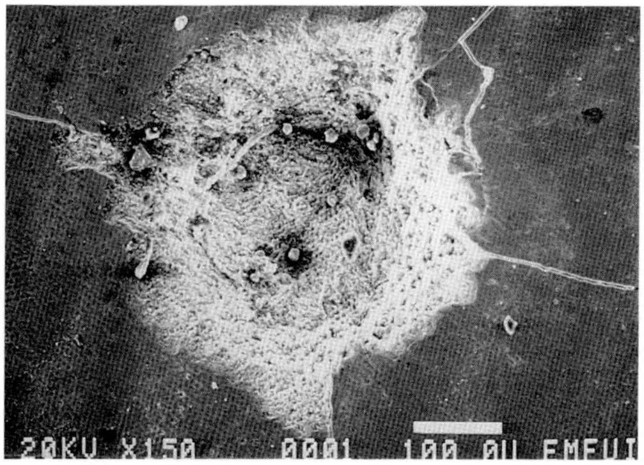

Fig 19.11 Scanning electron micrograph of Ho:YAG laser crater in enamel. Single pulse = 1 J.

limited in its predictive abilities. The importance of confirming the accuracy of the theoretical model predictions with actual experimental data is obvious.

Experimental Studies

Thus far a number of lasers have been compared that could probably be used as a laser handpiece. The relationship between the volume of dental enamel removed within a single pulse and the laser energy density of various laser types is relative (Fig 19.10). It is obvious, for instance, that a change in laser pulse shape or duration will result in a certain deformation of the given curves, and so on. Nevertheless, a basis is required for comparison. As expected, the Er:YAG laser is a leader in ablation efficiency, while the Nd:YAG is lowest, even if special emission modes are used, such as Q-switching pulses as illustrated (see Fig 19.10). Although the Ho:YAG laser enjoys an advantage of a comparatively wide range of permissible energy densities, it still occupies an intermediate position in terms of preference. Results of the SEM analysis of a Ho:YAG laser cavity surface indicate that in the range of energy densities near the destruction threshold for enamel, a cavity surface is melted off and surrounding tissues are thermally damaged (Fig 19.11). This thermal effect decreases, however, when the energy density is subsequently increased. The range of permissible energy densities is limited by the occurrence of macrodefects and cracks. Therefore, the operating range of energy densities of a specific laser system intended for enamel and dentin ablation must be much higher than the damage threshold for those substances to prevent cracks and thermal damage to surrounding structures.

As seen in this example, the Ho:YAG laser in this respect is preferable. In con-

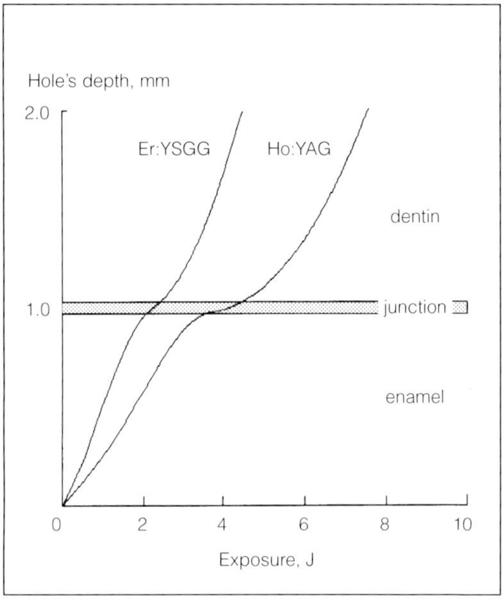

Fig 19.12 The relationship between laser crater depth and laser radiation exposure. Er:YAG laser = 110 J/cm^2; Ho:YAG laser = 1,200 J/cm^2.

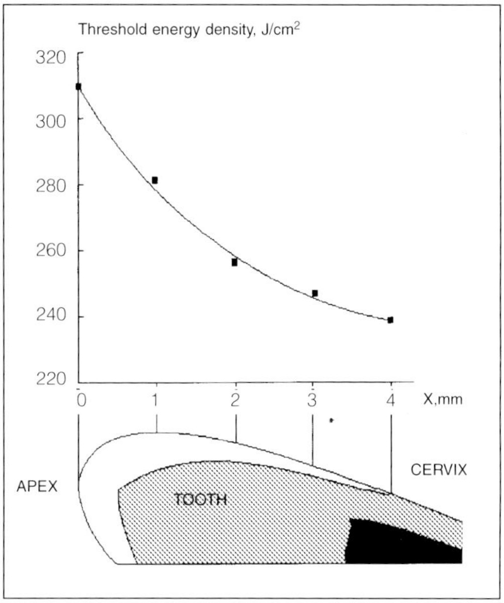

Fig 19.13 The relationship between the enamel damage threshold energy and location of the radiation on the tooth crown. Apex = cusp tip; cervix = cementoenamel junction.

trast, the Er:YAG laser operation requires much more accuracy, which can be considered a disadvantage for the dentist.

Laser Ablation Efficiency

Laser ablation efficiency is defined as the volume of tissue removed by a unit of radiant energy. The relationships between the hole depth and laser radiation exposure are nonlinear and the destruction depth varies from pulse to pulse (multipulsed operation mode) (Fig 19.12). This relationship is probably related to the modification of the cavity surface that occurs as a result of initial ablation as well as with the decrease in laser radiation density because of the displacement of the plane of processing away from the beam waist (focal spot). It is also remarkable that the slope of the curve (processing rate) depends on the type of the processed tissue (enamel, enamel-dentin junction, dentin). Magnitudes of the processing rate for Er:YAG laser for enamel and dentin are displayed in the Table. The processing rate for dentin is higher than that for enamel, which correlates inversely with the relative magnitudes of their damage thresholds. The influence of spray cooling on removal efficiency was also studied. Enamel removal efficiency is increased when spray cooling is used, while cooling has a negative effect on dentin removal efficiency.

There is also spatial nonuniformity of the enamel damage threshold (Fig 19.13).

Table. Magnitudes of Processing Rate for Er:YAG Laser

Tissue	Efficiency (x 10^{-3} mm^3/J)	
	Without Cooling	With Cooling
Enamel	12 ± 1	17 ± 2
Dentin	53 ± 5	36 ± 3

The nonuniformity is revealed in the relationship between the magnitude of the damage threshold and the location of the exposure on a tooth's crown surface. As seen, the laser destruction threshold for enamel increases in the direction from "cervix" (cementoenamel junction or cervical area) toward the "apex" (cusp tip). The nonuniformity of the damage threshold at various locations on the tooth surface is reflected in the nonuniformity of material removal efficiency as described. This factor is very significant and must be taken into account when using lasers in clinical practice.

In the relationship between the single pulse enamel removal efficiency of Er:YAG and Ho:YAG laser radiation and the location of the beam waist (focal spot), laser beam focusing under the enamel surface (prefocusing) improves the removal efficiency (Fig 19.14).

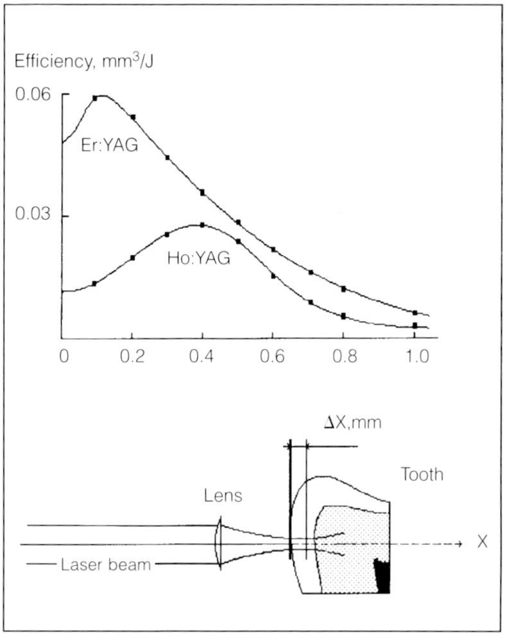

Fig 19.14 The relationship between enamel removal efficiency per pulse and laser focal spot location relative to the tooth surface.

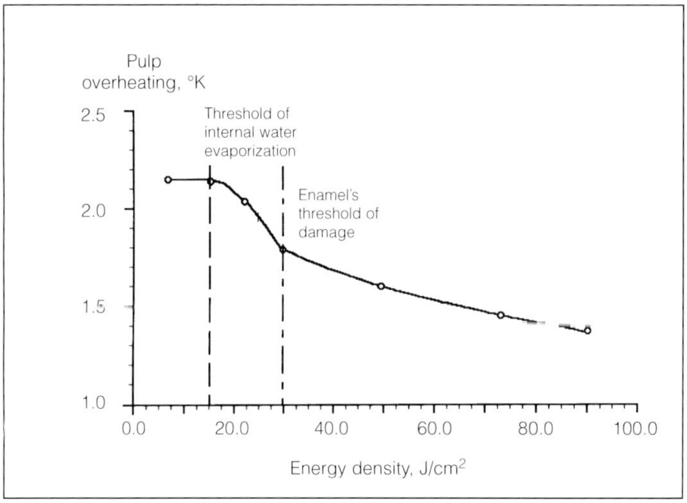

Fig 19.15 The relationship between pulp chamber overheating and Er:YAG laser radiation energy density.

The Tooth Pulp Temperature Response

We have also investigated the relationship between tooth pulp overheating and Er:YAG laser energy density under conditions when the radiation exposure energy is kept constant (Fig 19.15). Measurements were taken at the radiation exposure of 2.25 J while a tooth was placed in a thermostat. A decrease in tooth pulp overheating is observed when the energy density is increased. A reverse bend in the slope of the curve is seen at a point corresponding to the threshold energy density of laser destruction (30 J/cm^2). The magnitude of energy spent on material destruction exclusively (ie, specific ablation heat) can be estimated analyzing this relationship. As seen, under optimal focusing conditions, pulp overheating can be decreased by 40% due to the efficient escape of overheated decay products.

We considered several optical characteristics of dental hard tissues at different light intensities. The presented results display a modern level of knowledge of tooth optics. Still, there are many gaps in the extent of our knowledge, the resolution of which is the task for future researchers.

Acknowledgments

Some results presented in this chapter were obtained in close cooperation with our coworkers Andrey V. Belikov and Vladimir N. Grisimov, to whom we would like to express our deepest appreciation.

References

Altshuler GB, Grisimov VN. Effect of waveguide light propagation in human tooth [in Russian]. Dokl Acad Sci USSR 1990;3:1245–1248.

Altshuler GB, Grisimov V, Erofeev AV, et al. Human tooth as an optical device. SPIE Proc Holography Interferometry Opt Pattern Recognition Biomed 1991;1429: 95–104.

Chapter Twenty

New Concepts in Laser-Tissue Interaction

Guy Levy and Ioana M. Rizoiu

The main problem to be considered when analyzing the process of interaction between a laser beam and different organomineral structures is the complexity of tissue components. Any damaging side effects induced by the laser beam during the interaction process have to be minimized or avoided to protect the vitality of the cellular components (such as odontoblasts, fibroblasts, cementoblasts, or osteoblasts) of the organomineral structures. Considering that most of the time a laser beam interacts with the organomineral structures in a pure thermal mode, the most probable effect is tissue necrosis.

Major factors of control for the laser-induced thermal effect are: the proportion of organic and mineral substances in tissue; water content; vascularization; and tissue thermal properties, such as thermoconductivity and thermocapacity.

Optical Properties of Hard Tissues

The selection of an appropriate laser wavelength for specific tissues, such as organominerals, is of major importance for successful clinical intervention. Laser wavelengths with specific absorption for tissue components have the ability to control the interaction process by minimizing the thermal damage.

Because organomineral tissues are turbid or translucent types of materials, the diffuse and specular reflectance or transmittance properties are more appropriate for a description of the optical properties of these tissues. By definition, specular reflectance is the component of reflected light that is the result of a mirrorlike reflection off a sample (tissue) surface. The second type of reflectance, diffuse reflectance, is defined as light reflected in many directions by the surface of the sample. For transmittance, the specular component represents the light that travels directly through the sample in a straight line, not being affected by molecular or morphologic components of the tissue. On the contrary, the diffuse component of transmittance is totally controlled by tissue components that deviate the light from the main direction in many directions. For example, a transparent sample such as a pane of glass has almost a total specular

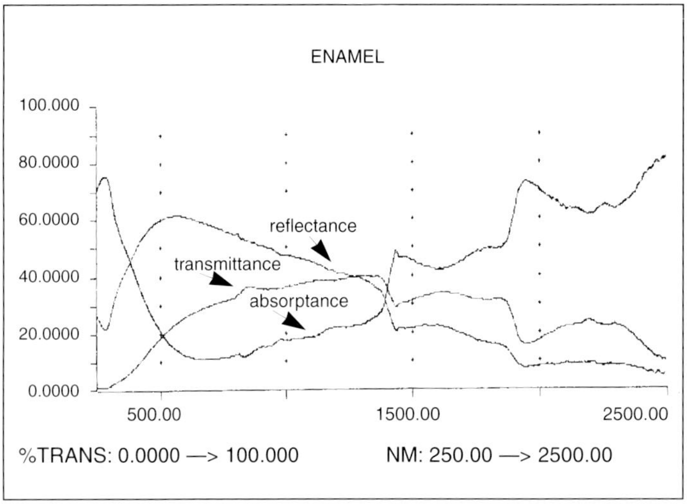

Fig 20.1 The spectra of absorptance, transmittance, and reflectance for sound enamel.

transmittance. As this glass becomes more frosted (translucent), the diffuse component of light becomes more evident.

Recent studies of the optical properties of dentin, enamel, bone, and hydroxyapatite were performed with spectrophotometry in a range of wavelengths from 250 to 2,500 nm (Wigdor et al, 1993). As the standard spectrophotometric methods proved to be inadequate because of the loss of light resulting from the scattering effects of these tissues, a traditional integrating sphere was the ideal accessory used for the experiments.

Enamel

Enamel is made of an extremely hard, translucent substance composed of 97% inorganic mineral material and approximately 3% organic substance, with a minimal water content.

The crystalline structure of parallel rods or prisms that extend from the dentin-enamel juncture to the surface of the anatomic crown are of a particular geometry and configuration. Seen in cross sections, the same rods of enamel are hexagonal, oval, or polygonal in shape with an average diameter of about 5 μm. Each rod of enamel is composed of microscopic crystals of hydroxyapatite embedded in a sparse framework of organic substance (Copenhaven et al, 1978). The high thermoconductivity ($k = 9.34 \times 10^3$ W/cm°C) of enamel is due to its structure and composition.

By following each spectrum of absorptance, transmittance and reflectance for sound enamel, major peaks or valleys that describe the way light penetrates the tissue can be easily identified (Fig 20.1). However, the spectra of absorptance show three major peaks at 283 nm, 1,434 nm and 1,944 nm. The peaks at 1,434 and 1,944 nm coincide with the absorption peaks for water. For reflectance and transmittance, the profile of the spectra is almost the reverse of the spectrum of absorption, so each peak in absorption is now a valley in transmittance or reflectance. The highest absorption in ultraviolet is approximately at the same level as the highest absorption in the infrared region. According to published data, wave-

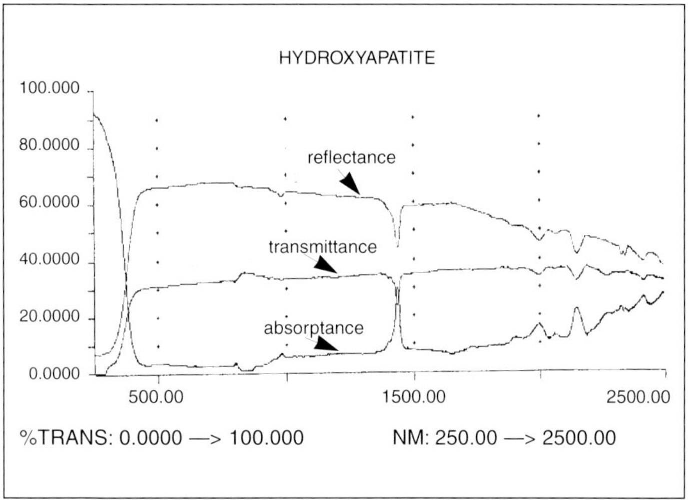

Fig 20.2 The spectra of absorptance, transmittance, and reflectance for hydroxyapatite.

lengths between 2,700 and 2,900 nm are strongly absorbed by water and hydroxyapatite (Wigdor et al, 1994).

Concerning the transmittance properties of enamel in the far infrared region, there are two wavelengths of interest. The first wavelength at 3,570 nm corresponds to a major peak of approximately 100% transmission. The transparency of enamel for this wavelength might be an interesting application for diagnosis. The second wavelength at 9,410 nm shows a major valley of transmittance, which is not higher than 5%. The region between 9,000 and 10,000 nm corresponds to strong absorption for hydroxyapatite and water. However, the CO_2 laser that operates in this region has a strong thermal impact on enamel.

The absorptance spectrum of hydroxyapatite presents a major peak at 1,434 nm and a few minor peaks at 1,994 nm, 2,145 nm, and 2,410 nm (Fig 20.2). It is important to note that in the ultraviolet region the absorptance reaches the highest level of 91%, corresponding to a wavelength at 250 nm. In a comparison of the absorptance spectra of hydroxyapatite and enamel, there are significant differences between the two. First, there is a decrease in absorptance background and diminution of the major peak at 1,434 nm for hydroxyapatite as compared to enamel. Also, some of the minor peaks of absorptance for hydroxyapatite at 2,145 and 2,410 nm are not present in the spectrum of enamel. At 1,434 nm, the peak absorptance for hydroxyapatite is narrower than the same peak for enamel. Based on the literature, there is no evidence that hydroxyapatite has a peak absorptance at 1,434 nm, so more investigations are needed.

The spectra of reflection and transmittance for hydroxyapatite are the reverse of the absorptance spectrum. Also, the level of reflectance for hydroxyapatite between 500 and 2,500 nm is almost twice as high as its transmittance level.

The transmittance spectrum for hydroxyapatite in the far infrared region shows a valley similar to that of enamel at 950 nm. Between 5,000 and 9,000 nm, a plateau at approximately 90% transmission characterizes the hydroxyapatite as a nonabsorbent material. The fast drop in transmission from 9,000 to 9,500 nm is

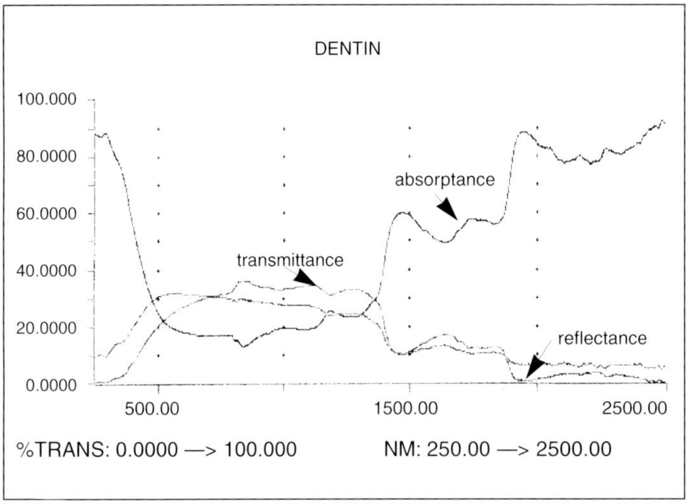

Fig 20.3 The spectra of absorptance, transmittance, and reflectance for dentin.

the most important change in the optical properties of hydroxyapatite in the far infrared region.

Dentin

Dentin consists of 70% inorganic mineral substance and 30% organic substance and water. The specificity of this tissue is given by the dentinal tubules that communicate with the pulpal surface, cementum, and enamel. Since the odontoblasts are arranged in a layer on the pulpal surface, their cytoplasm is located inside the dentinal tubules (Copenhaven et al, 1978). However, the process of dehydration of dentin will affect not only the hard tissue but the first layer of odontoblasts. Most of the time, this process is detrimental to the vitality of the entire pulpal tissue.

The thermoconductivity of dentin is much lower ($k = 5.69 \times 10^3$ W/cm°C) than that of enamel. The slow diffusion of heat through this tissue increases the chances of burning and carbonization during exposure to any powerful sources of light.

The two major peaks of absorptance at 1,471 and 1,942 nm represent the same peaks found for enamel and correspond to water absorptance (Fig 20.3). In addition to these peaks, dentin shows a few other minor peaks of absorptance at 1,184 nm, 1,737 nm, 2,164 nm, and 2,264 nm. The two minor peaks at 1,184 and 1,737 nm might be of interest for future investigation of new laser wavelengths in the near infrared region. High levels of absorptance for dentin are located in two different regions of the spectrum: the ultraviolet region from 250 to 300 nm and the middle infrared region from 1,942 to 2,500 nm. The reflectance and transmittance spectra of dentin are the reverse of the absorptance spectrum. Also, for the two regions of high levels of absorptance, transmittance is almost 0% and reflectance 10% higher.

For the far infrared region, the spectrum of transmission (T) for dentin shows three specific valleys at 3,000 nm (66%T), 5,880 nm (53%T), and 9,090 nm (35%T). The lowest level of transmission for this tissue is at 9,090 nm and corresponds to the CO_2 laser wavelength region; therefore, it is expected to have very good absorption properties and minimal thermal damage.

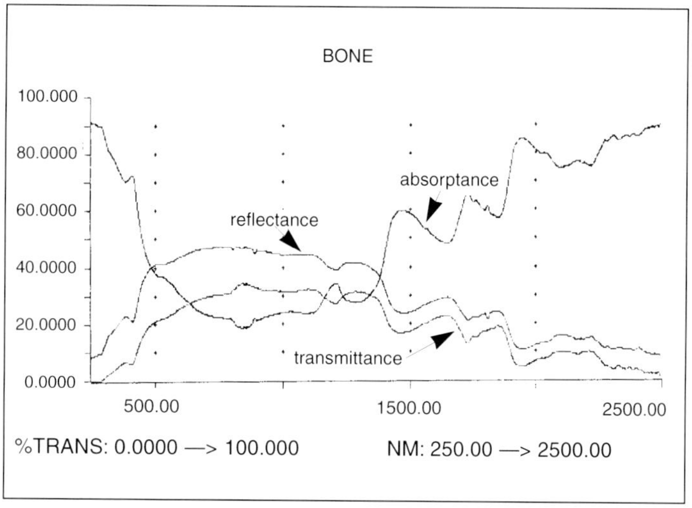

Fig 20.4 The spectra of absorptance, transmittance, and reflectance for cortical bone.

However, the thermal effect induced by the CO_2 laser beam in the interaction with the dentin is well known.

As a consequence of thermal stress, dentin develops multiple microcracks. Also, the pulpal cells in contact with the dentinal tissue can be easily affected by the heat produced during the interaction process.

Bone

Bone is composed of cells and an intercellular matrix of organic and inorganic substances. The organic fraction consists of collagenous fibrils that make up the lamellae of the bone matrix. The inorganic fraction of bone is responsible for its rigidity and represents approximately 65% of the dry weight. This fraction is basically composed of calcium phosphate and calcium carbonate with small amounts of magnesium, hydroxite, fluoride, and sulphate. Calcium is present mainly in the form of hydroxyapatite crystals with a needle-like shape and an average dimension of 1.5 nm × 30.0 nm. The crystals are bound mainly to the collagenous fibrils at the surface and within the fibrils (Rhodin, 1974).

Cortical bone is composed of organic and mineral substances in the same proportion as dentin so it is expected to show similar optical properties. Major peaks of absorptance are shown at 410 nm, 1,210 nm, 1,457 nm, 1,727 nm, and 1,944 nm (Fig 20.4). In comparison with dentin, bone has an additional peak of absorptance at 410 nm in the ultraviolet region and two peaks are within 30% higher at 1,210 nm and 1,727 nm, respectively. The two regions of high absorptance for dentin are reproduced in the spectrum of bone and correspond to the ultraviolet and middle infrared regions. Again, for spectra of reflectance and transmittance, each peak or valley of absorptance is reversed.

Laser Interaction with Biologic and Nonbiologic Structures

The interaction between laser radiation and matter is a complex process that begins with a temperature increase in the interaction zone. An important factor is that the peak temperature achieved in the interaction zone is always dictated by the thermal properties of the material. For a pulsed laser beam, the peak temperature of the interaction zone is higher than the peak temperature attained with continuous wave (cw) laser radiation. If the peak power, defined as the energy contained in a single laser pulse divided by its pulse width, is high enough, different physical processes such as thermal explosion, plasma cloud excitation, bubble cavitation, and ultrafast photovaporization can be induced. During the interaction of the photons with organomineral tissues, the optical properties of the tissue, such as absorption, transmission, and scattering, change according to the laser fluence. As a result of the modification of tissue optical properties, the superficial layer of the tissue shows an increase in absorption in a short time. Also, the temperature increases as the absorption increases.

A consequence of the high absorption and high temperature in the interaction zone is the initiation of a photochemical destructive process. During the photochemical destructive process, a low-temperature plasma cloud is created and maintained; the plasma cloud has an overheating effect on the tissue. As the heat is diffused into the surrounding tissue, the photochemical destructive process occurs well beyond the spot where the interaction takes place. The result of these processes is the formation of two layers with different optical and thermal properties. The first layer (superficial layer) modified by the laser beam has a dark color (new optical properties), high absorption coefficient, and low thermoconductivity. The second layer (underlayer) is a layer of normal tissue with typical thermal and optical properties. The formation of the two layers precedes any ablation process. In general, this concept can describe any tissue ablation process that occurs in a pure thermal mode. If the tissue shows no absorption for the laser wavelength, then processes previously described cannot be induced.

Interaction with Biologic Structures in the Presence of Fluid

Since most of the time interaction of a laser beam with matter is a thermal process, researchers have proposed various methods of cooling to control the temperature and thermal damage. For pulsed laser radiation the use of a coolant was justified, not only to avoid the increase of temperature produced by each laser pulse but also the expansion of heat between pulses. Studies have demonstrated that the thermal envelope created in a zone of tissue surrounding the interaction zone will continue to increase until full recovery of temperature has been achieved (Boehm et al, 1977).

In 1975, Boehm and Chen concluded that optimization of laser treatments involved minimizing the damage envelope and, because of this, cooling and precooling of the irradiated area was recommended. Since then, other researchers have understood the benefits of a medium to cool the interaction zone during laser emission. Nitrogen has been used to cool and precool tissues irradiated with a CO_2 laser beam. Wakaki (1979) experimented with nitrogen cooling to cut feline skin with a continuous wave CO_2 laser beam. Improvement of the quality of the laser cut and the period of healing demonstrated that cooling is an efficient method for control of heat expansion and tissue thermal damage.

In an in vitro experiment, Miserendino et al (1989) showed that after exposure of human enamel to a CO_2 laser at a power from 8 to 10 W and a duration of 10 to 25 sec, the pulp chamber temperature recovery to the pretreatment level requires 3 to

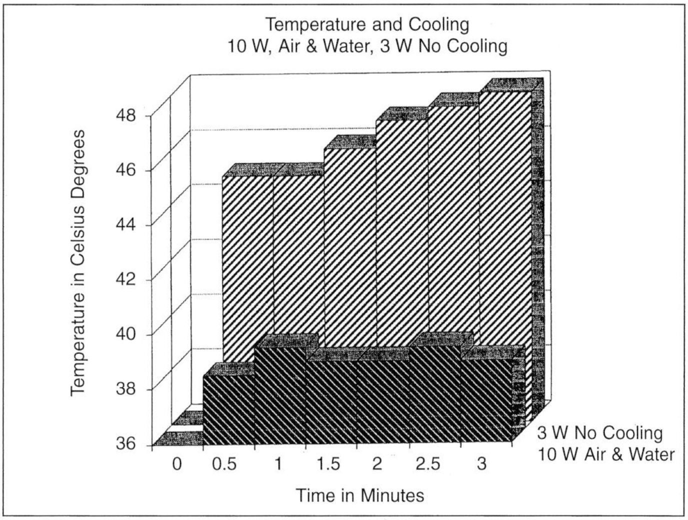

Fig 20.5 Temperature increase in the pulp chamber.

5 minutes. They also noted a cratering of the enamel surface at low power settings as a consequence of the induced thermal stress.

Levy (1991) proposed another method to control the elevation of temperature. The idea was to use the Nd:YAG pulsed laser beam with a coolant transparent to the laser beam and composed of a mixture of air and water at adjustable pressures. This technique proved to be efficient in controlling the heat generated during exposure of dental hard tissues. Later, Rizoiu et al (1994) has demonstrated that the Nd:YAG pulsed laser beam at a power level of 10 W with air-and-water cooling elevated the temperature inside the pulp chamber by 2.5°C, as compared with 12°C obtained at a power level of 3 W without air-and-water cooling (Fig 20.5).

In a histologic evaluation of the pulp reaction after exposure of enamel to a Nd:YAG pulsed laser beam and concurrent cooling, Miserendino et al (1994) have shown that there is no damage with an exposure of 12 W for 5 sec. The results of this study indicated no statistical difference between data obtained for the laser groups and data for the groups treated with the bur.

Other studies proved that a liquid medium is not only a way to control the expansion of heat during laser exposure but also an inducer of mechanical processes of interaction during root canal laser treatment.

Pressure wave signals emitted during the interaction of a Nd:YAG pulsed laser beam with root canal walls in a water medium were detected with a piezoceramic probe. The signals measured for different power densities proved to be correlated and to generate a linear type of function. Compared with conventional techniques, this process of interaction enhanced the removal of dentin on the canal walls and the disruption of bacteria (Levy et al, 1993).

Vapor Cavitation and Physical Processes Induced During Interaction. The induction of a vapor cavitation effect by lasers is not a new concept. In 1972, Lauterborn confirmed experimentally the vapor cavitation or optic cavitation induced by laser in a liquid medium. They also demonstrated that the process has many advantages, such as: easy to locate in place and time where the bubble cavities are generated; easy total control of the number of bubbles with the emission of the pulses; and easy to reproduce.

Since that time, different laser wavelengths have been tested to produce cavitation in liquids. An interesting study was conducted in Marseilles, France (Giovanneschi, 1986), with a double-frequency Nd:YAG laser focused inside capillary tubes filled with water. The whole cycle of cavitation was measured and analyzed. According to the measurements for a tube of 300-μm diameter, the initiation of the bubble occurs approximately within 200 nsec while the whole cycle of cavitation from initiation to collapse is accomplished within 85 μsec.

Besides the analysis of the bubble dynamics, the same experimental work included studies of the energy density needed to induce the bubble as well as the pressure created on the walls of the capillary tubes at bubble collapse.

For many applications, the most interesting step of a vapor cavitation phenomenon is the collapse of the bubble when pressure waves develop and transport mechanical energy inside the liquid into the surrounding area. Also, there is a linear dependency between the pressure, the diameter of the bubble and the laser energy. In a liquid medium, the cavitation phenomenon can be easily induced because of the liquid's specific properties, such as incompressibility.

The cavitation effect is easily induced by focusing a laser beam inside a liquid. The energy density is minimal and the pressure generated during the implosion affects the walls of the tube containing the liquid.

Models of Laser–Hard Tissue Interaction in Fluid

The laser ablation of tissue in fluid can be modeled in different ways. Each model is based on different laser parameters and tissue and fluid properties. An accurate modeling of these processes is difficult without a rigorous mathematical theory that relates to the experimental model and the experimental parameters. It is possible to qualitatively describe these processes, and several models representing the stages of the laser interaction process with hard tissue in the presence of fluid are presented.

In the first model, it is assumed that the tissue and fluid do not absorb the laser wavelength. The fluid acts as an ideal tissue coolant, and the laser energy is transferred directly to surrounding tissues. Adjacent tissues, however, may exhibit higher absorption properties and therefore generate heat once the laser radiation reaches them. Therefore, surrounding tissues are affected thermally and no ablation process occurs. From the moment that laser energy begins to affect surrounding tissues, the cooling fluid delivered in the interaction zone loses its ability to control heat generated along the energy pathway. This model describes a typical situation when laser beam energy is not absorbed at the tissue application point but penetrates adjacent tissues.

A second model is presented for tissue showing high absorption properties and a coolant transparent to the laser wavelength. An example to help analyze this model is the interaction of an Nd:YAG pulsed laser beam and dentin in the presence of an air-and-water spray. At high power settings (>12 W), the Nd:YAG pulsed laser beam creates a thin, superficial layer of carbonized dentin. This layer of carbonized dentin has new thermal and optical qualities as well as new morphologic properties. The new optical qualities of the carbonized layer increase absorption and reduce reflection properties of this layer. Also, the thermoconductivity of this layer is low and allows a fast rise in temperature in a short time. When the carbonization is set and the porosity of the structure is high enough, the penetration of water inside this layer is facilitated and ultrafast water vaporization processes are initiated. Within the carbonized layer, the temperature is very high and the water vaporization process is initiated instantaneously without energy supplements from the laser beam. The high pressure water vapors create microexplosions inside the carbonized layer, which is fragmented and ejected. This process will allow another noncarbonized layer of dentin to be exposed to the laser beam and a new cycle to be initiated.

Thus, the cycle of interaction encompasses:

1. The initial laser beam penetration and energy deposition inside the first layer of dentin
2. Heat generation and expansion
3. Carbonization of the first layer of dentin
4. Penetration of water inside the carbonized layer
5. Explosive vaporization of water inside the carbonized layer
6. Fragmentation and ejection of the carbonized layer
7. Normal (unlased) dentinal surface exposure

The third model describes the interaction when both the medium and cooling fluid highly absorb the laser wavelength. The critical parameter is the depth of beam penetration in the fluid (water). Beam penetration affects the amount of laser energy consumed by the fluid and the amount absorbed by the tissue. If the beam does not modify the tissue, then the fluid will not penetrate into the surface to help accelerate the ablation process. Such is the case when laser energy is applied to a tooth's enamel surface. Enamel has a mineral structure with a very low water content. However, when the laser beam is applied with concurrent fluid spray (air and water), and the depth of penetration in water is less than 1 µm (Er:YAG, 2.94 µm), the tissue structure will not be modified as efficiently. Although the structure of enamel remains compact, the fluid cannot penetrate the tissue.

According to Hibst and Keller (1993), the water contained in the dentin and enamel of the tooth structure may cause tissue fragmentation and particle ejection during its ultrafast vaporization, initiated with an Er:YAG laser. They postulate that water vapor pressure will affect tissue fragment velocity when it is ejected from the interaction zone. Large particles of tissue (enamel) that could not be accelerated to escape from the interaction zone would melt (at temperatures >1,500°C) and redeposit on the walls of the crater. Studies by Levy and Rizoiu (1994) have demonstrated highly efficient hard tissue ablation without visible thermal effects or debris depositions on the wall of the tooth crater. These results were achieved by applying different middle infrared laser wavelengths at a high repetition rate and with concurrent fluid spray.

The fourth model represents the interaction of middle infrared laser wavelengths and organomineral structures in the presence of a highly absorbent cooling fluid. The parameters of these laser wavelengths are listed in the Table. All these laser wavelengths operate at a higher repetition rate (> 30 Hz) than the 2,940-nm wavelength. In all cases represented by this model, repetition rates higher than 30

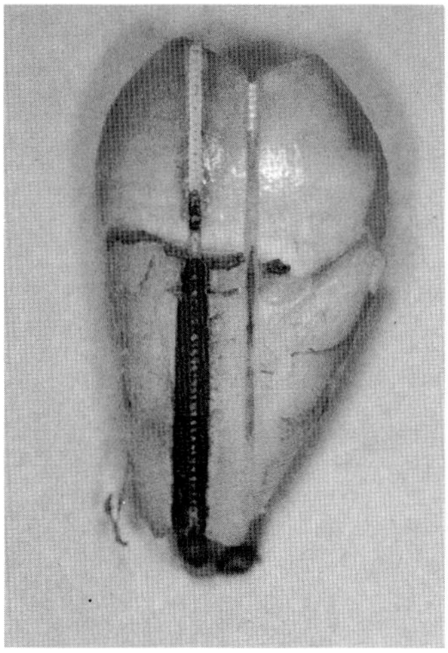

Fig 20.6 Tooth structure with two cuts. The first cut (left) was performed with middle infrared laser beam and no additional fluid. The second cut (right) was performed with a middle infrared laser beam and air-and-water spray. Power level = 3 W.

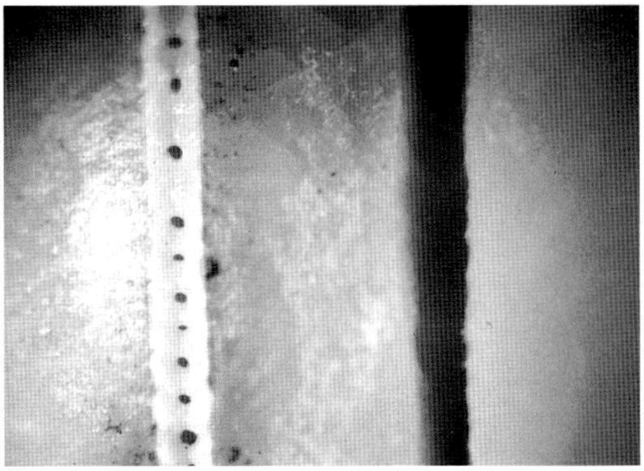

Fig 20.7 Detail of the two cuts in Fig 20.6.

Table. Middle Infrared Lasers

Parameters	YAG:Er	YSGG:Cr, Er	YALO(3):Er	YAG: Cr, Tm, Er
Wavelength (nm)	~2,940	~2,788	~2,714	~2,692
Maximum repetition rate (Hz)	<10	<100	<30	<100

Hz yielded dramatically improved abalation of hard tissues.

Improved ablation efficiency can be explained by greater beam penetration in water and changes in the tissue surface structure in the first stage of interaction (Fig 20.6). As the fluid continuously flows over the modified enamel surface, an ultrafast photovaporization of the water causes tissue fragmentation and removal. The fluid inside the modified layer of enamel plays a critical role in the ablation process.

Our preliminary investigation of the effects of cooled and uncooled mid-infrared laser on tooth hard structures is illustrative of the influence of a fluid cooling medium on the interactive process. When cooled ablation is compared to uncooled laser ablations of tooth surface enamel and root dentin, the effects of water on the ablation and modification of the respective structures become evident (Figs 20.6 and 20.7).

Compared to the third model, the very high pressure released during the transformation of water into vapor transfers to the ablated fragments high kinetic energies, which prevents tissue particles redeposition on the walls of the cut.

Middle Infrared Laser Radiation in the Presence of Fluid

The previous descriptions of different models of interaction were created to provide a better understanding of the processes that occur when a laser beam interacts with tissue in the presence of fluid. Analysis of the models and their applicability in the dental field demonstrated that middle infrared lasers are the most promising for hard tissue procedures.

Different middle infrared laser wavelengths (2,692 nm, 2,714 nm, and 2,788 nm) have been used in experiments on hard tissues to investigate morphologic changes produced after tissue ablation; efficiency of tissue ablation; and thermal effects.

Efficiency of Ablation and Morphologic Changes in Enamel. An in-vitro study (Levy and Rizoiu, 1994) with laser wavelengths of 2,788 nm, 2,714 nm, and 2,692 nm at a repetition rate of 30 Hz, pulse duration of 150 µsec, spot size of 700 µm, and a power level of 4 W was performed to determine the efficiency of ablation of enamel.

Samples of enamel were prepared by sectioning freshly extracted human molars with a diamond blade. The samples were then attached to a support for the beam to be focused on the surface of enamel. An electromagnetic engine was used to move the sample at a constant speed (0.519 mm/sec) in front of the laser beam. Three-millimeter long sections were prepared with one stroke of the laser beam and concurrent air-and-water spray (30 PSI air, 2.5 PSI water). The cross section of the cut had a triangular shape. The base of the triangle (w = 0.46 mm) was identified as the width of the cut. The depth of the cut (d = 0.87 mm) represents the height of the triangle. These measurements were used to

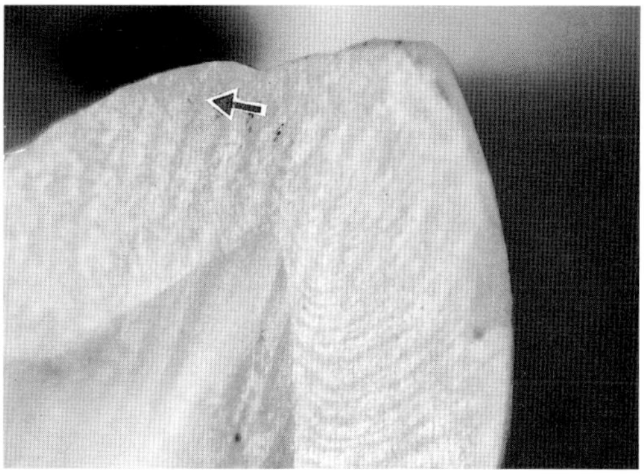

Fig 20.8 Coronal part of a first molar cut with middle infrared laser and concurrent air-and-water spray. Power level, 2 W; magnification, × 25.

calculate the following: the speed of volume ablation (A = 0.10385 mm^3/sec); the efficiency of ablation per joule (B = 0.025 mm^3/J); and the efficiency of ablation per pulse (C = 3.46 10^{-3} mm^3/pulse).

According to the calculations for enamel, the speed of ablation at a power level of 4 W is so high that 1 mm^3 of tissue is removed in less than 10 sec. The energy threshold of enamel ablation was established at 25 mJ and represents a power density of 6.5 J/cm^2. To compare these results, a study proved that a volume of enamel $10^{-4}$$cm^3$ was ablated with an Er:YAG laser (repetition rate 1 Hz) pulse duration between 500 µsec and 3 msec and energy per pulse up to 3 J) The threshold of enamel ablation was established at 1 J and represents a power density of 100 J/cm^2 (Bolshakov et al, 1989).

A microscopic examination of the morphologic changes and thermal effects produced on enamel was performed after cutting with the middle infrared laser. The coronal part of first molars was cut transversally with the laser and examined. The microscopic examination (Fig 20.8) showed a clean cut with minimal debris and no evidence of thermal modification of the enamel crystals. At the enamel-dentin

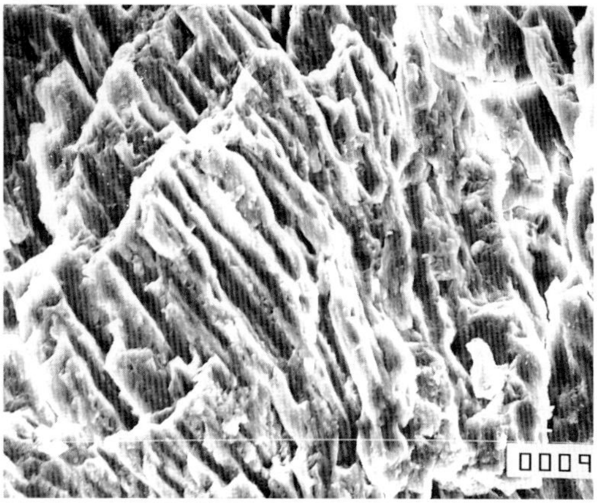

Fig 20.9 SEM view of the structure of laser-cut enamel. The crystalline structure visualized at this magnification shows no signs of thermal or mechanical damage. Cleavage steps created at levels where the columns were broken are also easy to identify. The structure is compact with no displacement of the prisms and no modification of the interprismatic distances. The amount of debris is minimal. Power level, 4 W; magnification, × 200.

juncture level, the cut was clean with a minimal amount of debris, no melting, and no signs of thermal or mechanical damage. The ability to ablate enamel with minimal thermal damage was reported by other investigaors as well. According to Hibst and Keller (1993), the crater wall appearance of the tooth ablated with an Er:YAG laser shows an amorphous mass deposit. They explain the presence of the amorphous material as an effect of the laser energy heating up the particles of tissue that could not escape from the zone of interaction. The process is called secondary debris heating, and large amounts of laser energy are consumed to melt (>1,300°C) the mineral material. The examination at high magnifications was performed with scanning electron microscopy (SEM).

The SEM examination of enamel at low magnification showed minimal morphologic modifications. The columnar geometry of the crystalline structure of this tissue was preserved. Along the columnar structure, a breakage of the rods was visible. A minimal amount of debris and the absence of any melted material indicated that the process of cutting is a cleavage and not a melting or a fragmentation.

At higher magnification (Fig 20.9), it was found that the enamel rods were truncated during the cutting process. Additionally, the interprismatic spaces were clean and free of cracks. Based on other studies performed with an Er:YAG laser, the electron microscopic analysis of enamel structure showed that a black amorphous product is sometimes present on the surface of the crystals. In conclusion, the Er:YAG laser produces minimal thermal modification of the crystalline structure of enamel.

Efficiency of Ablation and Morphologic Changes in Dentin. An experimental study was performed to determine the efficiency of ablation for dentin. Middle infrared laser wavelengths (see Table) delivered with a concurrent air-and-water spray were used. The laser was set at different powers between 0.5 and 5.5 W, with a repetition rate of 30 Hz, pulse duration of 140 µsec, and a spot size of 710 µm. The irradiation was performed with one stroke of the laser beam by moving the sample with an electromagnetic engine at a constant speed of 0.467 mm/sec.

The volume of dentin ablated per joule was found to be constant (0.0384 mm^3) and not related to the level of power. The speed of ablation in cubic millimeters per second as a function of the laser power yielded a linear function (Fig 20.10). A statistical analysis showed a linear correlation between the experimental data and the coefficient of correlation was 0.97.

The microscopic examination showed a very clean cut, with minimal debris and no thermal modification of the tissue.

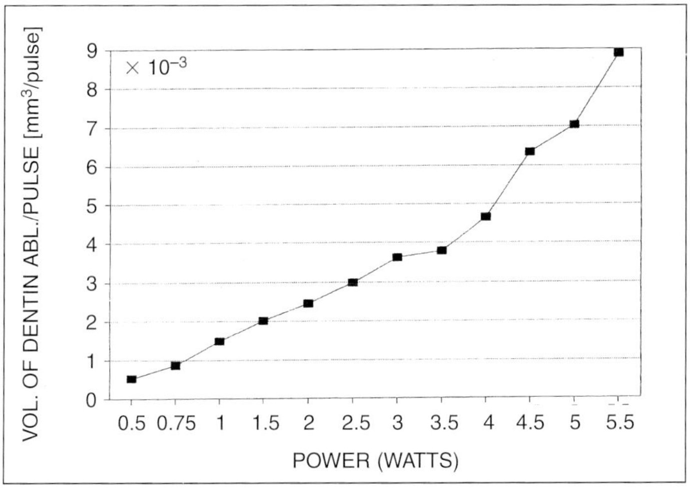

Fig 20.10 Volume of dentin ablated per pulse as a function of laser power.

The SEM examinations at magnifications of ×1,000 and ×3,500 show a minimal amount of debris on the ablated surface. When the cuts were performed longitudinally, the dentinal tubules were sectioned and no debris was found to cover the tubules or located inside the tubules. The intertubular substance was smoothly cut without any thermal modification. At ×3,500 (Fig 20.11) magnification for a transversel laser cut, there was no smear layer or debris covering the opened dentinal tubules.

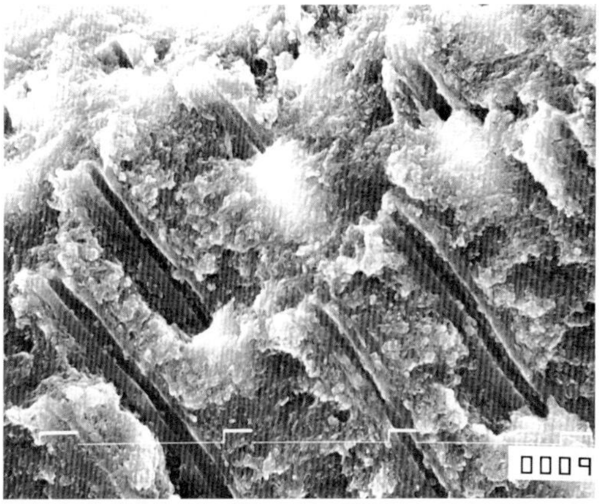

Fig 20.11 SEM view of dentin laser-cut with middle infrared laser radiation and concurrent air-and-water spray. Open dentinal tubules are cut longitudinally with no debris or mechanical and thermal damage. Power level, 4 W; magnification × 3,500.

Efficiency of Ablation and Morphologic Changes in Bone. With the use of different experimental middle infrared laser wavelengths, the efficiency of ablation of cortical bone was determined (Rizoiu and Levy, 1994). Samples of fresh bovine cortical bone were exposed to the pulsed laser beam delivered with a concurrent air-and-water spray. The cuts were performed with one stroke of the laser beam while moving the samples at a constant speed of 0.467 mm/sec. The procedure was repeated at ten different power settings between 0.5 W and 4.7 W. The length of the cut was 24 mm for all samples. Following the experiment, depth and width of the cuts created by the laser were measured and examined with light microscopy and SEM.

The results showed that the volume of ablation per joule is always constant and equal to 0.0437 mm^3/J. According to the calculations, at a power level of 4.5 W, 1 mm^3 of cortical bone was ablated within 5

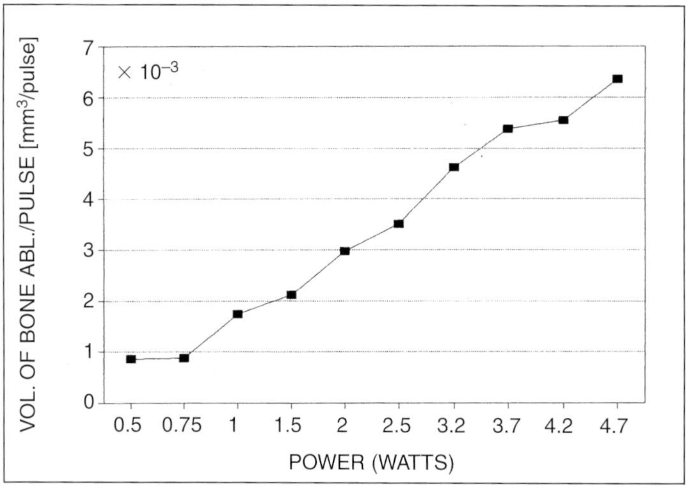

Fig 20.12 Volume of bone ablated per pulse as a function of laser power.

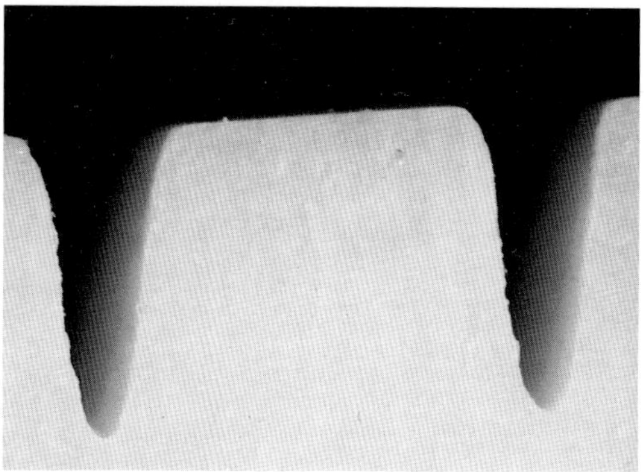

Fig 20.13 Cortical bone cut with middle infrared laser radiation and concurrent air-and-water spray (cross section). Power level = 4.7 W; magnification, × 50.

sec of exposure to the laser. The volume of bone ablated per pulse as a function of the average laser power yielded a linear function with a coefficient of correlation of 0.99 (Fig 20.12).

The light microscopic examination of the cuts indicated that the cut of the cortical bone has a triangular shape with a base the width of the cut and the apex representing the bottom of the cut (Fig 20.13). The study exhibits potential applications for a middle infrared laser wavelength to ablate bone in a nonthermal mode.

Conclusions

A laser beam interacts with matter by transferring its energy, which is converted into heat. For thermal modification and matter evaporation to occur, the temperature of the irradiated area has to pass a threshold to induce the substance phase change.

Continuous wave lasers are most commonly used for this process because they maintain a constant deposition of energy that produces a temperature high enough to induce the expected effect. For pulsed lasers, the pulse duration and repetition rate have to be selected according to the conductivity and diffusivity of heat inside the matter. Thermal processes induced by a laser beam interacting with matter are described in three stages: the first stage is when the absorbed energy is high enough to exceed the internal energy so the induced thermodynamic changes modify the lattice; the second stage is initiated when the internal temperature increases to the level of the melting point of matter and a change of phase (solid to liquid) occurs; and the third stage starts when the increasing temperature causes another phase change (liquid to vapor).

The complete process is laser-induced matter photovaporization. This process requires large amounts of laser power density (10^6 to 10^8 W/cm^2), which in industry is used to process different metals. Because of the high powers needed to process either biologic or industrial materials, the cost of the device and procedure are too high compared with conventional techniques.

The technique proposed in this chapter demonstrates that an interaction between the laser beam and a third fluid medium can be induced to produce photomechanical ablation of tissue or other solid-state material. In fact, the laser interaction is initiated after structural modifications of the superficial layer of material. The additional fluid is then involved in the interaction process but not until the fluid penetrates the microcracks and microporosities of the modified layer. Because water is incompressible and an ultrafast phase change (liquid to vapor) creates a tremendous increase in pressure, the photodisruption of matter occurs at relatively low levels of power density (400 to 800 W/cm^2).

This new approach of laser-matter interaction will open tremendous opportunities and practical applications not only in the biomedical field but also in industry. A promising future for this application will be established by the reduced size and cost of medical and industrial lasers.

References

Boehm RF, Chen MJ. Temperature in human teeth due to laser heating. Proc Am Soc Med Eng 1975; WA/BIO-8.

Boehm RF, Rich J, Janke S. Thermal stress and surface cracking associated with laser use on human teeth. Proc Am Soc Med Eng 1977;WA/BIO-3.

Bolshakov EN, Dolgikh RA, Zazulevskaya LY, et al. Experimental grounds for Er:YAG laser application to dentistry. SPIE 1989;1353:160–168.

Copenhaven WM, Kelly DE, Wood RL. Bailey's Textbook of Histology. Baltimore: Williams & Wilkins; 1978: 461–465.

Giovanneschi P. Contribution a l'etude de la cavitation a bulles isolees initiees par un rayonnement laser de grande intensite. Thesis, University of Sciences Marseilles, 1986:147–148.

Hibst R, Keller U. The mechanism of Er:YAG laser induced ablation of dental hard substances. SPIE 1993; 1880:156–161.

Lauterborn W. High speed photography of laser induced breakdown in liquids. Applied Physics Letter 1972;21: 27–29.

Levy G. Surgical Treatment Method and Instrument. U.S. Patent no. 5,020,995; 1991.

Levy G. Efficiency of dentin ablation using infrared pulsed laser radiation to induce vapor cavitation effects (abstract). Presented at the American Society for Laser Medicine and Surgery, April 8, 1994, Toronto.

Levy G, Rizoiu I. Morphological changes of dentin and enamel after ablation with an experimental laser beam (abstract). SPIE 1994. Presented at OE LASE '94, January 23, 1994, Los Angeles.

Levy G, Rizoiu I, Wigdor H. Photoacoustic effect induced in the root canal during exposure to a Nd:YAG pulsed laser beam. Presented at the American Society for Medicine and Surgery, April 18–20, 1993, New Orleans.

Miserendino LJ, Levy GC, Abt E, Rizoiu IM. The histologic effects of a thermally-cooled Nd:YAG laser on the dental pulp and supporting structures of rabbit teeth. J Oral Surg Oral Med Oral Pathol 1994;76:93–100.

Miserendino LJ, Neiberger EJ, Walia H, Luebke N, Brantley W. Thermal effects of continuous wave CO_2 laser exposure on human teeth: an in-vitro study. J Endodontics 1989;15:302–305.

Rhodin JAG. Histology. A Text and Atlas. New York: Oxford University Press, 1974:190–193.

Rizoiu I, Levy G. Interaction of an experimental laser on bone. Efficiency of ablation and thermal effects (abstract). SPIE 1994. Presented at OE LASE '94, January 23, 1994, Los Angeles.

Rizoiu I, Levy G, Wigdor H. A new model for temperature studies in dental pulp simulating the in-vivo condition. Presented at the American Society for Laser Medicine and Surgery, April 18–20, 1994, New Orleans.

Wakaki M. In Kaplan (ed): Laser Surgery. Jerusalem: Academic Press; 1979:27–41.

Wigdor H, Rizoiu I, Levy G. Light interaction with dental hard tissues spectrophotometry. Presented at the American Society for Laser Medicine and Surgery, New Orleans, April 18–20, 1994.

Glossary

Ablation Surgical removal of tissue by vaporization or other thermal mechanisms.

Absorption Conversion of radiant energy to other forms as it passes into a material.

Active medium Any material within the optical cavity of a laser that emits radiant light energy by transition from a higher energy (excited state) to a lower level when stimulated or pumped by an external power source.

Angstrom Unit of length equal to 10^{-10} meter.

Aperture A hole or opening through which light passes.

Argon laser A gas laser that emits light in the blue-green spectrum.

Attenuation The loss of optical intensity (average power) in a beam of light as it passes through matter.

Attenuation coefficient The rate of loss or decrease in average power of a laser beam as it passes through a specific material.

Average power In pulsed lasers, the power of the laser expressed in watts, which is determined by the product of the pulse energy (joules) and the pulse frequency (hertz).

Beam A unidirectional concentrated column of light.

Beam splitter An optical device that divides light into two separate beams.

Birefringence An optical property of a material that causes separation of a light beam into two divergent beams as it penetrates the material. Doubly refracting crystals (ie, calcite) are birefringent materials.

Carbon dioxide laser A gas laser that emits energy within the infrared spectrum.

Chromatic Having the properties of color (ie, hue and saturation).

Coherence A property of laser light. Radiant energy in which the waves travel in phase spatially and temporally. Radiation in which the distance between waves remains constant.

Collimation Alignment of a beam of radiant energy into nondivergent parallel waves.

Color The visible quality of an object or light that may be quantified in terms of hue, saturation, lightness (objects), and brightness (light sources).

Continuous wave laser A laser that emits radiation as a constant, uninterrupted stream rather than as short pulses or bursts.

Diode An electron tube or a semiconductor device that passes current in only one direction.

Diode laser A laser that uses a semiconductor as a source for emission.

Divergence Deviation or dispersion of a light beam away from a parallel direction. Deflection or moving apart of a collimated beam.

Doppler effect The change in frequency in reflected radiation that occurs when an object is in motion is a result of the doppler effect. Movement of the object away from the source of radiation will result in a reflection of a lower frequency as compared to a stationary object. Movement toward the radiant source results in a higher reflected frequency.

Dye laser A laser that emits light of changable frequency by using liquids of various colors as the active medium. Tunable dye lasers use dye solutions to produce laser output that can be adjusted over a range of wavelengths.

Efficiency For lasers, efficiency is determined by the percentage or ratio of power input to power output of the system.

Electromagnetic spectrum The entire range of all wavelengths and frequencies of radiant energy.

Electron probe microanalysis A process or method used to analyze the composition of minute samples. Spectral analysis of a material's emission resulting from its exposure to an electron beam.

Emission Release of radiant energy.

Energy For lasers, energy (joules) is equal to power (watts) multiplied by time (seconds).

Energy density The amount of energy that is distributed over a surface area or volume. Energy density or fluence is usually expressed in joules per square centimeter.

Excimer laser A variety of gas halide lasers that emit radiation in the ultraviolet range (120 to 560 nm). Examples include ArCl, ArF, XeCl, and XeF.

Excited state Elevation of an atom or molecule above its resting energy level. An unstable state that results from absorption of a quantum of energy by pumping energy into a system.

Fiber optic A transparent strand or bundle of fibers (usually glass) that is capable of transmitting light or radiant energy along its length.

Flash-lamp A high-intensity light source used for pumping solid-state lasers.

Fluence The radiant energy (joules) per surface area (square centimeters). (See *Energy density.*)

Flux The rate of flow of radiant energy expressed in joules per second.

Focal length The distance from a condensing lens to its point of maximum focus.

Focal point, focal spot, focus The position of maximum concentration of a beam of light when it passes through an optical condensing lens.

Focused mode In laser surgery, the positioning of the laser handpiece at a distance from the surface of the tissue or target that results in exposure of the highest energy density; using the laser handpiece at its focal length or smallest spot diameter.

Gas laser A laser that has a gas as its active medium. Examples include argon, CO_2, and helium:neon.

Ground state The resting or lowest energy level of an atom, molecule, or system.

He:Ne An abbreviated term for a helium:neon laser. In surgical lasers that emit invisible radiation, He:Ne lasers are combined with the active beam to allow visual focusing on the target tissue. He:Ne lasers emit continuous red monochromatic light.

Ho:YAG laser A pulsed laser emitting radiation at 2,100 nm.

Infrared spectrum Radiation that falls between 700 and 1,000 μm wavelength within the electromagnetic spectrum.

Irradiation The exposure of radiant energy on an object.

Joule A unit of energy or work equal to an exposure of 1 W of power for 1 sec.

Laser An acronym for "light amplification by stimulated emission of radiation." A device that has an optical cavity containing material (solid, liquid, or gas) that emits radiant energy of a specific wavelength when the material is stimulated by a power source to a higher energy level (excited state). The light or radiant energy emitted becomes intensified by oscillation within the optical cavity, and has the unique properties of being monochromatic, collimated, and coherent.

Maser An acronym for "microwave amplification by stimulated emission of radiation." The maser was the forerunner of the laser and operates by the same mechanism.

Medium Any material or substance contained within the optical cavity of a laser that can be stimulated to emit radiant energy.

Micrometer or micron (μm) A unit of measurement equal to 10^{-6} m.

Monochromatic Radiant light energy of a single or narrow band of wavelengths. Radiation of one color or wavelength.

Nanometer (nm) A unit of measurement equal to 10^{-9} m.

Nd:YAG laser A laser that has a solid crystal rod composed of yttrium-aluminum-garnet and is doped with neodymium as the active medium.

Optical cavity A cylindrical space containing a solid, gas, or liquid material that has reflective mirrors or surfaces at each end. The optical cavity serves as a resonator by reflection of photons along the length of the cavity.

Photoablation Removal of material by its interaction with light energy. (See *Ablation*.)

Photoacoustic effect Generation of an audible shock wave produced by absorption of laser energy in a material. The absorbed light energy becomes transformed into mechanical kinetic energy within the material, which results in rapid expansion accompanied by an audible microexplosion.

Photochemical effect Chemical reactions produced or stimulated by interaction of laser light with substances.

Photocoagulation In surgery, use of the laser to provide hemostasis through thermal effects on hemoglobin and denaturation of blood proteins. Sealing of small vessels also occurs by coagulation and tissue welding effects.

Photodisruption Fragmentation, or separation of target tissue, by the conversion of optical energy into mechanical forces or high-pressure acoustic waves. A characteristic of lasers capable of very short widths (10^{-9} sec) and high pulse energies (ie, Q-switched YAG). A nonthermal, nonspecific tissue interaction.

Photon A unit or quantum of radiant energy. According to quantum mechanics, it is the smallest quantity or particle of radiant energy having both mass and energy.

Picosecond In lasers, a duration of time or interval from 10^{-10} to 10^{-13} sec. One picosecond is equal to 1×10^{-12} sec.

Plasma A state of matter composed of free electrons, ions, and charged particles in a highly energized gaseous phase.

Polarization Orientation of light waves into an organized pattern that results in propagation of the beam in a single plane or orientation within three-dimensional space.

Population inversion The conversion of the active medium of a laser from its lower or resting energy level to its energized state. The condition required for stimulated emission to occur.

Power density A measure of the distribution of a laser's output over a given surface area. Units for power density are typically reported in watts per square centimeter for a given surface area or focal spot size.

Pulse duration In pulsed lasers, the time interval in which the laser emission occurs. (See also *Pulse width*.)

Pulse frequency See *Pulse repetition rate*.

Pulse repetition rate (PRR) In pulsed lasers, the frequency of pulses expressed in hertz or pulses per second (PPS). Another term for pulse frequency.

Pulsed mode Laser radiation that is released intermittently as short bursts of energy, as opposed to a continuous laser output.

Pulse width The time or duration of a laser pulse. (See *Pulse duration.*)

Pumping The process used to excite or elevate the active medium of a laser to a higher level sufficient to produce or stimulate emission. Any method that delivers energy to the laser medium.

Q A term or expression of the level of energy within the optical cavity, or resonator of a laser.

Q-switched laser A laser capable of emitting pulses of high energy and very short duration (nanosecond range) by the use of a shutter device.

Quantum The smallest value or quantity of radiant energy. (See *Photon.*)

Quantum mechanics In physics, the laws governing the properties of atomic particles and radiation.

Quartz A naturally occurring, crystalline material useful in the manufacture of lenses and fiberoptics for the transmission of laser light.

Radiation Transmission of energy through space or matter in the form of waves or particles.

Recrystallization In nonmetals, the return of a crystalline material from the fused to the solid state. A thermal process involving the re-solidification of a molten crystalline material.

Reflection The change in direction of a light beam or radiant energy when it contacts the surface of an object without penetration. (See *Absorption*, *Transmission*, and *Scatter.*)

Resonator The optical cavity of a laser, usually in the form a cylinder, bound at each end by mirrors, where one is totally reflective and the other partially reflective.

Ruby laser The first laser, developed by Maiman in 1960. A solid-state optically pumped laser that emits in the visible range (694.3 nm).

Scatter The change in direction of a light wave or beam of radiant energy when it either contacts a surface or enters a material without interaction. (See *Absorption*, *Reflection*, and *Transmission.*)

Semiconductor A material with electrical conductivity that lies between that of conductors and insulators. A partially conductive material whose conductivity can be modified by the addition of impurities to the material.

Semiconductor laser A laser that has a light-emitting diode as the source of coherent radiant energy or active medium. (See *Diode Laser.*)

Shutter A device or mechanism that regulates the time a laser emits radiant energy. In pulsed lasers, the mechanism used to control the intermittent release of energy.

Solid-state laser A laser that has a solid material, usually a crystal rod doped with trace elements, as its active medium. Diode or semiconductor lasers are usually excluded from this group, although they are by definition solid-state lasers.

Spontaneous emission The release of energy that occurs when an atom, ion, or molecule changes from a high-energy state (excited level) to a lower level.

Stimulated emission Release of radiant energy from a particle in its activated or high energy state by interaction with photons or radiant energy of the same frequency. Stimulated emission is the basis for laser operation.

Superpulsed Laser emission of ultrashort pulse duration and high pulse energy. Peak powers in superpulsed mode may be several times that of continuous mode.

Transmission The passage of radiation through a material without interaction. (See *Absorption*, *Reflection*, and *Scatter.*)

Tunable laser A laser that can be regulated or adjusted to emit radiation within a range of frequencies. (See *Dye laser.*)

Watt A unit of power. One watt of power applied over 1 sec will produce 1 J of energy.

Wave The path by which radiant energy travels through space, having both direction and amplitude, as in a sinusoidal curve.

Waveguide A cylindric hollow tube or fluid-filled device used for directing laser light.

Wavelength The shortest distance between two points that are in phase (same relative position) within an electromagnetic wave.

Xenon flash-lamp A high-intensity light source used for pumping solid-state lasers.

X-ray diffraction A method of analysis that uses x-rays to determine the crystal structure of materials.

X-ray microprobe analysis A method of analysis that uses scanning electron microscopy and spectroscopy.

YAG laser A variety of solid-state lasers with a crystal rod composed of yttrium-aluminum-garnet, which is doped with other elements such as erbium, holmium, or neodymium for the active medium. (See also *Nd:YAG, Ho:YAG,* and *Er:YAG lasers.*)

Units of Measurement, Equivalents, Formulas, and Constants

Time

millisecond	(msec)	=	10^{-3} sec
microsecond	(μsec)	=	10^{-6} sec
nanosecond	(nsec)	=	10^{-9} sec
picosecond	(psec)	=	10^{-12} sec

Length

millimeter	(mm)	=	10^{-3} m
micron	(μm)	=	10^{-6} m
nanometer	(nm)	=	10^{-9} m

Units of Measure

Energy (J) = 10^7 ergs (W × sec)
Fluence (energy density) = J/cm^2
Flux (irradiance) (E) = Joules (W × sec)
Frequency (v, Hz) = cycles/sec
Pi (π) = 3.1415925
Planck's constant (h) = 6.6256×10^{-27} erg-sec
Power (W) = energy/time (J/sec)
Power density (PD) = W/cm^2
Pulse repetition rate (PRR) = pulses/sec
Velocity of light (c) = 2.997925×10^{10} cm/sec
Velocity of a particle (v) = m/sec
Wavelength (λ) = unit distance

Formulas

Energy density = W × seconds / area in cm^2 = J/cm^2
Power density (PD) = W / area in cm^2 = W/cm^2
Surface area of a circle (A) = $\pi r^2 = \pi (d/2)^2$
Photon energy* (p) = hv or $p = h\ 1/\lambda$
Frequency of emission† (v) = $E_1 - E_2/h$
Wavelength (λ) = $v\ c$

*Planck's law states that the energy of a photon (p) is proportional to the frequency of radiation (v) or is inversely related to its wavelength (λ) by a constant proportion (h), which is Planck's constant.

†Bohr's law or Bohr's frequency rule states that the frequency of radiation emitted by a system (atom or molecule) in transition from a higher energy state (E_1) to a lower energy state (E_2) can be quantified according to the above formula.

Laser Precautions*

The application of laser radiation to both hard and soft tissue is becoming widespread. It serves as a replacement of the dental drill by eliminating noxious stimuli, noise, and vibration. The CO_2 laser ablates soft tissue and incises small tumors in the oral cavity. The adverse reactions are various forms of thermal damage to dentin and enamel. There is a disruption of the microscopic organization of the enamel matrix, and the heat actually causes the enamel to melt and flow. The char is visible on the surface, and the carbonization forms beneath the melted enamel. The charred pathologic tissue is subsequently removed by copious irrigation with normal saline and periodontal curettes. Recrystallized dentin is removed via surgical bone curettes. Very little research has been done with the Nd:YAG laser in the oral cavity. The effects of a Q-switched Nd:YAG laser through successive pulses acts as a drill.

Because of the great vascularity of the oral cavity, the laser is an effective tool for the control of hemorrhage. The following safety precautions should be heeded by practitioners when using the laser.

B12.1 Beam Alignment

The coaxial alignment of the aiming He:Ne beam and the surgical laser must be checked before any surgical procedure. This can be checked by using a moistened tongue depressor and firing the laser.

B12.2 Laser Control

To prevent the inadvertent damage that noncontrolled laser energy can cause, the laser should be placed in the standby mode when not in use.

B12.3 Reflected Energy

Because of the potential for reflected laser energy to cause damage, polished instruments should not be used, only anodized or frosted ones.

*From ANSI Z-136.3, For The Safe Use of Lasers in Health Care Facilities. Appendix B12 Dentistry. Reprinted by permission of Laser Institute of America, Orlando, FL.

B12.4 Fire Protection

The risk of fire is always a concern when lasers are in use. Therefore, when using any laser, noncombustible materials should be used. Also, it is very helpful to drape the surgical field with moistened towels to prevent combustion. All combustible materials must be kept in closed cabinets and any combustible fluid that is used in the surgical preparation must be fully dried before surgery.

B12.5 Eye Protection

The ocular tissue of all personnel (ie, surgeon, assistant, and patient) is probably the tissue most susceptible to damage from the laser. Protective lenses specific to the particular wavelength being used must be worn. Members of the surgical team must not look directly at the laser beam, even when wearing protective lenses.

B12.6 Anesthesia

When general anesthesia is used, nasotracheal intubation is preferred. Because of the proximity of the oral cavity to the endotracheal tube, laser use in the mouth can be very damaging. Moist throat backs must be used to protect the tube from accidental laser damage. Tubes should be either noncombustible or wrapped with reflecting tape. Extreme care must be taken by the surgeon even when the previous precautions are taken to keep the laser beam far from the endotracheal tube. Any exposure of the anesthetic agent to the laser beam can cause combustion in the bronchial system, which is life-threatening. When nasotracheal intubation is not possible and the tube rests in the oral cavity, it must be isolated and kept far from the surgical field.

B12.7 Tissue Damage

The amount of tissue damage is a function of power density and time. These variables must be respected when the laser is used for making incisions. The shortest time of tissue exposure for the desired result is advisable. To prevent carbon arcing, the tissue should be regularly wiped clean of carbon.

B12.8 Tissue Protection

The tissues of the oral cavity can be damaged irreversibly if exposed to unintentional laser energy. It is strongly advised that these tissues be protected from the laser. Enamel can be demineralized if exposed to the laser; therefore, when the laser beam is close to this tissue, metal retractors must be placed between the tooth and tissue. The alveolar bone can also be damaged if the laser is allowed to penetrate through the overlying gingiva. Great care must be taken not to overexpose the tissue, which may lead to adverse bone involvement.

B12.9 Plume Control

Large amounts of smoke are produced by laser energy impacting on the tissue. This plume of smoke is both noxious and potentially damaging if inhaled. Elimination of this plume with a smoke evacuator is essential.

Curriculum Guidelines and Standards for Dental Laser Education

I. Preamble

The curriculum guidelines for dental laser education were developed through a consensus process with members from dental academia, industry, and private practice. This document was developed at a workshop on the development of standards for dental laser education and laser instructor certification held at the University of California, San Francisco, on July 25 and 26, 1992. The purpose of the workshop was to develop a consensus among dental professionals who teach, use, or manufacture lasers in dentistry to define the standard of education for dental practitioners who use lasers.

The document was developed using recommendations from a wide range of information that exists on the use of lasers, which is appropriately referenced. The format of this document is in the style of curriculum guidelines as published by the American Association of Dental Schools. A working draft is currently being circulated among dental laser educators, researchers, practitioners, organized dentistry, and members of industry. After further discussion, modification, and review, the final document will be widely distributed and updated annually. Any questions concerning the guidelines may be addressed to the authors of this document in care of the organizer. Suggestions for the improvement of this standard and endorsement of this document are invited.

II. Statement of Authorship

These guidelines were developed by consensus among dental professionals for use in dental laser education. They are intended to provide guidance to practitioners and educators and to reassure the public on the issues of education, competency, and quality of care in the use of lasers in dentistry. They should not be interpreted as recommendations for restricting the application of this technology in dentistry. Adherence to these guidelines is in no way intended to restrict, limit, or regulate the use of lasers as a device.

III. Introduction

Laser applications in dentistry have specific indications and contraindications for use in treatment. An understanding of the fundamentals of laser optics and dental tissue interactions is essential. Therefore, practitioners must have a foundation in laser applications in dentistry to use these devices in the treatment of dental diseases in their patients.

Lasers are devices that have specific applications for the treatment of dental diseases. As with all medical devices, their manufacture and distribution are regulated by the Food and Drug Administration. These regulations control dental laser manufacturers but do not regulate the dental practitioner in the use of these devices. Hospitals and institutions have their own credentialing programs for use of specific devices, including lasers, in their facilities. Currently, there is ambiguity regarding the use of lasers in the private dental office. Dental lasers, as devices, *do not* comprise the basis for a dental specialty, but do require a level of education for their safe use in dentistry. It is the responsibility of the dental practitioner to be educated in the safe use of lasers in the dental setting. The curriculum outlined in this document is provided as a guide to education in laser use in dentistry.

IV. Statement of Purpose

This document provides guidelines for practitioners to assure safe and efficacious use of lasers for the health and welfare of the patient. Additionally, it establishes the standards of education in the use of lasers in dentistry and defines standards for the demonstration of competency in the safe and effective use of lasers by dental professionals.

V. Overview

There are four levels of education outlined in this document. Category 1 courses are commensurate with continuing education level courses designed to provide general information on lasers in dentistry. Category 1 courses are informational and do not have an assessment of the student's proficiency in laser use in dentistry. Category 2, 3, and 4 courses have specific educational goals, behavioral objectives, and examination of proficiency. Category 2 courses provide a basic level of education with didactic, laboratory, and clinical exercises that must be satisfactorily completed before using lasers clinically. Category 3 courses are an advanced level of education that have didactic, laboratory, and clinical observation, as well as a clinical case study requirement. Category 4 courses define the educational requirements for instructors of laser education in dentistry.

VI. Primary Education Goals

The goal of these curriculum guidelines and standards of education is to enhance student and practitioner understanding and knowledge of the application of laser technology in dentistry.

Students and practitioners must have training with demonstrated proficiency knowledge and skill for use of lasers in dentistry. Training must include specific objectives and requirements described below with demonstration of knowledge and proficiency. Competency should include both written and clinical examinations. Education and evaluation of competency of practitioners must be done under the supervision of and assessed by a trained teacher. Students and practitioners must have knowledge about the safe use of lasers in dentistry.

Practitioners' use of lasers must be limited to those devices in which the manufacturer has met the Center for Devices and Radiologic Health of the Food and Drug Administration requirements for that product. Manufacturers must meet the requirements and regulations of the Food and Drug Administration. Manufacturers should provide both an operator's manual and recommended clinical usage, supported by preclinical and clinical research where appropriate. Practitioners should follow the specific indications for use of the device with a sound knowledge of the indications and contraindications of use of the device. Dentists and dental hygienists as practitioners must limit their use of lasers to those procedures that are in accordance with the standards and practice of the profession and within the scope of practice of the practitioner based on competence as established by education, training, and experience. Dental auxiliaries within their scope of education, training, and experience must also have specific safety training and demonstrated proficiency in proper laser safety.

Students must have a knowledge of physics, laser-tissue interaction, and specific laser safety requirements for the dental operatory and treatment areas. Students must have a knowledge of the device and basic laser and biologic interactions including the safety recommendations outlined in the American National Standard for the Safe Use of Lasers (ANSI Z-136.1) and American National Standard for the Safe Use of Lasers in Health Care Facilities (ANSI Z-136.3). Students must have knowledge of basic laser physics and laser-tissue interaction. Students must also have a knowledge of specific tissue interactions of laser wavelengths and interactions with oral tissues and an understanding of fundamental laser properties including beam characteristics, wavelength, absorption, reflection, transmission, emission modes, and delivery systems. Students must also demonstrate knowledge of photothermal, photochemical, photoacoustic events, and effects of spot size, power, time, wavelength, energy density, and repetition rate on dental tissues.

Students must also have knowledge of and demonstrate laser safety technique and application in the dental setting. Students must have knowledge in dental clinical applications with contraindications, indications, specific inclusion and exclusion criteria, as well as oral tissue interactions and techniques for specific treatment with knowledge of laser dentistry delivery systems and specific laser devices. Students must know the treatment objective such as coagulation or excision. Students must have information on specific clinical usage and suggested settings for specific treatment objectives supported by research. Students and practitioners must be able to recognize successful treatment outcomes and to manage adverse effects. Students must know specific labeling and clinical use of the device. Additionally, students must have knowledge of the incident report mechanism.

It is the responsibility of the dental practitioner to follow the standard of education as defined by these guidelines.

The following curriculum guidelines are taken from currently available dental laser education programs and adapted from the recommendations put forth by the American Society for Laser Medicine and Surgery, Inc.

Category 1. Guidelines for General Dental Laser Courses

The curriculum for general dental laser courses may be slide/audio, video, or lecture format. General dental laser courses are intended to be educational, informational, and primarily didactic. It is suggested that Category 1 courses be 3 to 4 hours in length. This level of education is intended for students, dentists, dental hygienists, and dental auxiliaries.

I. Introduction and welcome
   A. Self-graded pre-test (optional)

II. Fundamentals of lasers
   A. Production of laser light
      1. Quantum theory
      2. Stimulated emission
   B. Electromagnetic spectrum
      1. Laser wavelengths
   C. Qualities of laser light
      1. Spatial and temporal beam coherency
      2. Optical components of laser light
      3. Monochromaticity and collimation of laser light
   D. Summary of laser effects on tissue
      1. Photoablation, coagulation, excision
      2. Laser effects on oral tissue
      3. Radiation, transmission, absorption
      4. Thermal effects

III. Review of types of lasers, delivery systems, special device characteristics, and clinical applications in dentistry
   A. Argon laser
   B. CO_2 laser
   C. Nd:, Ho:, Er:YAG lasers
   D. Other lasers
   E. Laser operating parameters
      1. Energy density
      2. Power
      3. Repetition rate
      4. Total energy

IV. Discussion of laser safety
   A. OSHA and ANSI requirements
   B. Eye protection
   C. Hazard prevention
   D. Endotracheal anesthesia
   E. Laser safety in the dental setting
      1. Limited access and posting of laser rooms
   F. FDA regulations
   G. OSHA standards

V. Laser safety principles and protocol
   A. Laser safety
   B. Proper training
   C. Limited access
   D. Warning and safety mechanisms
   E. Hazard reporting and incident reporting
   F. Laser use documentation

VI. Infection control
   A. Identification of biologic hazards
   B. Plume hazards
   C. Sterilization
   D. Post-test examination (optional)

Category 2. Guidelines for Basic Level Education Dental Laser Courses

The curriculum for a basic level of education in laser usage includes specific device instruction with proficiency in didactic and laboratory knowledge. Laboratory exercises and clinical demonstration must be at least 40% of the total teaching hours for this level course. Students and practitioners must demonstrate competency by written and clinical simulation examination to begin using lasers on patients. Mandatory proficiency must be demonstrated and examined on a specific laser device. Additional device instruction and education requires demonstrated proficiency at the Category 2 level. It is recommended that no fewer than 6 to 8 hours be devoted to the didactic components of the curriculum. This is the level of education that defines the standard of care for the dental practitioner. Successful completion of this level of education is essential for students, dentists, and dental hygienists. Dental auxiliaries are encouraged to demonstrate competency in the safety aspects of the clinical simulation proficiency examination.

I. Introduction and welcome
    A. Self-graded pre-test (optional)

II. Fundamentals of lasers
    A. Production of laser light
        1. Quantum theory
        2. Stimulated emission
    B. Electromagnetic spectrum
        1. Laser wavelengths
    C. Qualities of laser light
        1. Spatial and temporal beam coherency
        2 Optical components of laser light
        3. Monochromaticity and collimation of laser light
    D. Summary of laser effects on tissue
        1. Photoablation, coagulation, excision
        2. Laser effects on oral tissue
        3. Reflection, transmission, absorption
        4. Thermal effects

III. Review of types of lasers, delivery systems, special device characteristics, and clinical applications in dentistry
    A. Argon laser
    B. CO_2 laser
    C. Nd:, Ho:, Er:YAG lasers
    D. Other lasers
    E. Laser operating parameters
        1. Energy density
        2. Power
        3. Repetition rate
        4. Total energy

IV Discussion of laser safety
    A. OSHA and ANSI requirements
    B. Eye protection
    C. Hazard prevention
    D. Endotracheal anesthesia
    E. Laser safety in the dental setting
        1. Limited access and posting of laser rooms
    F. FDA regulations
    G. OSHA standards

V. Laser safety principles and protocol
    A. Laser safety
    B. Proper training
    C. Limited access
    D. Warning and safety mechanisms
    E. Hazard reporting and incident reporting
    F. Laser use documentation

VI. Infection control
    A. Identification of biologic hazards
    B. Plume hazards
    C. Sterilization
    D. Post-test examination (optional)

VII. Clinical summary of laser usage
    A. Discussion of indications and contraindications of laser use in dentistry
    B. Alternate methods of treatment and results
    C. Laser treatment and results
        1. Method of treatment

2. Specific equipment and facility requirements
3. Long-term results, assessing treatment outcomes
4. Pathologic samples, case studies of specific procedures

D. Follow-up care
1. Results of treatment
2. Side effects and complications

VIII. Practice management
A. Practice organization and management
B. Financial and insurance considerations
C. Malpractice considerations, jurisprudence, ethics
D. Recordkeeping, hazard documentation, informed consent

IX. Complete bibliography
A. General bibliography for lasers in dentistry
B. Subject bibliography for specific dental applications

X. Current research and future developments

XI. Laboratory exercise
A. Specific hands-on demonstration
B. Laser setup and operation
C. Simulated clinical experience on bovine tissues or other suitable biologic tissues or inanimate objects
D. Post-test clinical simulation

XII. Clinical observation and demonstration

XIII. Conclusion
A. Written post-test
B. Course evaluation
C. Certificate of attendance

Category 3. Guideline for Advanced Training and Clinical Case Studies Dental Laser Courses

Students and practitioners must have demonstrated proficiency measured by one or more of the following:

1. In-office mentor preceptor program
2. University or other accredited dental education program
3. Scientific session educational program

It is suggested that no fewer than 8 to 10 hours with an additional requirement for reviewed clinical case studies to be completed and evaluated within 6 months of completion of the didactic and laboratory portions of the curriculum. It is suggested that clinical proficiency be demonstrated by no fewer than five selected case studies with appropriate documentation (radiographs, dental charting, treatment record, intraoral photographs, results of diagnostic tests, and appropriate treatment documentation and follow-up). The curriculum guidelines suggest a mentor or preceptor program with a student-to-instructor ratio no greater than 5:1. These curriculum guidelines contain the essential elements of Category 2 courses with an additional requirement for individual clinical case studies. This level of education is above and beyond the standard of care for the dental practitioner and represents an advanced level of training and demonstrated clinical competency. This level of education is intended for dentists and dental hygienists to demonstrate an advanced level of clinical competency within the scope of their practice.

I. Introduction and welcome
A. Self-graded pre-test (optional)

II. Fundamentals of lasers
   A. Production of laser light
      1. Quantum theory
      2. Stimulated emission
   B. Electromagnetic spectrum
      1. Laser wavelengths
   C. Qualities of laser light
      1. Spatial and temporal beam coherency
      2. Optical components of laser light
      3. Monochromaticity and collimation of laser light
   D. Summary of laser effects on tissue
      1. Photoablation, coagulation, excision
      2. Laser effects on oral tissue
      3. Reflection, transmission, absorption
      4. Thermal effects

III. Review of types of lasers, delivery systems, special device characteristics, and clinical applications in dentistry
   A. Argon laser
   B. CO_2 laser
   C. Nd:, Ho:, Er:YAG lasers
   D. Other lasers
   E. Laser operating parameters
      1. Energy density
      2. Power
      3. Repetition rate
      4. Total energy

IV. Discussion of laser safety
   A. OSHA and ANSI requirements
   B. Eye protection
   C. Hazard prevention
   D. Endotracheal anesthesia
   E. Laser safety in the dental setting
      1. Limited access and posting of laser rooms
   F. FDA regulations
   G. OSHA standards

V. Laser safety principles and protocol
   A. Laser safety
   B. Proper training
   C. Limited access
   D. Warning and safety mechanisms
   E. Hazard reporting and incident reporting
   F. Laser use documentation

VI. Infection control
   A. Identification of biologic hazards
   B. Plume hazards
   C. Sterilization
   D. Post-test examination (optional)

VII. Clinical summary of laser usage
   A. Discussion of indications and contraindications of laser use in dentistry
   B. Alternate methods of treatment and results
   C. Laser treatment and results
      1. Method of treatment
      2. Specific equipment and facility requirements
      3. Long-term results, assessing treatment outcomes
      4. Pathologic samples, case studies of specific procedures
   D. Follow-up care
      1. Results of treatment
      2. Side effects and complications

VIII. Practice management
   A. Practice organization and management
   B. Financial and insurance considerations
   C. Malpractice considerations, jurisprudence, ethics
   D. Recordkeeping, hazard documentation, informed consent

IX. Complete bibliography
   A. General bibliography for lasers in dentistry

   B. Subject bibliography for specific dental applications

X. Current research and future developments

XI. Laboratory exercise
   A. Specific hands-on demonstration
   B. Laser setup and operation
   C. Simulated clinical experience on bovine tissues or
      other suitable biologic tissues or inanimate objects
   D. Post-test clinical simulation

XII. Clinical observation and demonstration

XIII. Essential elements of clinical case studies
   A. Diagnostic tests: tooth vitality, radiographic analysis, pocket depth measurement
   B. Treatment objective
   C. Treatment sequence
   D. Treatment and immediate postoperative evaluation
   E. Postoperative patient instructions
   F. Follow-up care (1 week, 1 month)
   G. Management of complications
   H. Assessing treatment outcome

XIV. Conclusion
   A. Written post-test
   B. Course evaluation
   C. Certificate of attendance

4. Guidelines for Instructor Training Courses

Although there are not any currently available courses that meet this standard, the goal is to as quickly as possible have all Instructors who teach laser use in dentistry meet this standard. To be an instructor of a Category 2 or 3 course, instructors must have attained that level of competency which has been demonstrated. Educators must have specific training in education, established educational skills, appropriate laser experience, and a knowledge base of both basic and clinical sciences. Instructors must be trained through an approved dental school, accredited dental program such as Advanced Education in General Dentistry or General Practice Residency in dentistry, and have specific educational requirements. The specific curriculum must meet the standards of the academic institution. Competency of the instructor must be demonstrated by written and clinical simulation examination with demonstrated proficiency in the education and administration of an educational program in laser applications in dentistry.

Bibliography

American Association of Dental Schools. Curriculum guidelines. J Dent Educ 1992;56:409–414.

American National Standard for the Safe Use of Lasers. ANSI Z-136.1—1986. Toledo, OH: The Laser Institute of America; 1986.

American National Standard for the Safe Use of Lasers in Health Care Facilities. ANSI Z-136.3—1988. Toledo, OH: The Laser Institute of America; 1988.

American Society for Laser Medicine and Surgery, Inc. Standards of Training for Physicians for the Use of Lasers in Medicine and Surgery. Wausau, WI, April 28, 1991.

Furr, KA (ed): CRC Handbook of Laboratory Safety, ed 3. Boca Raton, FL: CRC Press, Inc; 1991.

Gel D, O'Brien SJ, Vangsness CT, White JM, Wigdor HA (eds): Curriculum guidelines and standards for dental laser education. Lasers Ortho Dental Vet Med Proc SPIE 1993;1880:88–100.

Laser Institute of America. Laser Safety Committee. Guide for the Selection of Laser Eye Protection, ed 2. Orlando, FL: Laser Institute of America; 1989: ISBN 0-912035-08-0.

Office of the Federal Register. National Archives and Records Administration. Code of Federal Regulations, Food and Drugs. Washington DC: U.S. Government Printing Office; 1990:800–1299.

Smith JF (ed): Laser Safety Guide, ed 8. Toledo, OH: Laser Institute of America; 1992.

U.S. Department of Labor. Occupational Safety and Health Administration. Guidelines for Laser Safety and Hazard Assessment. Washington DC: U.S. Government Printing Office; 1991: Publication no 8-1.7.

Winburn DC. Practical Laser Safety, vol. 11. New York: Marcel Dekker, Inc; 1985: ISBN 0-8247-7348-9.

Authors of the Curriculum Guidelines and Standards for Dental Laser Education

Robert Barr
Eric Batterton
Raymond Braham
George Burbach
Kevin Chittim
Ronald E. Cole
Penny Ferwerda
Tony Fiorillo
Jack Foster
Bob Gregg
Alan Goldstein
Harold Goodis
Bahram Javid
Joel Kudler
Kim Kutsch
Arlen Lackey
Delwin McCarthy
Terry D. Myers
Wendy Ochs
Kevin O'Grady
Edward Pallante
Harvey Passes
Dennis Pietrini
Donna Plotkin
John W. Rice
Chuck Rose
May Ann Shulman
Mark T. Weiser
Joel M. White
Michael Yessik
Elissa Zasloff

Inquiries, comments, suggestions, and endorsements should be directed to the organizer:

Joel M. White, DDS, MS
USCF, Box 0758
707 Parnassus Avenue
San Francisco, CA 94143
(415) 476-0918
FAX (415) 476-0858

Index

Pages on which illustrations appear are indicated in *italics*; pages on which tables appear are indicated with the letter *t*.

A

Ablation
  bone
    Er:YAG laser, *167*, 167–168
    interaction with laser, 311–312, *312*
  defined, 315
  dental tissues, thermally induced, 61
  dentin
    efficiency of, interaction with laser, 310–311, *311*
    excimer laser, 176, *177*
  efficiency, 295t, 295–296, *295–296*
  enamel, interaction with laser, 309–310, *309–310*
  excimer laser, efficiency measurements, 268–270, *269*
  hard tissue
    decomposition, 61–62
    excimer laser, 266–268
  hydroxyapatite, with lasers, 62
  laser
    effect on enamel, 75–80, *76*, 77t, *78–80*
    efficiency of, 62t, 62–63, 295t, 295–296, *295–296*
    interaction with tissue, 51, *52*
  measurements, excimer laser, 174–175
  oral soft tissue, Er:YAG laser, 168
  rates, Er:YAG laser, 161–162, *162*
Absorption, defined, 315
Active medium, defined, 315
Administrative controls, for laser safety, *99–100*, 99–101
Airborne contaminants, control of, 98–99, *98–99*
Alloys, welding of, 235–236
American National Standards Institute
  laser guidelines, 106–107
American Society for Lasers in Medicine and Surgery, standards of practice, 109
Anesthesia, safety issues, 322
Angstrom, defined, 315
Animal experiments, Er:YAG laser, 166–168
ANSI. *See* American National Standards Institute
Antibacterial investigation, excimer laser, 266–268
Aperture, defined, 315
Aphthous ulcers, CO_2 laser and, 148
ArF laser, 271, *272*, 273, *274*
Argon laser, *29*, 37–38
  caries, prevention, 223, *223*
  clinical applications of, in restorative dentistry, 217–230
  curettage, 130–133, *132*
  defined, 315
  esthetic dentistry, 228, *228*
  frenectomy, 137
  gingival retraction, 133–134, *134*
  gingivectomy/gingivoplasty, 135–136, *136*
  glass-ionomer base material, photopolymerization of, 229, *229*
  hemangioma, traumatic, excision of, 141, *141*
  implant recovery, 142, *142*
  instruments, characteristics of, 130, 130t
  interaction with restorative materials, 217–219
  interproximal caries detection, 219–221
  lateral incisor, restoration of, 224–225, *225*
  oral lesion therapy, 137–139, *138*
  photopolymerization of composite resins, 224–229
  preventive dentistry, 222–223

restoration
Class V composite resin, geriatric patient, 226, *226*
molar, conservative Class II, 227, 227–228
root planing, 130–133, *132*
surgical applications of, 129–143
surgical characteristics of, *114*, 121–122, *122*
tissue interactions, 129–130
transillumination, 220, *221*
ASLMS. *See* American Society for Lasers in Medicine and Surgery
Attenuation
coefficient, defined, 315
defined, 315
Average power, defined, 315

B

Bacteria
excimer laser, effects on, 175–176, 178–179, *179–181*
Beam
alignment, safety issues, 321
defined, 315
generation, 30–31, *31*
profile, *31–32*, 32–33
splitter, defined, 315
Biologic tissue, laser interaction with, 39–55, 299–313, 303–312
ablation, 51, *52*
argon laser, 129–130
bone, 303, *303*
clinical manifestations of, 51–54
dentin, *302*, 302–303
enamel, *300–301*, 300–302
fluid, in presence of, 304–306, *305*
hard tissue
in fluid, 306–308, *308*, 308t
optical properties of, 299–303
hemostasis, 53–54
incision, 51, *52*
laser irradiation, tissue effects of, 42–50, *43*
middle infrared laser radiation, 309–312
models of, 58–62
Nd:YAG laser, 200–201
optical properties of tissues, 40–42, *40–43*
photochemical interaction, 44–45
photoelectrical interactions, 50
photomechanical interactions, 50
photothermal interactions, 45–50, 48t, *49*
physical processes induced during interaction, 305–306
sterilization, 53–54
tissue welding, 53–54
vapor cavitation induced during interaction, 305–306
wavelength specificity, 40–42, *40–43*
Biopsy
CO_2 laser, 145–147, *146–147*
fibroma, trauma, Ho:YAG laser, *191*, 191–192
hemangioma, Nd:YAG laser, 211, *212*
pyogenic granuloma, Nd:YAG laser, 209–211, *210*
Biostimulation therapy, 247–257, *248*, 255–256
Birefringence, defined, 315
Bone
ablation
Er:YAG laser, *167*, 167–168
interaction with laser, 311–312, *312*
laser interaction with, 303, *303*
morphologic change, interaction with laser, 311–312, *312*

C

Carbon dioxide laser. *See* CO_2 laser
Caries
detection, interproximal, argon laser, 219–221
prevention, argon laser, 223, *223*
Ceramic materials, welding of, 231–241, *232*
Certification
in laser technology, 111
laser technology, 111
Chemical effects, of laser on hard tissue, 61
Chromatic, defined, 315
CO_2 laser, 31–32
aphthous ulcers, 148
biopsies, 145–147, *146–147*
clinical applications of, 145–160
coagulation, 150
crown lengthening, 151–153, *153*
defined, 315
development of, 19–20, *19–20*
distal wedge reduction, 153–154
frenectomy, 151, *152*
gingival troughing, 157
gingivectomy/gingivoplasty, 154, *155*
granulation tissue, removal of, 150
hemorrhagic disorders, 157, *158*
herpetic lesions, 148–150
hypersensitivity, 154
implants (stage II), exposure of, 150, *151*
malignant lesions, 157
premalignant lesions, 147–148, *149*
preprosthetic surgery, 155–156, *156*
tongue lesions, 147
tuberosity reduction, 153–154
vesiculobullous lesions, 147–148, *149*
white lesions, 147–148, *149*
Coagulation
CO_2 laser, 150
graft donor site, Nd:YAG laser, 207–208, *208*

Coherence, defined, 315
Collimation, defined, 315
Color, defined, 315
Combustion hazards of lasers, 93, 93t
Components of laser, 30–31, *31*
Constants, 320
Contact, noncontact modes, contrasted, 121
Continuous wave laser
  defined, 315
  hard tissue, 63–64, *64*
Control of laser
  measures for, 94t, 94–96
  safety issues, 321
Corrosion resistance, evaluation of, 238–241, *240*, 240–241t
Credentialing
  in laser technology, 111
Crown lengthening, CO_2 laser, 151–153, *153*
Curettage, argon laser, 130–133, *132*
Curriculum guidelines, for dental laser education, 110–111, 323–333

D

Decomposition, ablative, hard tissue, 61–62
Dental alloys, welding of, 235–236
Dental auxiliaries, educational requirements, in lasers, 109–110
Dental hard tissue. *See* Hard tissue
Dental laser education, curriculum guidelines, 110–111
Dental laser research, history of, 18t, 18–20
Dental materials, laser processing of, 231–245
  alloys, welding of, 235–236
  ceramic materials, welding of, 231–241, *232*
  corrosion resistance, evaluation of, 238–241, *240*, 240–241t
  double-beam laser modification, 233–235, *233–235*
  laser welding, Nd:YAG laser, 236–238, *237–239*, 238t
  titanium, welding, with Nd:YAG laser, 241–244, *242*, 244t
Dental pulp. *See* Pulp
Dentin
  ablation
    efficiency of, interaction with laser, 310–311, *311*
    excimer laser, 176, *177*
  laser interaction with, *302*, 302–303
  light propagation, *287–288*, 287–289
Development of laser dentistry, 17–19
Diode, defined, 315
Diode laser, 37
  defined, 316
Distal wedge reduction, CO_2 laser, 153–154
Divergence, defined, 316
Doppler effect, defined, 316
Dosimetry, *252*, 252–255
  photodynamic therapy, *252*, 252–255
Double-beam laser modification, 233–235, *233–235*
Dye laser, defined, 316

E

Education, about lasers, in dentistry, 103–112, 107–111
  course content, 110–111
  curriculum guidelines, 110–111, 323–333
  requirements, for dental auxiliaries and staff, 109–110
Efficiency, defined, 316
Electrical control measures, 97
Electrical hazards of lasers, 94
Electromagnetic spectrum, defined, 316
Electron microscopy, scanning, excimer laser, 271–274
Electron nonlinearity, and optics, 289
Electron probe microanalysis, defined, 316
Electron-oscillation nonlinearity, optics, 289
Emission, defined, 316
Enamel
  ablation
    efficiency of, interaction with laser, 309–310, *309–310*
    excimer laser, 176, *177*
  biologic tissue, laser interaction with, *300–301*, 300–302
  laser effects on, 75–80, *76*, 77t, *78–80*
  light propagation, *287–288*, 287–289
  morphologic change, interaction with laser, 309–310, *309–310*
  surface, light scattering, 284–286, *284–286*
Energy
  defined, 316
  reflected, safety issues, 321
Energy density, 35, *35*
  defined, 316
Environmental control measures, with lasers, 96–97
Environmental hazards of lasers, 91–93, 92t, *93*
Epulides fissurata, Ho:YAG laser, *193*, 193–195
Equivalents table, 320
Er:YAG laser, *64*, 65
  ablation rates, 161–162, *162*
  animal experiments, 166–168
  bone ablation, *167*, 167–168
  filling materials, removal of, 165, *165*
  hard and soft tissues, effects on, 161–171
  in-vitro experiments, 161–165
  morphology, *162–163*, 162–164

oral soft tissue ablation, 168
pulp
reaction, long-term, 166–167, *167*
temperature response, *296*, 297
temperature measurements, 164, *164*
Er:YSGG laser, 65, *65*
Esthetic dentistry, argon laser, 228, *228*
Excimer laser, 67–68, *68*
ablation
efficiency measurements, 268–270, *269*
measurements, 174–175
antibacterial investigation, 266–268
applications research, 262–265
ArF laser, 271, *272*, 273, *274*
bacteria
effects on, 175–176
growth, effects on, 178–179, *179–181*
defined, 316
dentin, ablation of, 176, *177*
enamel, ablation of, 176, *177*
hard tissue ablation, 266–268
interactions with hard tissue, analysis of, 261–282
investigations, preliminary, 174–176
irradiated surfaces, microscopic evaluation of, 175
light microscopy, 270
photoacoustic measurements, 276
plume dynamics, 274–276, *275–276*
pulpal chamber temperature, change in, 177, *177*
research
clinical/investigative, 173–186
current status, 265–279
root canal, 176, 179–183
scanning electron microscopy, 178, *178*, 271–274
shock wave imaging, 274–276, *275–276*
sterilization studies, *278*, 279
temperature measurements, 175
thermal camera measurements, 270–271
time-resolved spectroscopy, 277–279, *278*
transducer measurements, 277
transmission electron microscopic findings, 178
XeCl laser, 271, *272*, 273, *273*
Excited state, defined, 316
Eye protection, 97–98, *98*, 322. *See also* Ocular hazards

F

FDA. *See* Food and Drug Administration
Fiber optic, defined, 316
Fiber optic delivery systems, 117–121, *119*
Fibroma, Ho:YAG laser, *191*, 191–192
Filling materials, removal of, Er:YAG laser, 165, *165*
Fire, control measures, 97, 322
Flash-lamp
defined, 316
pulsing, 36
Fluence, defined, 316
Fluid
laser interaction in presence of, 304–306, *305*
middle infrared laser radiation, 309–312
Flux, defined, 316
Focal length, defined, 316
Focal point, defined, 316
Focus, defined, 316
Focused mode, defined, 316
Food and Drug Administration, medical devices, 103–105
Formula table, 320
Frenectomy
argon laser, 137
CO_2 laser, 151, *152*
Nd:YAG laser, 205–207, *206*, 208–209, *209*

G

Gas laser, defined, 316
Gating, *34*, 34–35
Geometry, spot, with beam profile, *31–32*, 32–33
Geriatric patient, restorations, argon laser, 226, *226*
Giant cell tumor, lingual, Ho:YAG laser, *189*, 189–190
Gingival retraction, argon laser, 133–134, *134*
Gingival troughing, CO_2 laser, 157
Gingivectomy/Gingivoplasty
argon laser, 135–136, *136*
CO_2 laser, 154, *155*
Nd:YAG laser, 205–207, *206*
Glass-ionomer base material, argon laser, 229, *229*
Graft donor site, coagulation, Nd:YAG laser, 207 208, *208*
Granulation tissue, removal of, CO_2 laser, 150
Granuloma, pyogenic, Nd:YAG laser, 209–211, *210*
Ground state, defined, 316
Guidelines, for lasers in dentistry, 86t, 86–87, 88t

H

Hard tissue, 62t, 68–69, *69*
ablation
decomposition, 61–62

excimer laser, 266–268
hydroxyapatite, with lasers, 62
applications of lasers, 105
chemical effects of laser, 61
continuous wave laser, 63–64, *64*
Er:YAG laser, *64*, 65
effects on, 161–171
Er:YSGG laser, 65, *65*
excimer laser, 67–68, *68*
interactions with, analysis of, 261–282
Ho:YAG laser, 65–67, *66*, 196
laser ablation, efficiency of, 62t, 62–63
laser applications, 23–24, *24*
laser effects on, 57–70
laser treatment, 57–58, 58t
laser-induced destruction of, 290–291
mechanical effects of laser on, 60t, 60–61
Nd:YAG laser, 67, *67*
nonlinear optical characteristics of, 289–290
optical properties of, 58–60, *59–60*
laser interaction with, 299–303
pulsed CO_2 laser, 63–64, *64*
radiation, laser, control of, 63–68
TEA CO_2 lasers, *64*, 64–65
thermal effects of laser, 60
thermally induced ablation, 61
tissue-laser interaction, models of, 58–62
Tm:YAG laser, 65–67, *66*
Hazard classification, of lasers in dentistry, 87–94
Heat nonlinearity, optics, 289–290
Hemangioma
excisional biopsy of, Nd:YAG laser, 211, *212*
traumatic, excision of, argon laser, 141, *141*
Hemorrhagic disorders, CO_2 laser, 157, *158*
Hemostasis, laser interaction with tissue, 53–54
He:Ne laser, defined, 316
Herpes, lesions, CO_2 laser, 148–150
History of laser dentistry, 17–19
Holmium
characteristics of, 187–188
physics of, 188
Ho:YAG laser, 65–67, *66*
clinical application, 188–195
defined, 316
epulides fissurata, multiple, removal of, *193*, 193–195
hard tissue, use on, 196
holmium, characteristics of, 187–188
lingual benign giant cell tumor, *189*, 189–190
surgical characteristics of, *114*, 123–124, *124*
traumatic fibroma, Ho:YAG laser, *191*, 191–192
Hydroxyapatite, ablation of, with lasers, 62
Hypersensitivity, CO_2 laser, 154

I

Implants
exposure of, CO_2 laser, 150, *151*
recovery, argon laser, 142, *142*
Incision, laser interaction with tissue, 51, *52*
Incisor, lateral, restoration of, argon laser, 224–225, *225*
Infrared spectrum, defined, 316
Interproximal caries detection, argon laser, 219–221
Irradiated surfaces, microscopic evaluation of, excimer laser, 175
Irradiation
defined, 316
tissue effects, laser, 42–50, *43*

J

Joule, defined, 316

L

Laser. *See also* particular wavelengths
defined, 317
Lattice nonlinearity, optics, 289
Light
absorption, *28*, 30
amplification, by stimulated emission of radiation, *28*, 30
delivery systems, photodynamic therapy, *252*, 252–255
emission, *28*, 30
microscopy observations, excimer laser, 270
propagation, in enamel/dentin, *287–288*, 287–289
scattering, at enamel surface, 284–286, *284–286*
Linear optical characteristics of teeth, 283–289
Lingual benign giant cell tumor, Ho:YAG laser, *189*, 189–190

M

Malignant lesions, CO_2 laser, 157
Maser, 17, 317
Measurement, units of, 320
Mechanical effects, of laser on hard tissue, 60t, 60–61
Medical devices, Food and Drug Administration, 103–105
Medium, defined, 317

Micrometer, defined, 317
Microscopic evaluation, irradiated surfaces, excimer laser, 175
Middle infrared laser radiation, 309–312
Monochromatic, defined, 317
Morphology, Er:YAG laser, *162–163*, 162–164

N

Nanometer, defined, 317
Nd:YAG laser, 20, 67, *67*
- advantages of, 202
- clinical applications of, 199–216
- contact, noncontact, modes, 202
- defined, 317
- frenectomy, 205–207, *206*
  - maxillary midline, 208–209, *209*
- gingivectomy, 205–207, *206*
- graft donor site, coagulation of, 207–208, *208*
- hemangioma, 211, *212*
- periodontal therapy, 212–215, *213–214*
- physics, 200
- pulsed, scientific basis for, 202–211, *204*
- pyogenic granuloma, 209–211, *210*
- surgical characteristics of, *114*, 122–123, *122–123*
- tissue effects, 200–201
- variables, effect on laser, 201
- welding, 236–238, *237–239*, 238t
  - titanium, 241–244, *242*, 244t

Nonbiologic structure, laser interaction with, 303–312
Noncontact lasers, surgery, 113–117, *114–116*

O

Occupational Safety and Health Administration, laser safety guidelines, 106–107
Ocular hazards, of lasers, 88–90, *89*, 90t. *See also* Eye Protection
Operator, safety training requirements, 95–96
Optical cavity, defined, 317
Optical characteristics
- of hard tissue, 58–60, *59–60*
- nonlinear, hard tissues, 289–290
- of teeth, linear, 283–289
- of tissues generally, 40–42, *40–43*

Optics, dentistry and, 283–297
- ablation, laser, efficiency of, 295t, 295–296, *295–296*
- electron nonlinearity, 289
- hard tissues
  - laser-induced destruction of, 290–291
  - nonlinear optical characteristics of, 289–290
- heat nonlinearity, 289–290
- lattice nonlinearity, 289
- light
  - propagation, in enamel/dentin, *287–288*, 287–289
  - scattering, at enamel surface, 284–286, *284–286*
- teeth, linear optical characteristics of, 283–289
- thermophysical model, 291–297, *292–293*

Oral lesion therapy, argon laser, 137–139, *138*
Oral soft tissue ablation, Er:YAG laser, 168
OSHA. *See* Occupational Safety and Health Administration

P

Periodontal therapy, Nd:YAG laser, 212–215, *213–214*
Photoablation, defined, 317
Photoacoustic effect, defined, 317
Photoacoustic measurements, excimer laser, 276
Photochemical effect, defined, 317
Photochemical interaction, biologic tissue, laser, 44–45
Photochemotherapy, 248–252
- distribution, *250–251*, 250–252
- photosensitizers, 249–252, *250*

Photocoagulation, defined, 317
Photodisruption, defined, 317
Photodynamic therapy, 247–257, *248*
- basis of, 247–248, *248*
- clinical applications, 252–255
- light delivery systems, *252*, 252–255

Photoelectrical interactions, 50
Photomechanical interactions, 50
Photon
- defined, *28–29*, 29, 317

Photopolymerization
- of composite resins, argon laser, 224–229
- of glass-ionomer base material, argon laser, 229, *229*

Photosensitizers, photochemotherapy, 249–252, *250*
Photothermal interactions, biologic tissue, laser, 45–50, 48t, *49*
Physical processes, during biologic tissue, laser interaction, 305–306
Physics, laser, 27–38
- argon laser, *29*, 37–38
- beam
  - generation, 30–31, *31*
  - profile, *31–32*, 32–33
- CO_2 laser, 31–32

diode lasers, 37
energy, 35, *35*
density, 35, *35*
flash-lamp pulsing, 36
gating, *34*, 34–35
laser components, 30–31, *31*
light
absorption, *28*, 30
amplification, by stimulated emission of radiation, *28*, 30
emission, *28*, 30
Nd:YAG laser, 200
photons, defined, *28–29*, 29
power density, 33, 33t, *34*
pulsing, *34*, 34–35
Q-switching, *36*, 36–37
radiation, stimulated emission of, light amplification by, *28*, 30
solid-state lasers, *29*, 35–37
spot geometry, *31–32*, 32–33
Picosecond, defined, 317
Plasma, defined, 317
Plume
control, safety issues, 322
dynamics, excimer laser, 274–276, *275–276*
Polarization, defined, 317
Population inversion, defined, 317
Power density, 33, 33t, *34*
defined, 317
Precautions, laser, 321–322
Premalignant lesions, CO_2 laser, 147–148, *149*
Preprosthetic surgery, CO_2 laser, 155–156, *156*
Preventive dentistry, argon laser, 222–223
Procedural controls, for laser safety, *99–100*, 99–101
Profile, beam, *31–32*, 32–33
Protective equipment, personal, 97–101
Pulp
chamber temperature, change in, excimer laser, 177, *177*
laser effects on, 71–82, *72–73*, *73*, 74t, 74–75, *76*
reaction, long-term, Er:YAG laser, 166–167, *167*
temperature response, Er:YAG laser, *296*, 297
Pulse
duration, defined, 317
frequency, defined, 317
repetition rate, defined, 317
width, defined, 318
Pulsed CO_2 laser, hard tissue, 63–64, *64*
Pulsed mode, defined, 318
Pulsing, Nd:YAG laser, scientific basis for, 202–211, *204*
Pumping, defined, 318
Pyogenic granuloma, Nd:YAG laser, 209–211, *210*

Q

Q, defined, 318
Q-switching, *36*, 36–37
defined, 318
Quantum, defined, 318
Quantum mechanics, defined, 318
Quartz, defined, 318

R

Radiation
defined, 318
laser, control of, 63–68
stimulated emission of, light amplification by, *28*, 30
Recrystallization, defined, 318
Reflected energy, safety issues, 321
Reflection, defined, 318
Regulation, of lasers in dentistry, 86t, 86–87, 88t, 103–112
Resins, composite, photopolymerization of, argon laser, 224–229
Resistance, corrosive, evaluation of, 238–241, *240*, 240–241t
Resonator, defined, 318
Root canal, excimer laser, 176, 179–183
Root planing, argon laser, 130–133, *132*
Ruby laser
defined, 318
development of, 18–19

S

Safety
administrative controls, *99–100*, 99–101
airborne contaminants, control of, 98–99, *98–99*
anesthesia, 322
beam alignment, 321
combustion hazards, 93, 93t
control measures, 94t, 94–96, 321
electrical, 97
environmental, 96–97
fire, 97
electrical hazards, 94
environmental hazards, 91–93, 92t, *93*
eye protection, 97–98, *98*, 322
fire precaution, 322
of lasers in dentistry, 83–124
specific recommendations, 95
ocular hazards, of lasers, 88–90, *89*, 90t
operator training requirements, 95–96
personal protective equipment, 97–101

plume control, 322
precautions, 321–322
procedural controls, *99–100,* 99–101
reflected energy, 321
safety officer, role of, 94–95
standards, of lasers in dentistry, 85–102, 86t, 86–87, 88t
tissue
damage, 322
hazards, 90–91
protection, 322
treatment controlled area, laser, *96,* 96–97
Scanning electron microscopy, excimer laser, 178, *178,* 271–274
Scatter, defined, 318
Semiconductor, defined, 318
Semiconductor laser, defined, 318
Shock wave imaging, excimer laser, 274–276, *275–276*
Shutter, defined, 318
Solid-state laser, *29,* 35–37
defined, 318
Spontaneous emission, defined, 318
Spot geometry, *31–32,* 32–33
Standards
for dental laser education, 323–331
for lasers, in dentistry, 103–112
of practice (ASLMS), 109
of safety, lasers in dentistry, 85–102
Sterilization
laser interaction with tissue, 53–54
studies, excimer laser, *278,* 279
Stimulated emission, defined, 318
Superpulsed, defined, 318
Surgery, 113–124
argon laser, *114,* 121–122, *122,* 129–143
contact *vs* noncontact modes, 121
fiberoptic delivery systems, 117–121, 119
Ho:YAG lasers, *114,* 123–124, *124*
Nd:YAG lasers, *114,* 122–123
noncontact lasers, 113–117, *114–116*
preprosthetic, CO_2 laser, 155–156, *156*

T

TEA CO_2 lasers, *64,* 64–65
Temperature
ablation, induced by, 61
camera measurements, excimer laser, 270–271
effects, of laser on hard tissue, 60
measurements
Er:YAG laser, 164, *164*
excimer laser, 175
pulp
chamber, change in, excimer laser, 177, *177*
Er:YAG laser, *296,* 297
Thermophysical model, optics, 291–297, *292–293*
Time-dependent tissue effects of laser, 51–53
Time-resolved spectroscopy, excimer laser, 277–279, *278*
Tissue
biologic, laser interaction with. *See* Biologic tissue, laser interaction with
welding
argon laser, 139–141, *140*
laser interaction with tissue, 53–54
Titanium, welding, with Nd:YAG laser, 241–244, *242,* 244t
Tm:YAG laser, 65–67, *66*
Tongue
benign giant cell tumor, Ho:YAG laser, *189,* 189–190
lesions, CO_2 laser, 147
Training programs, for lasers and dentistry, 107–111
essential elements of, 108t, 108–109
Transducer measurements, excimer laser, 277
Transillumination, argon laser, 220, *221*
Transmission, defined, 318
Transmission electron microscopy, excimer laser findings, 178
Trauma, fibroma, Ho:YAG laser, *191,* 191–192
Troughing, gingival, CO_2 laser, 157
Tuberosity reduction, CO_2 laser, 153–154
Tumor, benign giant cell, lingual, Ho:YAG laser, *189,* 189–190
Tunable laser, defined, 318

U

Units of measurement, 320t

V

Vapor cavitation, during biologic tissue–laser interaction, 305–306
Vesiculobullous lesions, CO_2 laser, 147–148, *149*

W

Watt, defined, 318
Wave, defined, 318
Waveguide, defined, 319
Wavelength
defined, 319
research in, 22, 23, *23*

specificity, biologic tissue, 40–42, *40–43*
Welding
of alloys, 235–236
of ceramic materials, 231–241, *232*
of dental alloys, 235–236
Nd:YAG laser, 236–238, *237–239,* 238t
tissue
argon laser, 139–141, *140*
biologic tissue, laser interaction with, 53–54
of titanium, with the Nd:YAG laser, 241–244, *242,* 244t
White lesions, CO_2 laser, 147–148, *149*

X

XeCl laser, 271, *272,* 273, *273*
Xenon flash–lamp, defined, 319
X-ray
diffraction, defined, 319
microprobe analysis, defined, 319

Y

YAG laser, defined, 319

Z

Z-136.3 standard, of American National Standards Institute, 106